THIRD EDITION

RECOGNITION & INTERPRETATION OF

ECG Rhythms

Ginger Murphy Ochs, RN, BSN, CEN
Clinical Nurse
University of California San Diego Medical Center
San Diego, California

Melvin A. Ochs, MD, FACEP
Director, Emergency Department
Scripps Memorial Hospital of Chula Vista
Medical Director
San Diego County
Division of Emergency Medical Services
San Diego, California

APPLETON & LANGE
Stamford, Connecticut

Copyright © 1997 by Appleton & Lange
A Simon & Schuster Company
Copyright © 1990 by Appleton & Lange; Copyright © 1982 by Capistrano Press, Ltd.

97 98 99 00 01 / 10 9 8 7 6 5 4 3 2 1

Prentice Hall International (UK) Limited, *London*
Prentice Hall of Australia Pty. Limited, *Sydney*
Prentice Hall Canada, Inc., *Toronto*
Prentice Hall Hispanoamericana, S.A., *Mexico*
Prentice Hall of India Private Limited, *New Delhi*
Prentice Hall of Japan, Inc., *Tokyo*
Simon & Schuster Asia Pte. Ltd., *Singapore*
Editora Prentice Hall do Brasil Ltda., *Rio de Janeiro*
Prentice Hall, *Upper Saddle River, New Jersey*

Library of Congress Cataloging-in-Publication Data

Ochs, Ginger Murphy.
    Recognition and interpretation of ECG rhythms / Ginger Murphy Ochs,
Melvin A. Ochs—3rd ed.
        p.   cm.
    Rev. ed. of: Interpretation of the electrocardiogram / Karen
Milazzo Jones, Ginger Murphy Ochs. 2nd ed. c1990.
    Includes bibliographical references.
    ISBN 0-8385-4323-5 (pbk: :alk. paper)
    1. Arrhythmia—Diagnosis.   2. Electrocardiography.   I. Ochs,
Melvin A.   II. Jones, Karen Milazzo   Interpretation of the
electrocardiogram.   III. Title
    [DNLM: 1. Arrhythmia—diagnosis.   2. Electrocardiography.   WG 140
016r   1997]
RC685.A65J66   1997
616.1'2807547—dc21
DNLM/DLC
for Library of Congress   96-29695

Acquisitions Editor: Kimberly Davies
Production Editor: Jeanmarie M. Roche
Designer: Mary Skudlarek

ISBN 0-8385-4323-5

90000

9 780838 543238

PRINTED IN THE UNITED STATES OF AMERICA

Contents

Preface

The positive feedback from grateful students and teachers of ECG courses made the decision to do the revision for this new edition an easy one! Their comments reinforced our own feeling that we had achieved an ideal combination in the text's systematic approach, balanced with that other essential—an abundance of practice strips. Although Karen Jones was not available to work on the new edition, I decided to take on the task of updating and expanding the text. I felt, however, that I needed a co-author with whom to exchange ideas and to assist with the revision. As luck would have it, my husband, who is a board certified practicing emergency department physician, was available. This is our first collaborative effort in publishing. I hope you find the third edition of *Interpretation of the Electrocardiogram,* now titled *Recognition and Interpretation of ECG Rhythms,* as useful as the previous editions.

This book has been beneficial to many instructors who have taught basic ECG interpretation to a wide range of students including ECG technicians, nurses, medical students, physician assistants, and paramedics. We believe that the two greatest strengths of this book are its systematic approach to ECG interpretation and the large number of strips that are provided to practice rhythm interpretation.

The biggest change we made in this edition was to change the "normal" QRS measurement from "0.12 second or less" to "less than 0.12 second". This change is consistent with standards used in the American Heart Association's Textbook of Advanced Cardiac Life Support. In revising the text, this change did not cause any major changes in dysrhythmia interpretation. Despite reviewer suggestion, however, we chose not to identify P waves as P' when they did not originate in the S-A node. Although it is understood that the only true P wave must originate in the S-A node, which is the dominate pacemaker of the heart, we do not feel that this designation is a common practice in the basic ECG courses. Additionally, we have added 50 new strips in keeping with our philosophy that individuals learn ECG interpretation best with lots of practice.

We again wish to thank the staffs of the Emergency Department and the ICU at Scripps Memorial Hospital of Chula Vista for their help in collecting interesting ECG strips for our use. I would also like to thank my husband for agreeing to do this project with me and our daughters, Jennifer and Jessika, for understanding why we were preoccupied on some days.

Ginger Murphy Ochs

Introduction

ANATOMY AND PHYSIOLOGY OF THE HEART

The heart acts as a muscular pump propelling blood into the arterial system and collecting blood that is returned by the venous system. The physiologic role of this circulation is the delivery of oxygen (O_2) and essential metabolites to the tissues of the body and the removal of waste products such as carbon dioxide (CO_2). The heart is divided into right and left sides, each side consisting of an atrium (receiving chamber) and a ventricle (pumping chamber). The right atrium receives unoxygenated blood from three sources: the inferior vena cava, the superior vena cava, and the coronary sinus. Blood collected in the right atrium passes through the tricuspid valve into the right ventricle. During ventricular systole (contraction) the tricuspid valve is closed, and unoxygenated blood is pumped through the pulmonary valve into the pulmonary arteries and to the lungs. The oxygenated blood is then returned to the left atrium via four pulmonary veins, subsequently passing through the mitral valve into the left ventricle. The mitral valve closes, and during ventricular systole blood is ejected through the aortic valve and into the aorta, which in turn distributes oxygenated blood to the peripheral tissues (Fig. 1–1).

As blood passes through the systemic capillary bed that joins peripheral arteries and veins, its red blood cells surrender their O_2 to the tissues and accumulate CO_2. Conversely, as blood passes through the pulmonary capillaries, its red cells exchange CO_2 for O_2 from the inspired air within the pulmonary alveoli.

CORONARY ARTERIES

Adequate blood supply to the muscular and electrical systems of the heart is maintained by the coronary artery system. The two main coronary arteries originate from the aorta immediately beyond the aortic valve.

The right coronary artery proceeds to the anterior surface of the heart, winds around to the right into the groove between the right atrium and right ventricle, and descends posteriorly through the interventricular septum. It supplies the inferior wall of the left ventricle, the right atrium and ventricle, and part of the septum as well as the sinoatrial (S-A) and atrioventricular (A-V) nodes in the conduction system.

The left coronary artery divides into the left anterior descending and circumflex branches. The left anterior descending branch passes anteriorly down the groove between the two ventricles, supplying the anterior portion of the left ventricle and part of the interventricular septum. The circumflex

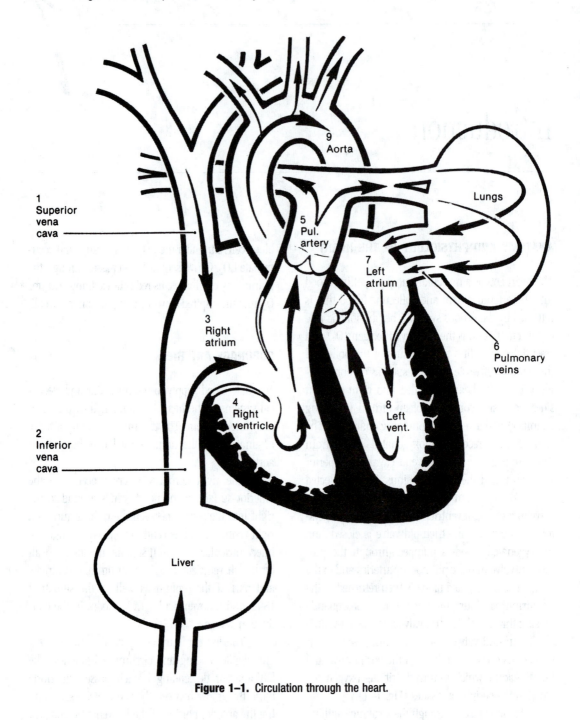

Figure 1–1. Circulation through the heart.

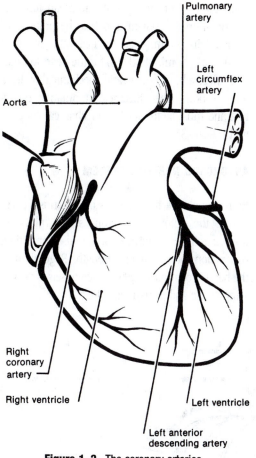

Pulmonary artery

Left circumflex artery

Aorta

Right coronary artery

Right ventricle

Left ventricle

Left anterior descending artery

Figure 1–2. The coronary arteries.

artery winds around the left side of the heart anteriorly between the left atrium and ventricle, and may reach the posterior portion of the A-V groove. In about 40% of people the circumflex supplies the S-A node instead of the right coronary artery (Fig. 1–2).

PROPERTIES OF CELLS

There are two types of cardiac cells, the characteristics of which are responsible for the mechanical and electrical activity of the heart.

1. *Myocardial cells* make up the bulk musculature of the heart and are the actual contracting cells. Normally, these cells have the property of contractility, responding to each electrical stimulus.
2. *Specialized cells* comprise the conduction system where the electrical activity preceding mechanical activity occurs. They have the following very important properties that control their function and therefore the activity of the heart.
   a. *Conductivity* is the ability to transmit impulses from one area to another. This is also a property of the muscular cells; however, conduction through the heart muscle is six times slower than through specialized cells.
   b. *Excitability (irritability)* is the capability of the cell to respond to a stimulus. An ionic imbalance across the cell membrane initiates irritability.
   c. *Automaticity* is the capacity to initiate an impulse or stimulus, a characteristic specific only to the specialized cells.
   d. *Rhythmicity* is the property of regularity of the intervals at which impulses are formed.
   e. *Refractoriness* is the property of being unresponsive to an impulse.

NORMAL CONDUCTION SYSTEM

Normally impulses originate in the specialized conduction cells of the S-A node located near the entrance of the superior vena cava in the right atrium. Since it fires more rapidly than any other site (60 to 100 times per minute), it is the dominate pacemaker of the heart. The S-A node artery (a branch of the right coronary artery in 60% of humans) supplies the S-A node. The impulse spreads through right atrial muscle via internodal pathways and through the interatrial pathways (Bachmann's bundle) to the left atrial muscle. This stimulates them to contract mechanically, thus ejecting blood into the ventricles. Located in the right atrium near the tricuspid valve is the A-V node. When the impulse reaches the A-V node, conduction is delayed (0.1 second) allowing time for the atria to eject blood into the ventricle. Since the junctional tissue around the A-V node has the property of automaticity, if the S-A node fails, the A-V junction can assume control at a rate of 40 to 60 per minute.

Traveling through the bundle of His and down the right and left bundle branches, the impulse reaches the His–Purkinje system, and conduction once again spreads rapidly. Each bundle branch supplies the inner portion of its respective ventricle. The bundle branches break up into a network of many tiny branches called the Purkinje fibers. It is these fibers that allow a rapid spread of the impulse through the ventricular mass. If the S-A node and A-V junction fail to initiate an impulse, the His–Purkinje system also has the property of automaticity and may pace the heart at a rate of 20 to 40 beats per minute. Thus, for the heart to function effectively, electrical and mechanical systems must work together. Electrical stimulation occurs first and must be followed by mechanical contraction (Fig. 1–3).

AUTONOMIC NERVOUS SYSTEM

Even though the heart has its own intrinsic pacemaker, the autonomic nervous system plays an important role in the rate of impulse formation, conduction, and pumping strength. Regulation of the heart is controlled by two different sets of nerves, sympathetic and parasympathetic.

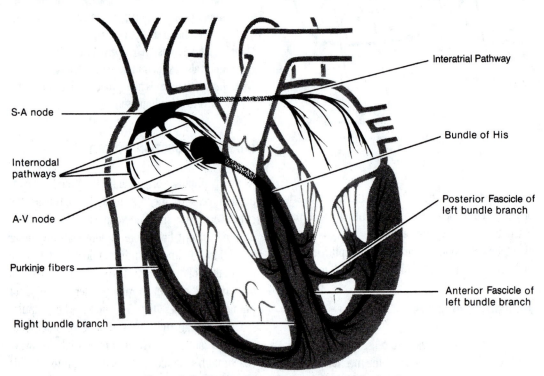

Figure 1–3. The normal conduction system of the heart.

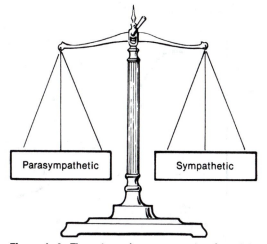

Figure 1–4. The autonomic nervous system in a state of balance.

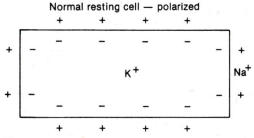

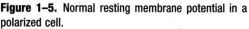

Figure 1–5. Normal resting membrane potential in a polarized cell.

1. *Sympathetic* nerve fibers innervate both the atria and ventricles. When stimulated there is an *increase* in heart rate, A-V conduction, cardiac contractility, and irritability.
2. *Parasympathetic* influence reaches the heart via the vagus nerve fibers. These innervate the S-A node, atrial muscle fibers, and the A-V node but have little or no effect on the ventricular musculature. Stimulation of the vagus nerve causes a *decrease* in heart rate, A-V conduction, contractility, and irritability. Normally the function of the heart is kept in a state of balanced control because of the opposite effects of the parasympathetic and sympathetic nerves (Fig. 1–4). However, both of these mechanisms can cause various dysrhythmias. If one system is blocked, the other will assume control; if one is stimulated, it will assume control.

ELECTROPHYSIOLOGY

Electrical activity in the cell is dependent upon the flow of sodium and potassium ions across the cell membrane. In the normal resting state of a cell there are more positively charged sodium ions (Na^+) outside the cell than there are positively charged potassium ions (K^+) inside the cell. This causes a relative negativity inside the cell in comparison to the outside. In this resting, or *polarized,* state the negative ions line up along the inside of the cell wall and the positive ions line up along the outside of the cell wall, thus creating a resting membrane potential (RMP). In this state the cell is ready to accept a stimulus (Fig. 1–5).

Cells in the conducting system undergo spontaneous leakage of positive ions across the cell membrane, slowly lowering the resting membrane potential (RMP) until it reaches the threshold value. At this point spontaneous depolarization occurs. As long as the RMP remains undisturbed, electrical current does not flow through the cell. However, any stimulus that increases the cell membrane permeability to sodium ions will result in a rapid sequence of changes. Sodium ions rush into the cell and potassium ions leak out, causing an ionic imbalance. This change in polarity causes a flow of electrical current from cell to cell. Successive stimulation from cell to cell is called *depolarization* (Fig. 1–6).

A fraction of a second after depolarization, the cell will return to its resting state. Na^+ is pumped out of the cell and K^+ flows back in. Electrical current is now flowing again because of the difference

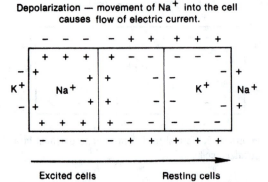

Depolarization — movement of Na⁺ into the cell causes flow of electric current.

Figure 1–6. Chainlike spread of depolarization (cell depolarized, cell in the process of depolarization, and cell in resting state ready to be depolarized). Movement of Na^+ into the cell causes flow of electric current.

in polarity. This return to a normal state is called *repolarization*. At this time the cell is again in a polarized state, ready to accept another impulse (Fig. 1–7). This whole sequence of changes (depolarization and repolarization) is called the *action potential* (Fig. 1–8).

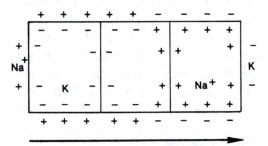

Repolarization

Cell returns to normal state

(Na⁺ moves out, K⁺ moves in)

Occurs in same direction as depolarization

Figure 1–7. Cells repolarizing in a chainlike fashion (cell completely repolarized, cell in the process of repolarizing, and cell waiting to be repolarized).

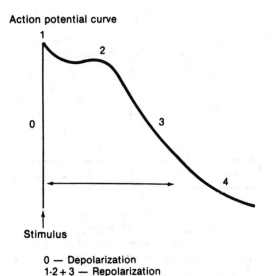

Action potential curve

0 — Depolarization
1-2 + 3 — Repolarization
4 — Resting membrane potential

Figure 1–8. Action potential curve demonstrating depolarization and repolarization.

REFRACTORY PERIODS

As stated earlier, the cell has the property of refractoriness or unresponsiveness. Refractoriness is divided into three periods of the cardiac cycle.

1. *Absolute refractory period* (ARP) is the time during the cardiac cycle in which the heart cannot respond to a stimulus. This occurs during depolarization and completed depolarization. At this time the cells are in the process of depolarizing or reversing their electrical charges. This absolute refractory period serves as a protective mechanism to the heart muscle, preventing it from responding to all the impulses fired by an excessively rapid pacemaker (Fig. 1–9).

2. *Relative refractory period* (RRP) is the period during the cardiac cycle in which the cell can respond to a strong stimulus. During this period, the repolarization phase is in process but not quite completed. Conduction can occur but at a slower rate and usu-

Absolute refractory period — cell cannot respond to a stimulus

During depolarization

Complete depolarization

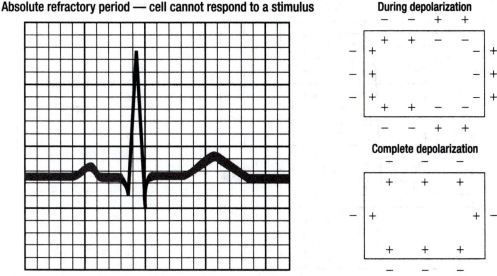

Figure 1–9. Ionic state of cardiac cells during absolute refractory period and representation on ECG.

ally presents as a bizarre complex. This occurs when some cells are polarized and others are depolarized. The polarized cells are ready to accept an impulse, and the depolarized cells are still refractory. If a stimulus occurs often enough and fast enough in the relative refractory period, serious dysrhythmias

such as ventricular tachycardia (VT) or ventricular fibrillation (VF) may occur. This phase is referred to as the vulnerable phase and corresponds to the T wave on the ECG (Fig. 1–10).

3. *Nonrefractory period* is the time when the heart is completely repolarized and ready to adequately and

During repolarization

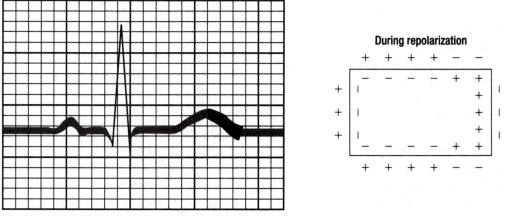

Figure 1–10. Ionic state of cardiac cells during relative refractory period and representation on ECG.

Non-refractory period — cell ready to accept an impulse

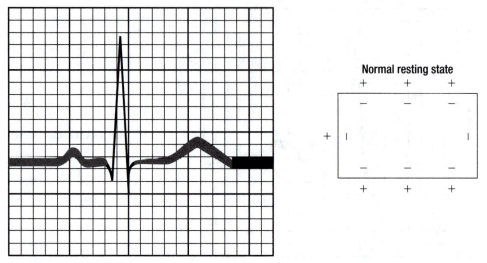

Figure 1–11. Ionic state of cardiac cells during the nonrefractory period and representation on ECG.

efficiently respond to another stimulus (Fig. 1–11). It is important to realize that the refractory period is not the same in all heart cells and that it may be altered by heart rate, specific drugs, and electrolyte disturbances (Fig. 1–12).

PACEMAKER RULES

1. S-A node
   a. Fires at a rate of 60–100/min
   b. Since it fires more rapidly than other sites, is the dominant pacemaker of the heart
2. Internodal pathways
   a. Supply right atrium
   b. Cause right atrium to depolarize
3. Interatrial pathway (Bachman's bundle)
   a. Supplies left atrium
   b. Causes left atrium to depolarize
4. A-V junction (area of bundle of His)
   a. Fires at a rate of 40–60/min
   b. Takes over if S-A node fails

   c. May become excitable and override the S-A node
   d. Delay of 0.1 second at A-V node allows time for atrial depolarization and contraction
5. His–Purkinje system
   a. Composed of
      (1) Bundle of His
      (2) Right and left bundle branches; left bundle branch subdivides into left anterior fascicle and posterior fascicle
      (3) Purkinje fibers
   b. Fires at a rate of 20–40/min
   c. Takes over if S-A node and A-V junction fail
   d. May become excitable and override the S-A node and the A-V junction

GRAPH PAPER

1. Voltage—measured on the vertical axis by a series of horizontal lines that are 1 mm apart
2. Duration—measured on the horizontal axis by a series of vertical lines; the interval between vertical lines equals 0.04 second (Fig. 1–13)

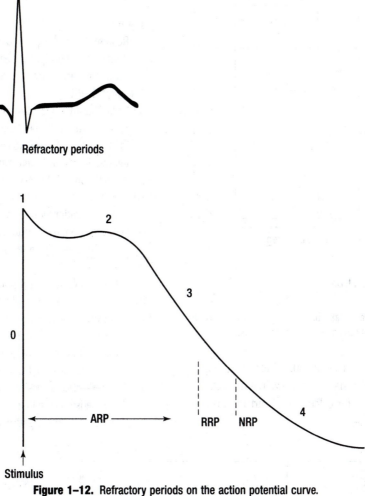

Refractory periods

Figure 1–12. Refractory periods on the action potential curve.

CALCULATING HEART RATES

Calculating heart rates is an essential tool to interpreting dysrhythmias. Once you understand the layout and measurement of the graph paper, rate calculations become easy. There are three possible methods for determining heart rates (Fig. 1–14). Method 1 is the most accurate, yet it is very time consuming to calculate and impractical when trying to get a quick estimate of the heart rate.

Method 2, on the other hand, can be completed very quickly, but its use is limited to regular rhythms (Table 1–1). Method 3 is the most practical and commonly used because calculations can be determined for both regular and irregular rhythms quickly.

In the self-evaluation section of Chapter 1, all three methods have been used so that you can gain

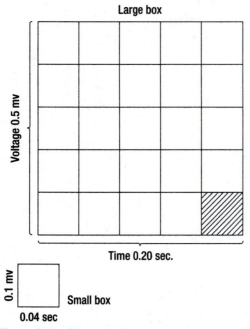

Large box

Voltage 0.5 mv

Time 0.20 sec.

0.1 mv

Small box

0.04 sec

Figure 1–13. Schematic of one large box from graph paper. Five small boxes equal one large box.

experience in practicing all three approaches. However, in the remaining self-evaluation sections, Method 3 is used for calculating heart rates unless otherwise indicated.

THE NORMAL ECG COMPLEX

1. P wave
   a. Represents atrial depolarization
   b. If present and upright in Lead II, normally indicates impulse originated in S-A node (Fig. 1–15)
2. PR interval (PRI)
   a. Normal duration: 0.12–0.20 second
   b. Measured from the beginning of the P wave to the beginning of the QRS complex
   c. Represents atrial depolarization and delay (0.1 second) through the A-V node (Fig. 1–16)
3. QRS complex
   a. Normal duration: less than (<) 0.12 second
   b. Measured from the beginning of the QRS (Q or R wave, whichever is present) to the end of the S wave
   c. Represents ventricular depolarization
   d. Q wave—first negative (downward) deflection
   e. R wave—first positive (upward) deflection above the isoelectric line
   f. S wave—first negative (downward) deflection following the R wave below the isoelectric line
   g. R′ wave—second positive (upward) deflection above the isoelectric line
   h. S′ wave—second negative (downward) deflec-

1 1500 divided by number of small boxes between 2 R waves	— most accurate — only used with regular rhythms — takes time to figure (see Table 1–1)	or memorize this scale
2 300 divided by number of large boxes between 2 R waves	— very quick — not too accurate with fast rates — only used with *regular* rhythms	1 lg. sq. = 300 2 lg. sq. = 150 3 lg. sq. = 100 4 lg. sq. = 75 5 lg. sq. = 60 6 lg. sq. = 50
3 10 multiplied by number of Rs in 6 seconds	— less precise — only method good for *irregular* rhythms — very quick estimate	

Figure 1–14. Three methods for calculating heart rates.

TABLE 1–1. QUICK REFERENCE TABLE FOR CALCULATING HEART RATE IF ECG RHYTHM IS REGULAR

Cycle Length (Seconds)	Number of 0.04 Sec Boxes	Rate	Cycle Length (Seconds)	Number of 0.04 Sec Boxes	Rate
0.16	4	375	0.84	21	72
0.20	5	300	0.88	22	68
0.24	6	250	0.92	23	65
0.28	7	214	0.96	24	63
0.32	8	188	1.00	25	60
0.36	9	168	1.04	26	58
0.40	10	150	1.12	28	54
0.44	11	136	1.20	30	50
0.48	12	125	1.28	32	47
0.52	13	115	1.36	34	44
0.56	14	107	1.44	36	42
0.60	15	100	1.52	38	40
0.64	16	94	1.60	40	38
0.68	17	88	1.68	42	36
0.72	18	83	1.76	44	35
0.76	19	79	1.84	46	33
0.80	20	75	1.92	48	31

tion following the R wave below the isoelectric line (Fig. 1–17)

4. ST segment
   a. Period between the completion of ventricular depolarization and beginning of ventricular repolarization
   b. Normally isoelectric; may be elevated or depressed with myocardial injury, ischemia,

ventricular aneurysm, and some medications (Fig. 1–18)

5. T wave
   a. Represents recovery phase (ventricular repolarization)
   b. Normally upright in Lead II; may be inverted or diphasic if myocardial ischemia or injury is present (Fig. 1–19)

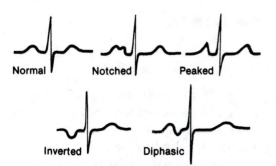

Normal   Notched   Peaked

Inverted   Diphasic

Figure 1–15. Variation in P wave configurations.

Prolonged   Shortened   Normal

Figure 1–16. Variation in PR Interval duration.

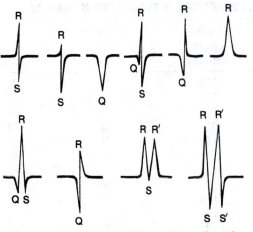

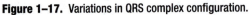

Figure 1–17. Variations in QRS complex configuration.

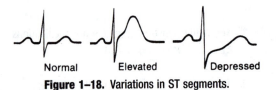

Figure 1–18. Variations in ST segments.

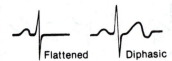

Figure 1–19. Variations in T wave configurations.

CLASSIFICATION OF DYSRHYTHMIAS

By Site

1. Sinus
2. Atrial
3. Junctional
4. Ventricular

By Mechanism

1. Tachycardia (greater than 100/min)
2. Bradycardia (less than 60/min)
3. Prematurity (ectopic)
4. Flutter
5. Fibrillation
6. Conduction defects

APPROACH TO DYSRHYTHMIA INTERPRETATION

1. Rhythm
   a. PP interval (PPI)
   b. RR interval (RRI)
2. Rate
   a. PP rate (PPR) atrial rate
   b. RR rate (RRR) ventricular rate
3. P wave configuration
4. PR interval (PRI) duration
5. QRS complex duration and configuration

Questions to Ask

Rhythm (Note: if the difference between intervals is less than .08 second, it is considered regular)

1. Is the PP interval regular or irregular?
2. Is the RR interval regular or irregular?
3. Are there any early complexes?
4. Are there any late complexes?
5. Is there a pattern of irregularity?

Rate

1. What is the exact atrial rate (PP rate)?
2. What is the exact ventricular rate (RR rate)?
3. Is it within normal limits?
4. Is it rapid?
5. Is it slow?
6. Is the atrial rate the same as the ventricular rate?

P Wave

1. Is it present?
2. What is the configuration? (upright in Lead II?)
3. Is there one P for every QRS?
4. Is the P in front of or behind the QRS?
5. Are there more Ps than QRSs? Fewer?
6. Do all the P waves look alike?
7. Can you plot P waves through the cycles?

PR Interval (PRI)

1. What is the exact duration of the PRI?
2. Is it short?
3. Is it prolonged?
4. Are all the PRIs constant?
5. If the PRI is not constant, is it getting progressively longer?
6. Is there a pattern to the changing PRI?

QRS Complex

1. What is the configuration?
2. What is the exact duration of the QRS complex?
3. Is it prolonged?
4. Do all QRSs look alike?
5. Does the QRS bear a fixed relationship to the P wave?

SELF-EVALUATION

Directions

Answer keys for the Self-Evaluation section begin on page 255.

1. **Matching.** Place the letter of the appropriate item(s) before each numbered statement. Some answers are used more than once, and not all answers will be used.
2. **ECG practice strips.** For the following ECG strips:.
   1. Label:
      a. P wave
      b. PRI
      c. QRS
      d. ST segment
      e. T wave
   (Place labels on each ECG strip.)
   2. Determine if PPI and RRI are regular or irregular.
   3. Calculate rates using appropriate method:
      a. PPR
      b. RRR
   4. Measure:
      a. PRI
      b. QRS
   (Place calculations for 2–4 in spaces provided.)
   *Note that all strips are Lead II and are 6 seconds long unless otherwise indicated.

MATCHING

_____ 1. Two types of cardiac cells
_____ 2. Ability to transmit impulses
_____ 3. Ability to respond to an impulse
_____ 4. Ability to initiate an impulse
_____ 5. Property of regularity
_____ 6. Intrinsic rate of S-A node
_____ 7. Intrinsic rate of A-V node
_____ 8. Intrinsic rate of ventricle
_____ 9. When stimulated, causes an increase in heart rate and pumping action
_____ 10. When stimulated, causes a decrease in heart rate and pumping action
_____ 11. Electrical stimulation of cells
_____ 12. Electrical recovery of cells
_____ 13. Time in the cardiac cycle during which the cardiac cells cannot respond to a stimulus
_____ 14. Time during the cardiac cycle in which the cardiac cells can respond to a strong stimulus
_____ 15. Time when the heart has completed repolarization and is ready to respond to another stimulus

a. excitability
b. myocardial
c. nonrefractory period
d. contraction
e. sympathetic nerves
f. depolarization
g. 20–40/min
h. automaticity
i. specialized
j. relaxation
k. 40–60/min
l. relative refractory period
m. parasympathetic nerves
n. rhythmicity
o. repolarization
p. 60–100/min
q. absolute refractory period
r. conductivity

_____ 16. On what part of the PQRST complex does the vulnerable period fall?
_____ 17. Two dysrhythmias that may be generated if a stimulus occurs during the vulnerable period
_____ 18. Dominant pacemaker of the heart
_____ 19. Two other parts of the heart that can pace the heart if the dominant pacemaker fails.
_____ 20. Duration in seconds of one small box on the ECG graph paper
_____ 21. Duration in seconds of one large box on the ECG graph paper
_____ 22. Two types of rhythms that are best calculated by counting the number of R waves in a 6-second strip and multiplying by 10
_____ 23. The fastest way to estimate heart rates for these rhythms is to divide 300 by the number of large squares between two R waves.
_____ 24. The most accurate way to calculate heart rates for these types of rhythms is to divide 1500 by the number of small boxes between two R waves.
_____ 25. Represents atrial depolarization
_____ 26. Represents ventricular depolarization

a. atrial fibrillation
b. S-A node
c. internodal pathways
d. 0.04 second
e. irregular
f. 0.20 second
g. T wave
h. 0.06 second
i. A-V junction
j. atrial tachycardia
k. regular
l. ventricular tachycardia
m. P wave
n. His–Purkinje system
o. QRS complex
p. ventricular fibrillation
q. S wave

_____ 27. Represents ventricular repolarization

_____ 28. Represents the time it takes for an impulse to pass from the S-A node through the atria and the delay through the A-V node

_____ 29. The delay at the A-V node allows time for this to occur

_____ 30. Measured from the beginning of the P wave to the beginning of the QRS complex

_____ 31. Measured from the beginning of the Q wave to the end of the S wave

_____ 32. Measurement of the normal PR interval

_____ 33. Measurement of the normal QRS complex

_____ 34. An initial negative (downward) deflection of the QRS complex

_____ 35. First positive (upward) deflection of the QRS complex

_____ 36. First negative (downward) deflection of the QRS complex following the first positive (upward) deflection

_____ 37. A negative (downward) deflection of the QRS complex following the first positive (upward) deflection

_____ 38. Second positive (upward) deflection of the QRS complex

a. T wave
b. ventricular filling
c. 0.12 second
d. P wave
e. 0.12–0.20 second
f. atrial filling
g. Q wave
h. S wave
i. S' wave
j. PR interval
k. less than (<) 0.12 second
l. R wave
m. R' wave
n. QRS complex
o. 0.10–0.24 second
p. PR segment

ECG PRACTICE STRIPS

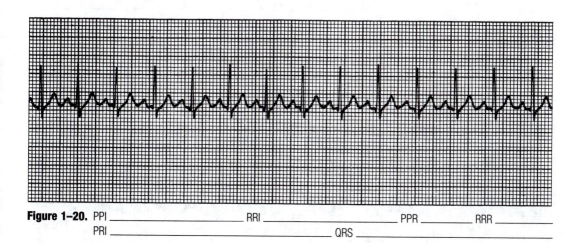

Figure 1–20. PPI _____ RRI _____ PPR _____ RRR _____
PRI _____ QRS _____

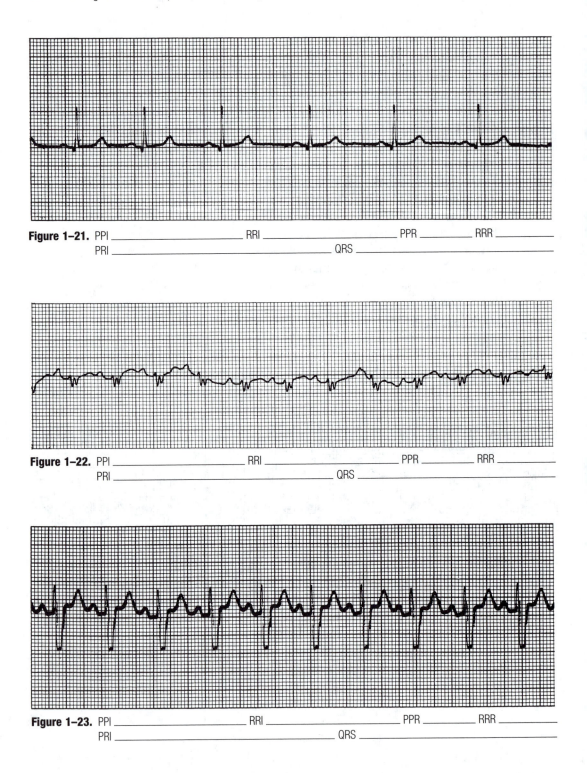

Figure 1–21. PPI _____ RRI _____ PPR _____ RRR _____
PRI _____ QRS _____

Figure 1–22. PPI _____ RRI _____ PPR _____ RRR _____
PRI _____ QRS _____

Figure 1–23. PPI _____ RRI _____ PPR _____ RRR _____
PRI _____ QRS _____

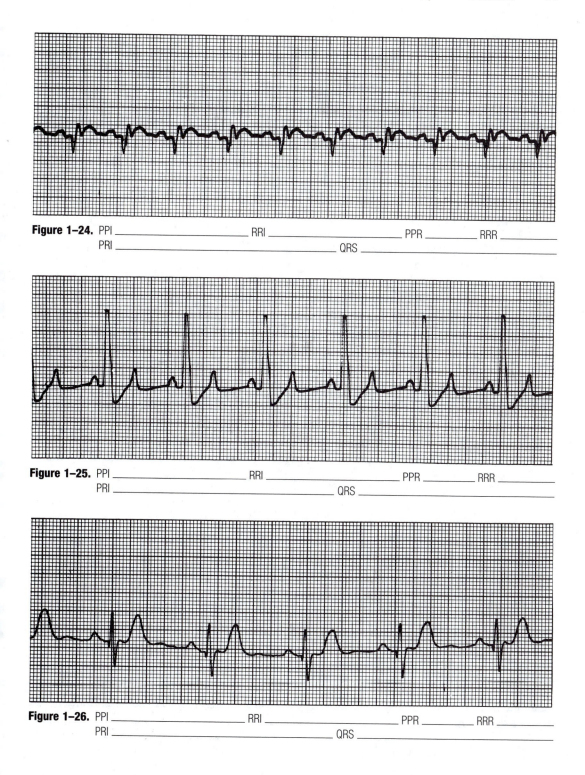

Figure 1–24. PPI _____ RRI _____ PPR _____ RRR _____
PRI _____ QRS _____

Figure 1–25. PPI _____ RRI _____ PPR _____ RRR _____
PRI _____ QRS _____

Figure 1–26. PPI _____ RRI _____ PPR _____ RRR _____
PRI _____ QRS _____

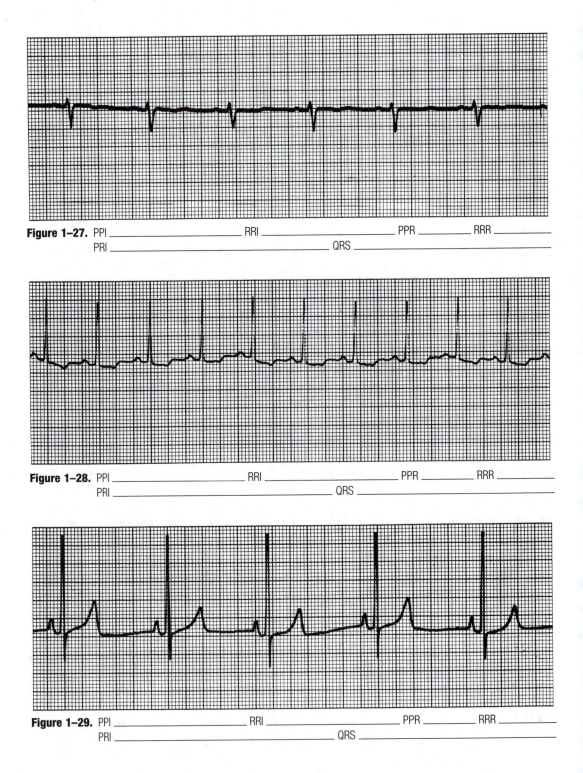

Figure 1–27. PPI _____ RRI _____ PPR _____ RRR _____
PRI _____ QRS _____

Figure 1–28. PPI _____ RRI _____ PPR _____ RRR _____
PRI _____ QRS _____

Figure 1–29. PPI _____ RRI _____ PPR _____ RRR _____
PRI _____ QRS _____

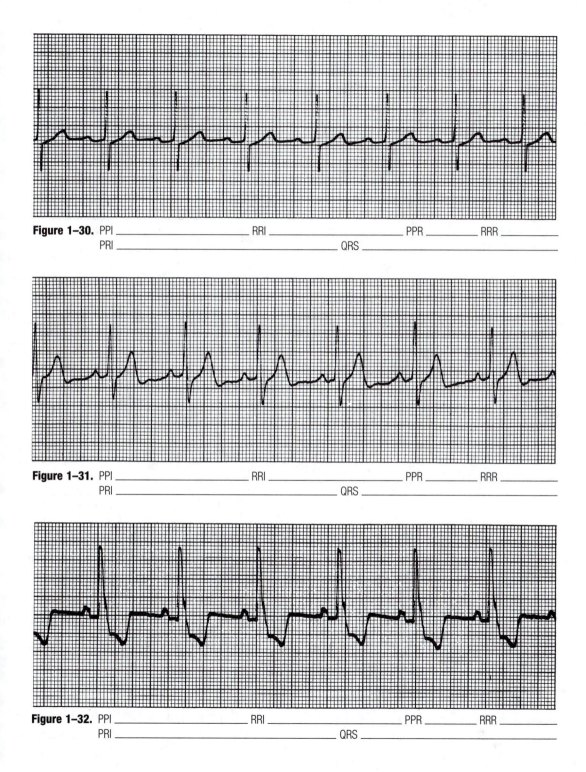

Figure 1–30. PPI _____ RRI _____ PPR _____ RRR _____
PRI _____ QRS _____

Figure 1–31. PPI _____ RRI _____ PPR _____ RRR _____
PRI _____ QRS _____

Figure 1–32. PPI _____ RRI _____ PPR _____ RRR _____
PRI _____ QRS _____

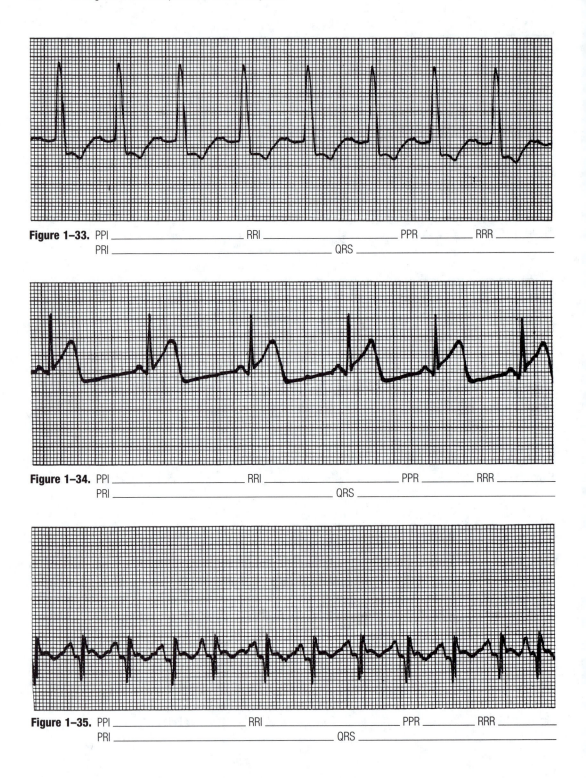

Figure 1–33. PPI _____ RRI _____ PPR _____ RRR _____
PRI _____ QRS _____

Figure 1–34. PPI _____ RRI _____ PPR _____ RRR _____
PRI _____ QRS _____

Figure 1–35. PPI _____ RRI _____ PPR _____ RRR _____
PRI _____ QRS _____

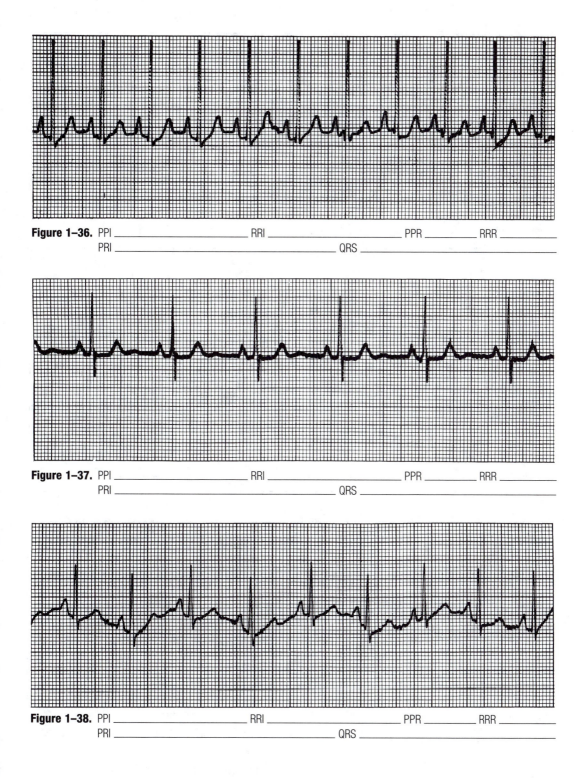

Figure 1–36. PPI _____ RRI _____ PPR _____ RRR _____
PRI _____ QRS _____

Figure 1–37. PPI _____ RRI _____ PPR _____ RRR _____
PRI _____ QRS _____

Figure 1–38. PPI _____ RRI _____ PPR _____ RRR _____
PRI _____ QRS _____

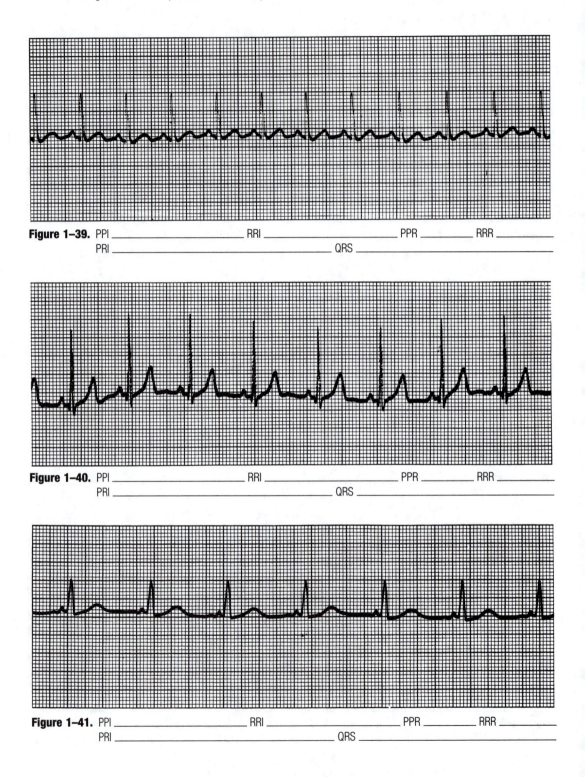

Figure 1–39. PPI _____ RRI _____ PPR _____ RRR _____
PRI _____ QRS _____

Figure 1–40. PPI _____ RRI _____ PPR _____ RRR _____
PRI _____ QRS _____

Figure 1–41. PPI _____ RRI _____ PPR _____ RRR _____
PRI _____ QRS _____

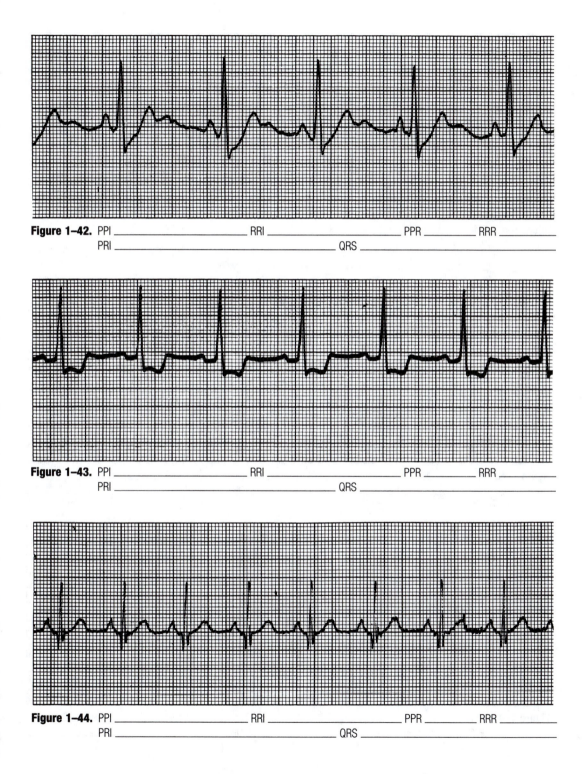

Figure 1–42. PPI _____ RRI _____ PPR _____ RRR _____
PRI _____ QRS _____

Figure 1–43. PPI _____ RRI _____ PPR _____ RRR _____
PRI _____ QRS _____

Figure 1–44. PPI _____ RRI _____ PPR _____ RRR _____
PRI _____ QRS _____

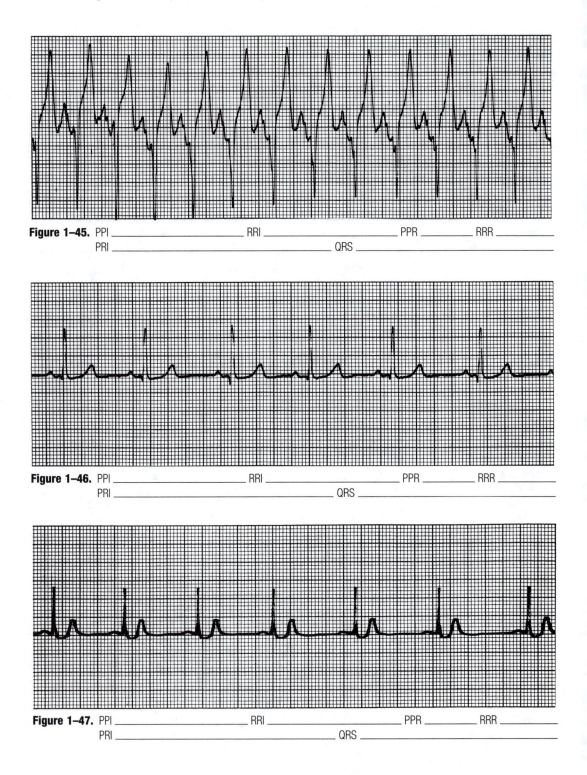

Figure 1–45. PPI _____ RRI _____ PPR _____ RRR _____
PRI _____ QRS _____

Figure 1–46. PPI _____ RRI _____ PPR _____ RRR _____
PRI _____ QRS _____

Figure 1–47. PPI _____ RRI _____ PPR _____ RRR _____
PRI _____ QRS _____

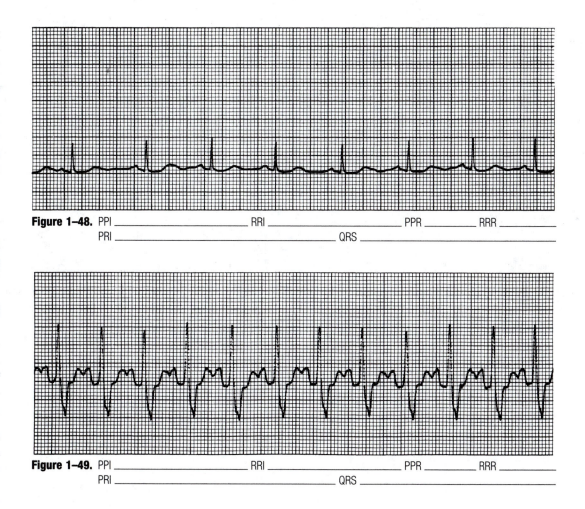

Figure 1–48. PPI _____ RRI _____ PPR _____ RRR _____
PRI _____ QRS _____

Figure 1–49. PPI _____ RRI _____ PPR _____ RRR _____
PRI _____ QRS _____

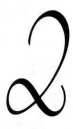

Sinus and Atrial Dysrhythmias

DYSRHYTHMIAS ORIGINATING IN THE SINOATRIAL (S-A) NODE

I. Normal Sinus Rhythm (NSR)
A. ECG features
1. *PP interval:* regular
2. *RR interval:* regular
3. *PP rate:* 60–100/min
4. *RR rate:* 60–100/min
5. *P wave:* upright in Lead II
6. *PRI:* 0.12–0.20 second
7. *QRS interval:* less than (<) 0.12 second
(Figs. 2–1 and 2–2)
B. Common etiology: normal
C. Clinical signs and symptoms: none

II. Sinus Bradycardia (SB)
A. ECG features
1. *PP interval:* regular
2. *RR interval:* regular
3. *PP rate:* less than 60/min
4. *RR rate:* less than 60/min
5. *P wave:* upright in Lead II
6. *PRI:* 0.12–0.20 second
7. *QRS interval:* less than (<) 0.12 second
(Figs. 2–3 and 2–4)
B. Common etiology
1. Damage to the sinoatrial (S-A) node
2. Increased parasympathetic tone

3. Hypoxemia
4. Normal in conditioned athletes
C. Clinical signs and symptoms
1. Seldom symptomatic, unless rate markedly decreased
2. Slow, regular pulse
3. Potential danger—may lead to blocks or escape rhythms

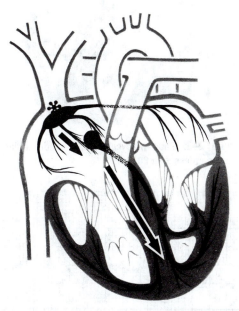

Figure 2–1. Normal sinus rhythm: S-A node initiates impulse at 60–100/min.

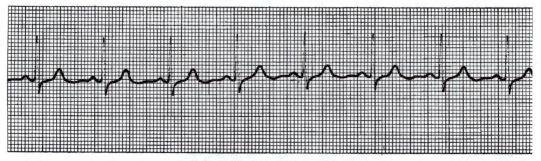

Figure 2–2. Normal sinus rhythm.

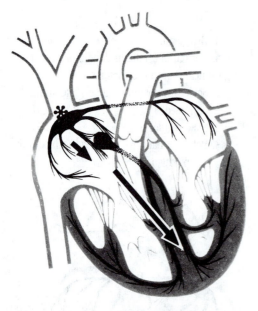

Figure 2–3. Sinus bradycardia: S-A node initiates impulse at less than 60/min.

III. Sinus Tachycardia (ST)

  A. ECG features
    1. *PP interval:* regular
    2. *RR interval:* regular
    3. *PP rate:* greater than 100/min
    4. *RR rate:* greater than 100/min
    5. *P wave:* upright in Lead II
    6. *PRI:* 0.12–0.20 second
    7. *QRS interval:* less than ($<$) 0.12 second
      (Figs. 2–5 and 2–6)
*Note: In rates greater than 160/min, it may be difficult to identify the P wave.
  B. Common etiology
    1. Pain
    2. Fever
    3. Hypoxemia
    4. Congestive heart failure (CHF)/pulmonary edema

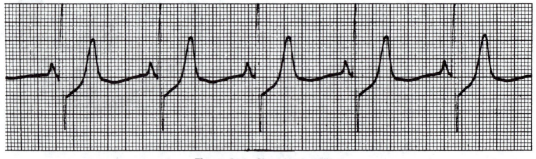

Figure 2–4. Sinus bradycardia.

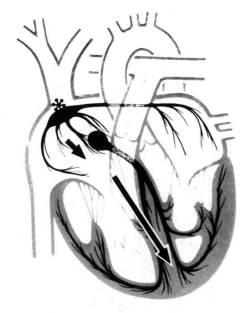

Figure 2–5. Sinus tachycardia: S-A node initiates impulse greater than 100/min.

 5. Shock
 6. Agitation
 7. Illicit drugs (cocaine, methamphetamines, etc.)
 8. Caffeine
 9. Nicotine
 C. Clinical signs and symptoms
  1. Vary with rate
  2. Rapid, regular pulse

 3. May sense palpitations
 4. May experience dyspnea
 5. May be asymptomatic
 6. In presence of myocardial infarction (MI), may be associated with ischemia and/or congestive heart failure

IV. Sinus Arrhythmia
 A. ECG features
  1. *PP interval:* irregular
  2. *RR interval:* irregular
  3. *PP rate:* varies (usually 60–100/min)
  4. *RR rate:* varies (usually 60–100/min)
  5. *P wave:* upright in Lead II
  6. *PRI:* 0.12–0.20 second
  7. *QRS interval:* less than (<) 0.12 second (Figs. 2–7 and 2–8)
 B. Common etiology
  1. Common in children and young adults
  2. Respirations
   a. Increase in heart rate with inspiration
   b. Decrease in heart rate with expiration
  3. Considered benign
 C. Clinical signs and symptoms
  1. Irregular pulse
  2. Usually asymptomatic
V. S-A Block or S-A Arrest (An entire PQRST complex is missing. Missing complex may be followed by an escape mechanism from the junction or ventricle.)

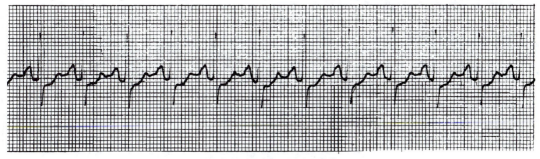

Figure 2–6. Sinus tachycardia.

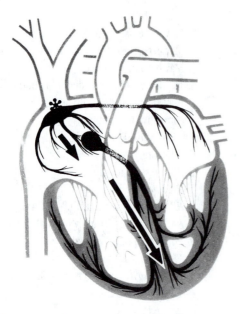

Figure 2–7. Sinus arrhythmia: S-A node initiates impulse irregularly.

A. ECG features
   1. *PP interval:* usually regular except for missing P wave
   2. *RR interval:* usually regular except for missing QRS complex

   3. *PP rate:* usually 60–100/min; may be bradycardic
   4. *RR rate:* usually 60–100/min; may be bradycardic
   5. *P wave:* normal and upright in Lead II; absent on blocked or arrested complexes
   6. *PRI:* 0.12–0.20 second on conducted complexes; absent on blocked or arrested complexes
   7. *QRS interval:* less than (<) 0.12 second on conducted complexes, absent on blocked or arrested complexes (Figs. 2–9 and 2–10)

B. Common etiology
   1. Insult to the S-A node
   2. Increased parasympathetic tone
   3. Hypoxemia
   4. Digitalis toxicity

C. Clinical signs and symptoms
   1. Patient usually unaware of dysrhythmia
   2. Patient may sense a skipped beat
   3. Pulse will have a prolonged pause
   4. If frequent, may develop signs and symptoms of decreased cardiac output due to bradycardic rate

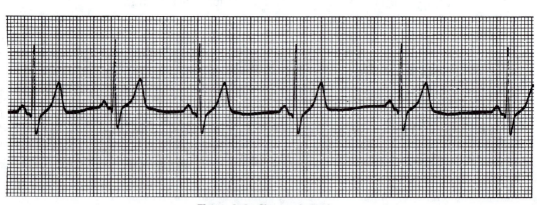

Figure 2–8. Sinus arrhythmia.

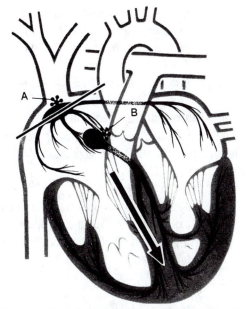

Figure 2–9. S-A block or S-A arrest: **A.** Impulse blocked or arrested in S-A node for one cycle. **B.** Escape junctional complex may come in (refer to Chapter 3).

DYSRHYTHMIAS ORIGINATING IN THE ATRIA

I. Premature Atrial Complex (PAC)

A. ECG features

1. *PP interval:* regular except for early beat (interval between the P wave before and the P wave after the PAC does not equal two times the normal PP interval. Sinus node is depolarized by PAC and resets, causing the next PP interval to have a normal duration.)

2. *RR interval:* regular except for early complex

3. *PP rate:* varies

4. *RR rate:* varies

5. *P wave:* may differ from sinus P wave; may be notched, peaked, diphasic, or lost in preceding ST segment or T wave

6. *PRI:* usually changes (may or may not be prolonged)

7. PACs do not have to occur in the same relationship to previous PQRST complex and, most often, do not.

*Note: Always identify underlying rhythm within which the PAC occurs.

8. *QRS interval:* less than (<) 0.12 second (Figs. 2–11 and 2–12)

B. Common etiology

1. Atrial stretch (may be seen with valve disease, early CHF, liver disease, pulmonary hypertension, stimulant medications, and illicit drugs)

2. Hypoxemia

3. Atrial stimulation (from catheter, pacemaker wire, etc.)

4. Frequent PACs may precede atrial flutter, atrial fibrillation, or supraventricular tachycardia

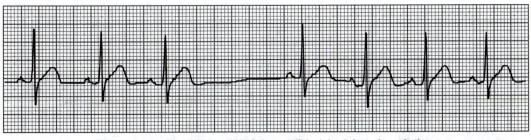

Figure 2–10. Sinus rhythm with S-A arrest/block back into sinus rhythm.

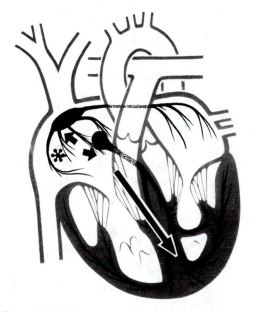

Figure 2–11. Premature atrial complex: Irritable focus in atrium initiates impulse early.

C. Clinical signs and symptoms
  1. Irregular pulse
  2. Patient usually unaware of PACs

II. Atrial Tachycardia

A. ECG features
  1. *PP interval:* regular
  2. *RR interval:* regular
  3. *PP rate:* 150–250/min
  4. *RR rate:* 150–250/min
  5. *P wave:* all P waves alike; shape of P waves same as PAC. Rapid rate may cause P wave to merge with proceeding T wave. If unable to distinguish P wave, interpreted as *supraventricular tachycardia (SVT)*
  6. *PRI:* 0.12–0.20 second
  7. *QRS interval:* less than (<) 0.12 second (Figs. 2–13 and 2–14)

*Note: Paroxysmal supraventricular tachycardia (PSVT) is the same as supraventricular tachycardia except that it starts and stops suddenly (Fig. 2–15).

B. Common etiology
  1. Atrial stretch (may be seen with valve disease, early CHF, liver disease, pulmonary hypertension, stimulant medications, and illicit drugs)
  2. Increased sympathetic tone
  3. Hypoxemia
  4. Digitalis toxicity
  5. Atrial stimulation (from catheter, pacemaker wire, etc.)

C. Clinical signs and symptoms
  1. Rapid, regular pulse
  2. May exhibit signs and symptoms of decreased cardiac output or CHF
  3. May be extremely dangerous in an MI
    a. Increased oxygen consumption
    b. Increased workload

III. Atrial Flutter

A. ECG features
  1. *PP interval:* regular
  2. *RR interval:* regular or irregular

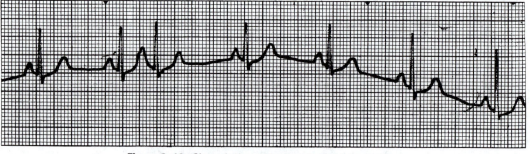

Figure 2–12. Sinus rhythm with premature atrial complex.

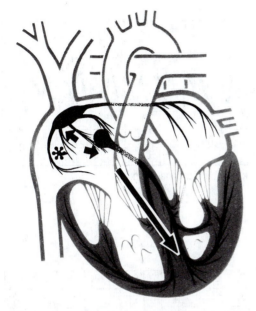

Figure 2–13. Atrial tachycardia: Irritable focus in atrium paces the heart at 150–250/min.

3. *PP rate:* 250–350/min

4. *RR rate:* varies

5. *P wave:* sawtooth appearance (called F waves); more than one F wave is present for each QRS

6. *PRI:* unable to measure

7. *QRS interval:* less than (<) 0.12 second (may be distorted by F wave; Figs. 2–16, 2–17, 2–18, and 2–19)

B. Common etiology

   1. Increased sympathetic tone

   2. Atrial stimulation (from catheter, pacemaker wire, etc.)

   3. Hypoxemia

   4. Valvular disease

   5. Hyperthyroidism

C. Clinical signs and symptoms

   1. Depend on ventricular rate

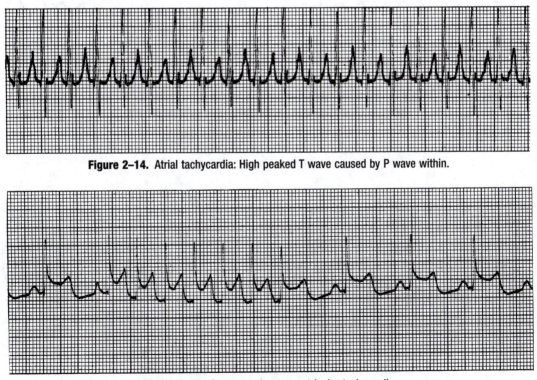

Figure 2–14. Atrial tachycardia: High peaked T wave caused by P wave within.

Figure 2–15. Paroxysmal supraventricular tachycardia.

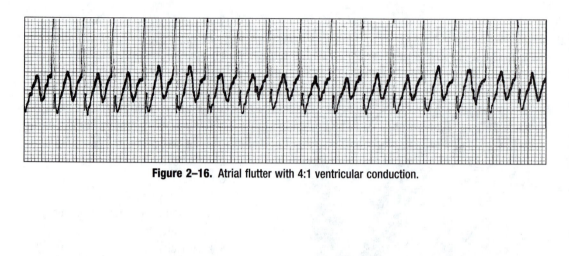

Figure 2–16. Atrial flutter with 4:1 ventricular conduction.

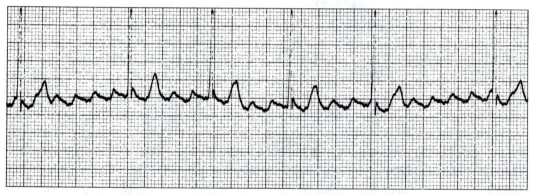

Figure 2–17. Atrial flutter with variable ventricular conduction.

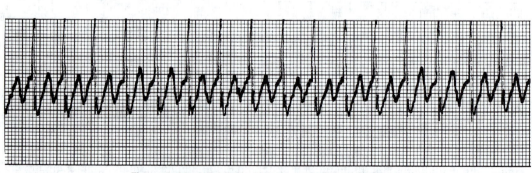

Figure 2–18. Atrial flutter with 2:1 ventricular conduction.

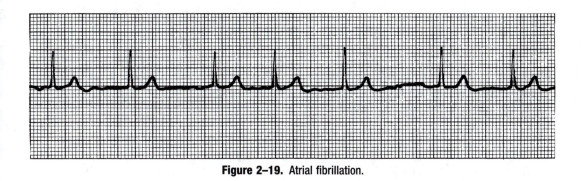

Figure 2–19. Atrial fibrillation.

  2. May experience palpitations, angina, or dyspnea
  3. May cause ischemia and/or CHF
IV. Atrial Fibrillation
  A. ECG features
   1. *PP interval:* grossly irregular
   2. *RR interval:* grossly irregular
   3. *PP rate:* greater than 400/min (unmeasurable)
   4. *RR rate:* varies
   5. *P wave:* no discernible P wave; atrial activity is characterized by undulations in the baseline that may be coarse or fine (called *F* waves)
   6. *PRI:* unable to measure
   7. *QRS interval:* less than (<) 0.12 second (Figs. 2–19, 2–20)

  B. Common etiology
   1. Increased sympathetic tone
   2. Arteriosclerotic heart disease (ASHD)
   3. Hypoxemia
   4. Hyperthyroidism
   5. Valvular disease
  C. Clinical signs and symptoms
   1. Irregular pulse
   2. May have pulse deficit (difference in apical rate and radial pulse)
   3. Depend on ventricular response
   4. May experience palpitations, angina, or dyspnea
   5. May cause decreased cardiac output
   6. May cause ischemia/CHF
   7. May develop emboli from atrial wall thrombus formation

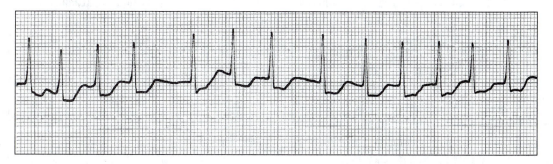

Figure 2–20. Atrial fibrillation. Note: the RRI appears more regular as the ventricular rate increases.

SELF-EVALUATION

Directions

Answer keys for the Self-Evaluation section begin on page 265.

1. **Matching.** Place the letter of the appropriate item(s) before each numbered statement. Some answers are used more than once, and not all answers will be used.
2. **ECG practice strips.** For simplicity and practicality, all rates have been calculated by using Method 3 (Fig. 1–14). Keep in mind that your measurements for PRIs and QRS complexes may vary slightly and still be correct. Use the systematic approach shown in Chapter 1 to interpret the ECG strips. It is important that you follow all steps and not take shortcuts.

For the following ECG strips:
1. Determine if the PPI and RRI are regular or irregular.
2. Calculate rates using the appropriate method:
   a. PPR
   b. RRR
3. Measure:
   a. PRI
   b. QRS
4. Interpretation

Place your answers in the spaces provided.

*Note that all strips are Lead II and are 6 seconds long unless otherwise indicated.

MATCHING

_____	1.	Represents atrial depolarization on the ECG	a. upright
_____	2.	Normal pacemaker of the heart	b. 0.12–0.20 second
_____	3.	In Lead II, shape of the P wave if impulse originates in the S-A node	c. S-A node
			d. regular
_____	4.	Rate for normal sinus rhythm	e. irregular
_____	5.	Dysrhythmia originating in S-A node that has a rate less than 60/min	f. inspiration
			g. expiration
_____	6.	Dysrhythmia originating in S-A node that has a rate greater than 100/min	h. P wave
			i. 60–100/min
_____	7.	Normal measurement of the PR interval	j. sinus bradycardia
_____	8.	Measurement of PR interval in NSR, sinus bradycardia, and sinus tachycardia	k. sinus tachycardia
			l. inverted
_____	9.	Where in the conduction system the impulse originates in a sinus arrhythmia	m. 40–60/min
			n. atrium
_____	10.	In a Lead II, shape of P wave in a sinus arrhythmia	o. greater than 0.20 second
_____	11.	RRI of a sinus arrhythmia	
_____	12.	RRI of a sinus bradycardia	
_____	13.	In a sinus arrhythmia, during this phase of the respiratory cycle the heart rate increases.	
_____	14.	In a sinus arrhythmia, during this phase of the respiratory cycle the heart rate decreases.	

_____ 15. A dysrhythmia in which an entire PQRST complex is missing
_____ 16. An early beat initiated by an irritable focus in the atrium
_____ 17. Shape of P wave in an atrial ectopic
_____ 18. Dysrhythmias originating in the atrium at a rate of 150–250/min
_____ 19. The part of the PQRST complex in which the P wave may fall in an atrial dysrhythmia
_____ 20. Supraventricular tachycardia that starts and stops suddenly
_____ 21. PR interval in an atrial tachycardia
_____ 22. Where in the conduction system an atrial impulse originates
_____ 23. Measurement of the QRS interval in an atrial tachycardia
_____ 24. Where in the cardiac cycle premature atrial complexes occur
_____ 25. A dysrhythmia in which the RRI is grossly irregular and no discernible P waves are present
_____ 26. Where in the conduction system the impulse originates in atrial fibrillation
_____ 27. In atrial fibrillation, the part of the conduction system that determines the number of impulses conducted to the ventricles

a. notched
b. T wave
c. PSVT
d. atrioventricular (A-V) node
e. 0.12–0.20 second
f. PAC
g. atrial fibrillation
h. peaked
i. atrial tachycardia
j. lost in preceding ST segment or T wave
k. atrium
l. less than (<) 0.12 second
m. S-A node
n. diphasic
o. early
p. late
q. greater than 0.20 second
r. 0.12 second or greater
s. S-A arrest/block

_____ 28. Atrial rate in atrial fibrillation
_____ 29. Ventricular rate in atrial fibrillation
_____ 30. Dysrhythmia that has a sawtooth appearance
_____ 31. Atrial rate in atrial flutter
_____ 32. Ventricular rate in atrial flutter
_____ 33. In atrial flutter, the part of the conduction system that determines the number of impulses conducted to the ventricle
_____ 34. If the atrial rate in atrial flutter is 300, determine the ventricular rate for each of the following:
_____ a. 3:1 ventricular conduction
_____ b. 2:1 ventricular conduction
_____ c. 4:1 ventricular conduction
_____ d. 1:1 ventricular conduction
_____ 35. PPI of flutter waves
_____ 36. A rapid, regular, atrial dysrhythmia in which P waves are not distinguishable
_____ 37. Where in the heart the impulse in a supraventricular dysrhythmia originates
_____ 38. Dysrhythmias that frequent premature atrial complexes lead to

a. S-A node
b. A-V node
c. atrium
d. atrial flutter
e. atrial fibrillation
f. supraventricular tachycardia
g. variable
h. greater than 400/min
i. 250–350/min
j. 300/min
k. regular
l. irregular
m. 75/min
n. 100/min
o. 150/min

ECG PRACTICE STRIPS

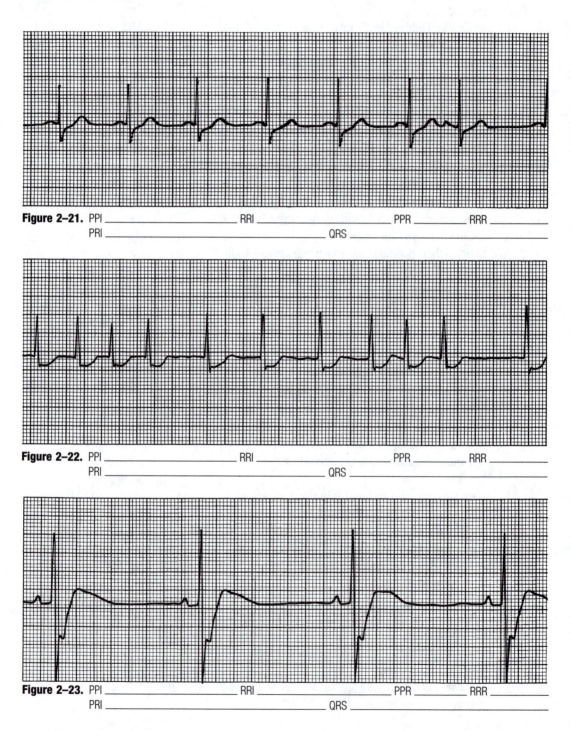

Figure 2–21. PPI _____ RRI _____ PPR _____ RRR _____
PRI _____ QRS _____

Figure 2–22. PPI _____ RRI _____ PPR _____ RRR _____
PRI _____ QRS _____

Figure 2–23. PPI _____ RRI _____ PPR _____ RRR _____
PRI _____ QRS _____

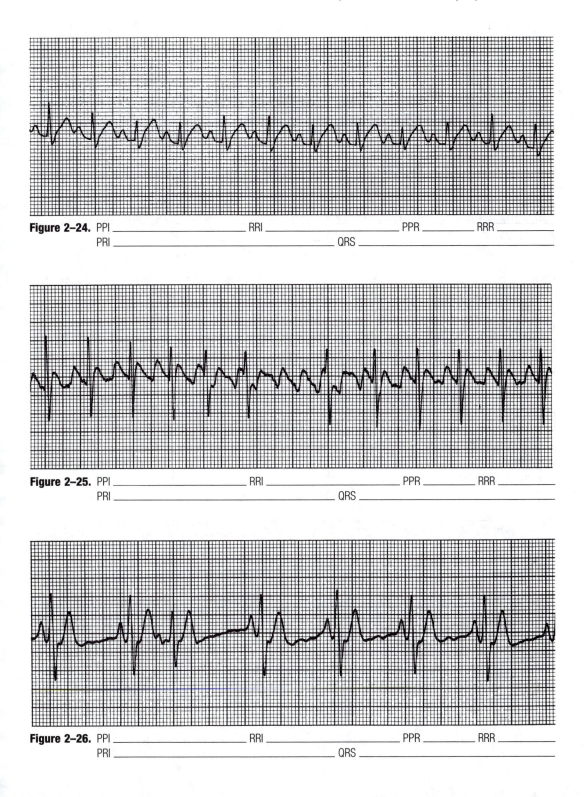

Figure 2–24. PPI _____ RRI _____ PPR _____ RRR _____
PRI _____ QRS _____

Figure 2–25. PPI _____ RRI _____ PPR _____ RRR _____
PRI _____ QRS _____

Figure 2–26. PPI _____ RRI _____ PPR _____ RRR _____
PRI _____ QRS _____

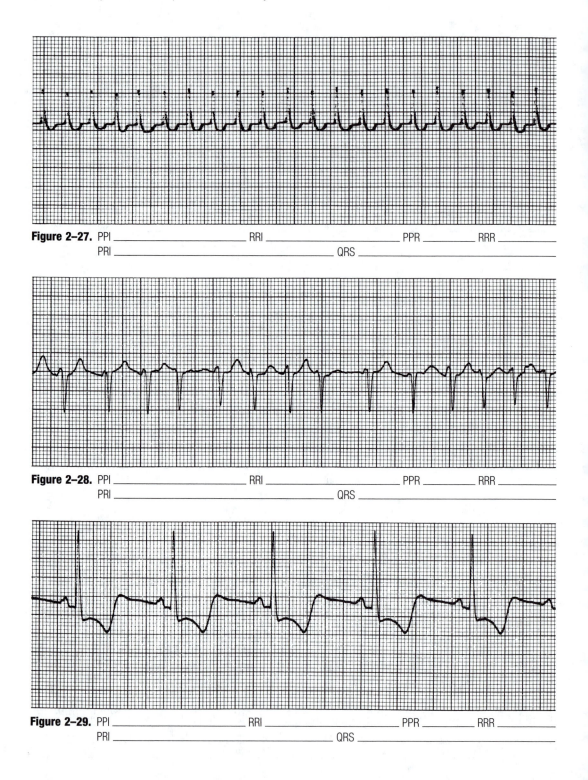

Figure 2–27. PPI _____ RRI _____ PPR _____ RRR _____
PRI _____ QRS _____

Figure 2–28. PPI _____ RRI _____ PPR _____ RRR _____
PRI _____ QRS _____

Figure 2–29. PPI _____ RRI _____ PPR _____ RRR _____
PRI _____ QRS _____

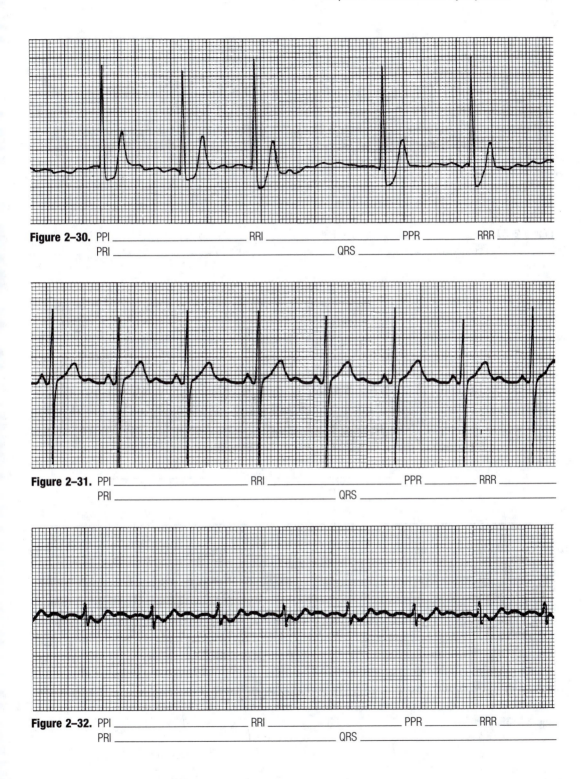

Figure 2–30. PPI _____ RRI _____ PPR _____ RRR _____
PRI _____ QRS _____

Figure 2–31. PPI _____ RRI _____ PPR _____ RRR _____
PRI _____ QRS _____

Figure 2–32. PPI _____ RRI _____ PPR _____ RRR _____
PRI _____ QRS _____

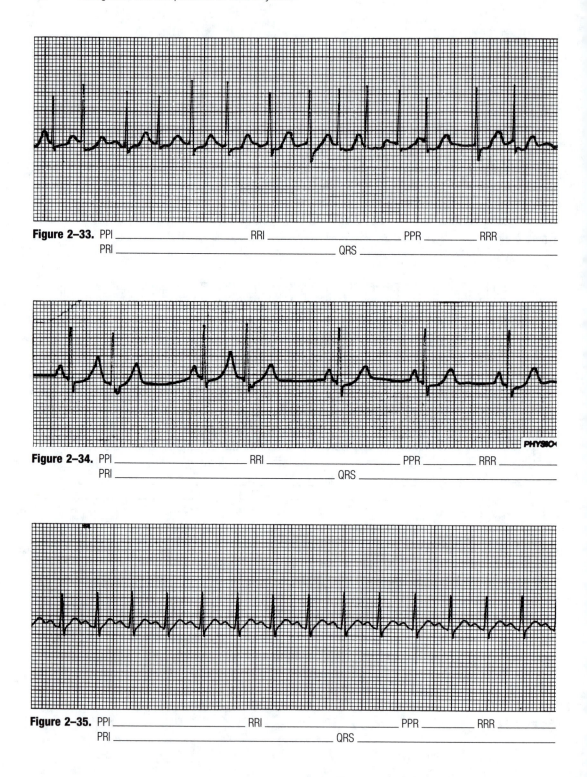

Figure 2–33. PPI _____ RRI _____ PPR _____ RRR _____
                PRI _____ QRS _____

Figure 2–34. PPI _____ RRI _____ PPR _____ RRR _____
                PRI _____ QRS _____

Figure 2–35. PPI _____ RRI _____ PPR _____ RRR _____
                PRI _____ QRS _____

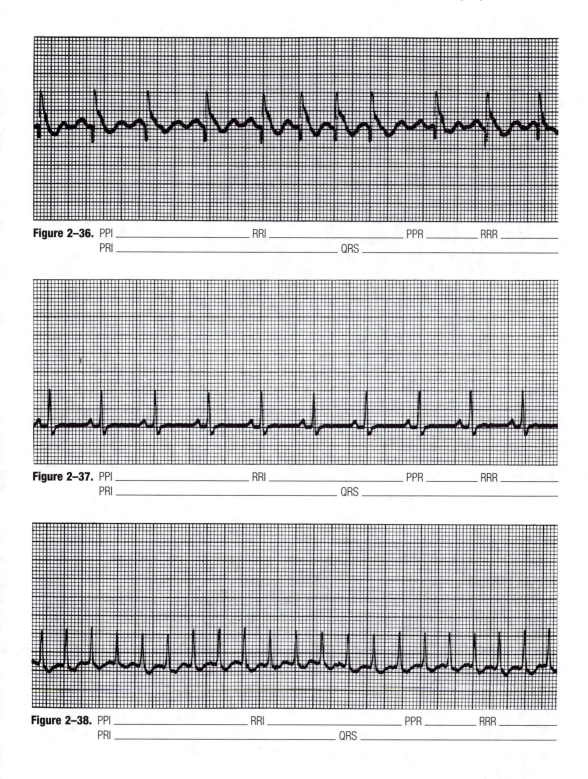

Figure 2–36. PPI _____ RRI _____ PPR _____ RRR _____
PRI _____ QRS _____

Figure 2–37. PPI _____ RRI _____ PPR _____ RRR _____
PRI _____ QRS _____

Figure 2–38. PPI _____ RRI _____ PPR _____ RRR _____
PRI _____ QRS _____

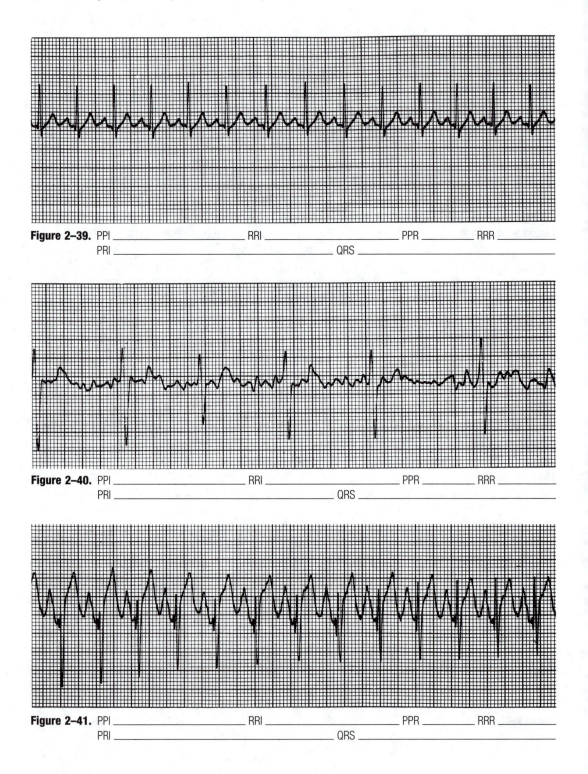

Figure 2–39. PPI _____ RRI _____ PPR _____ RRR _____
PRI _____ QRS _____

Figure 2–40. PPI _____ RRI _____ PPR _____ RRR _____
PRI _____ QRS _____

Figure 2–41. PPI _____ RRI _____ PPR _____ RRR _____
PRI _____ QRS _____

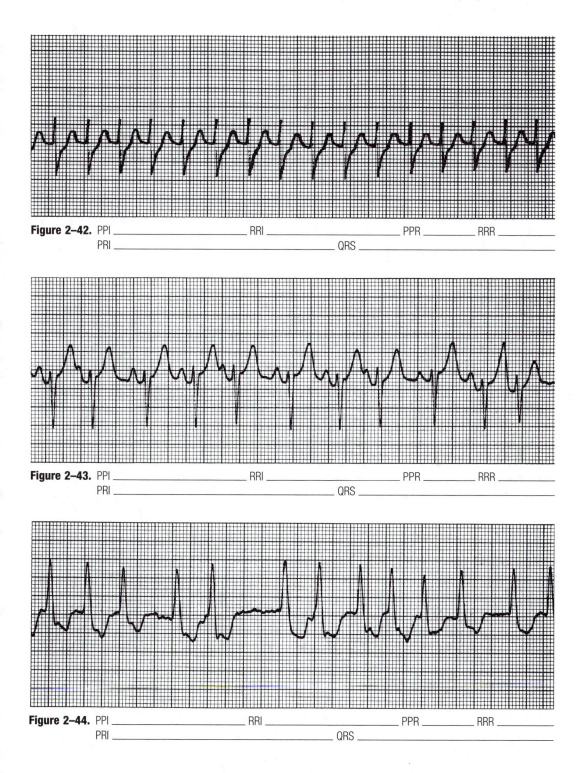

Figure 2–42. PPI _____ RRI _____ PPR _____ RRR _____
PRI _____ QRS _____

Figure 2–43. PPI _____ RRI _____ PPR _____ RRR _____
PRI _____ QRS _____

Figure 2–44. PPI _____ RRI _____ PPR _____ RRR _____
PRI _____ QRS _____

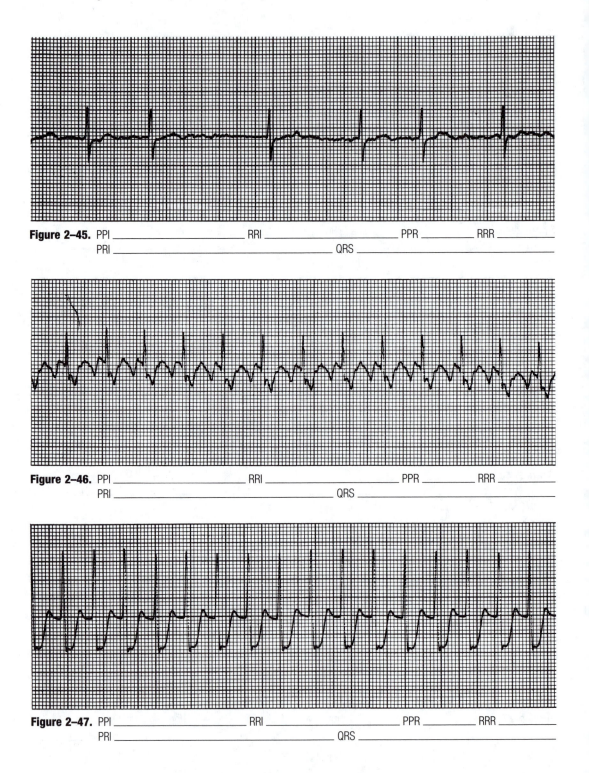

Figure 2–45. PPI _____ RRI _____ PPR _____ RRR _____
PRI _____ QRS _____

Figure 2–46. PPI _____ RRI _____ PPR _____ RRR _____
PRI _____ QRS _____

Figure 2–47. PPI _____ RRI _____ PPR _____ RRR _____
PRI _____ QRS _____

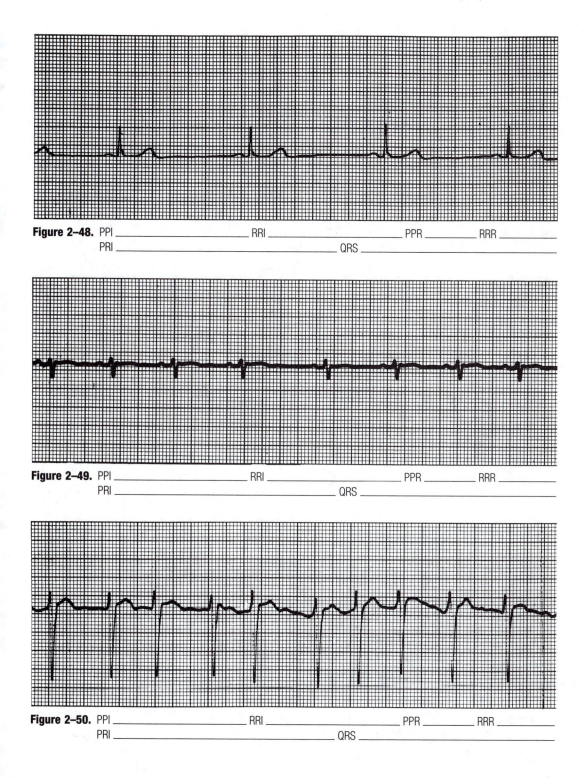

Figure 2–48. PPI _____ RRI _____ PPR _____ RRR _____
PRI _____ QRS _____

Figure 2–49. PPI _____ RRI _____ PPR _____ RRR _____
PRI _____ QRS _____

Figure 2–50. PPI _____ RRI _____ PPR _____ RRR _____
PRI _____ QRS _____

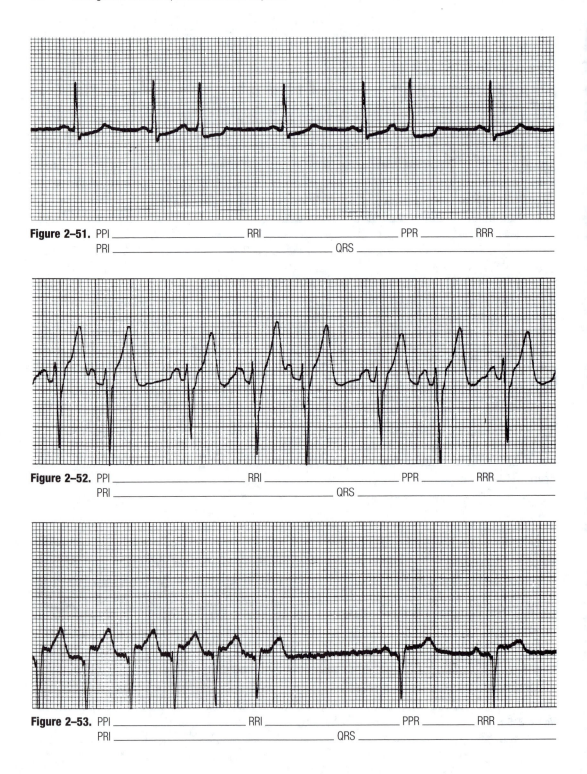

Figure 2–51. PPI _____ RRI _____ PPR _____ RRR _____
PRI _____ QRS _____

Figure 2–52. PPI _____ RRI _____ PPR _____ RRR _____
PRI _____ QRS _____

Figure 2–53. PPI _____ RRI _____ PPR _____ RRR _____
PRI _____ QRS _____

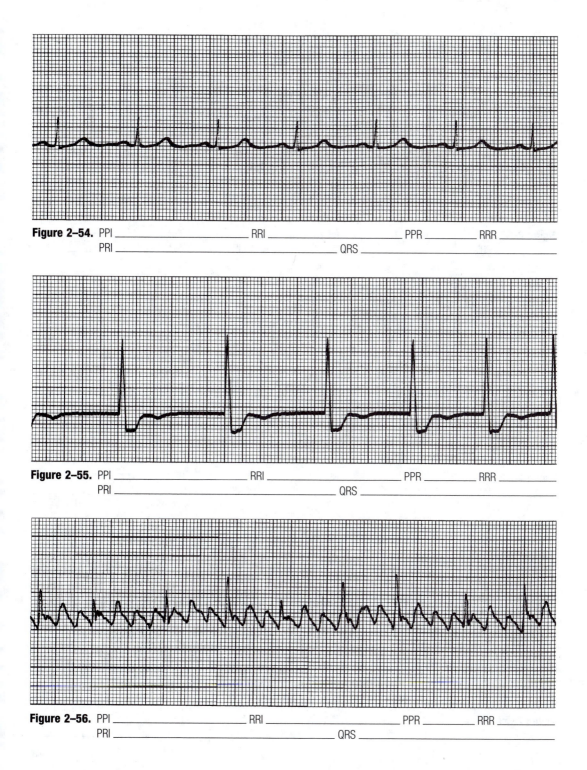

Figure 2–54. PPI _____ RRI _____ PPR _____ RRR _____
PRI _____ QRS _____

Figure 2–55. PPI _____ RRI _____ PPR _____ RRR _____
PRI _____ QRS _____

Figure 2–56. PPI _____ RRI _____ PPR _____ RRR _____
PRI _____ QRS _____

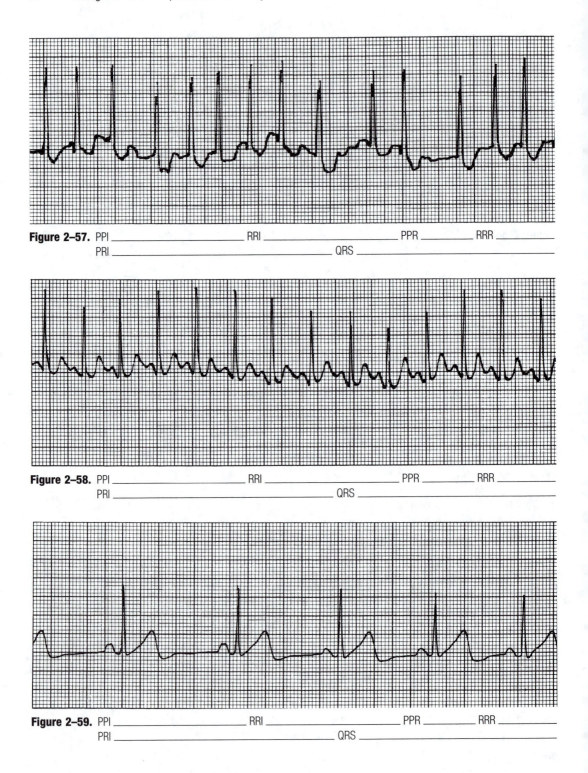

Figure 2–57. PPI _____ RRI _____ PPR _____ RRR _____
PRI _____ QRS _____

Figure 2–58. PPI _____ RRI _____ PPR _____ RRR _____
PRI _____ QRS _____

Figure 2–59. PPI _____ RRI _____ PPR _____ RRR _____
PRI _____ QRS _____

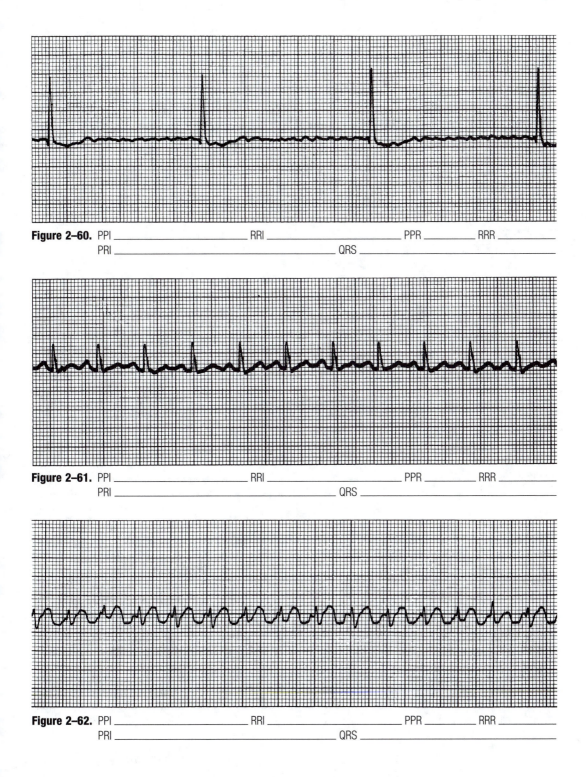

Figure 2–60. PPI _____ RRI _____ PPR _____ RRR _____
PRI _____ QRS _____

Figure 2–61. PPI _____ RRI _____ PPR _____ RRR _____
PRI _____ QRS _____

Figure 2–62. PPI _____ RRI _____ PPR _____ RRR _____
PRI _____ QRS _____

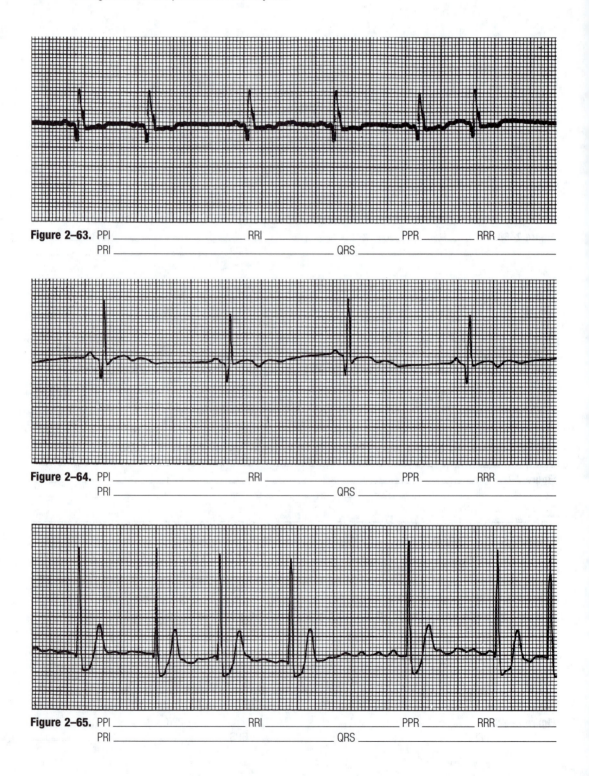

Figure 2–63. PPI _____ RRI _____ PPR _____ RRR _____
PRI _____ QRS _____

Figure 2–64. PPI _____ RRI _____ PPR _____ RRR _____
PRI _____ QRS _____

Figure 2–65. PPI _____ RRI _____ PPR _____ RRR _____
PRI _____ QRS _____

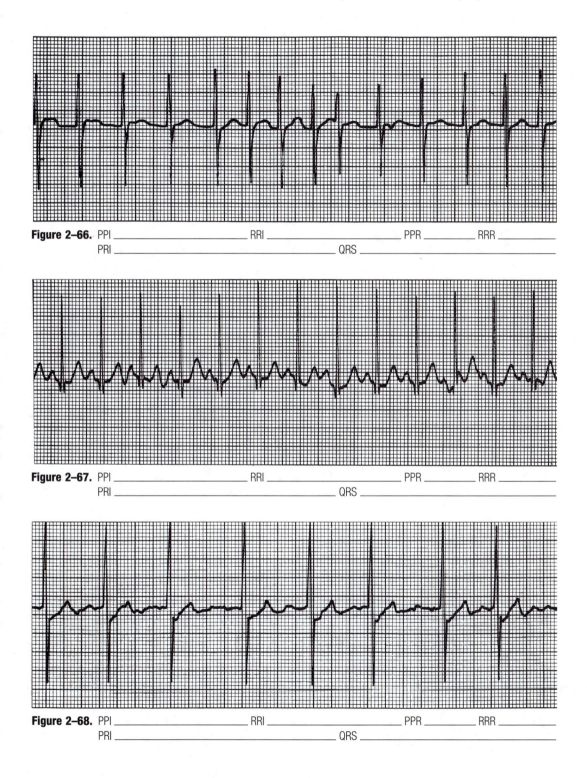

Figure 2–66. PPI _____ RRI _____ PPR _____ RRR _____
PRI _____ QRS _____

Figure 2–67. PPI _____ RRI _____ PPR _____ RRR _____
PRI _____ QRS _____

Figure 2–68. PPI _____ RRI _____ PPR _____ RRR _____
PRI _____ QRS _____

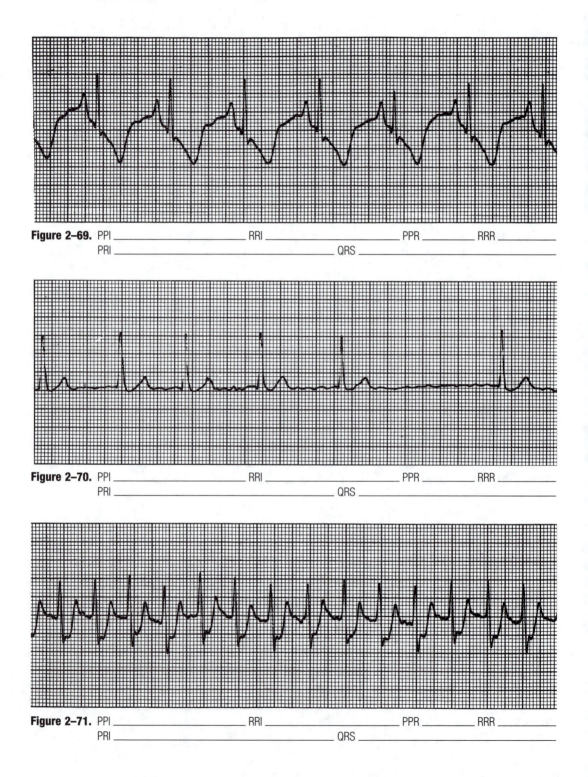

Figure 2–69. PPI _____ RRI _____ PPR _____ RRR _____
PRI _____ QRS _____

Figure 2–70. PPI _____ RRI _____ PPR _____ RRR _____
PRI _____ QRS _____

Figure 2–71. PPI _____ RRI _____ PPR _____ RRR _____
PRI _____ QRS _____

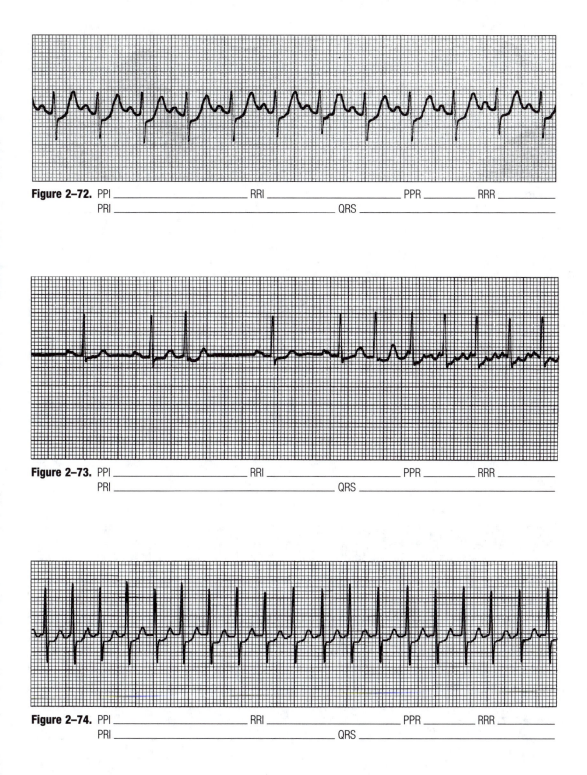

Figure 2–72. PPI _____ RRI _____ PPR _____ RRR _____
PRI _____ QRS _____

Figure 2–73. PPI _____ RRI _____ PPR _____ RRR _____
PRI _____ QRS _____

Figure 2–74. PPI _____ RRI _____ PPR _____ RRR _____
PRI _____ QRS _____

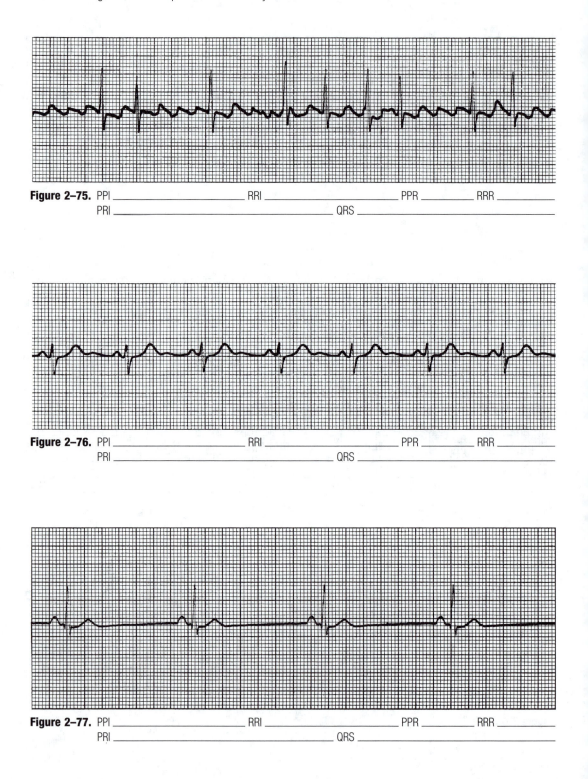

Figure 2–75. PPI _____ RRI _____ PPR _____ RRR _____
PRI _____ QRS _____

Figure 2–76. PPI _____ RRI _____ PPR _____ RRR _____
PRI _____ QRS _____

Figure 2–77. PPI _____ RRI _____ PPR _____ RRR _____
PRI _____ QRS _____

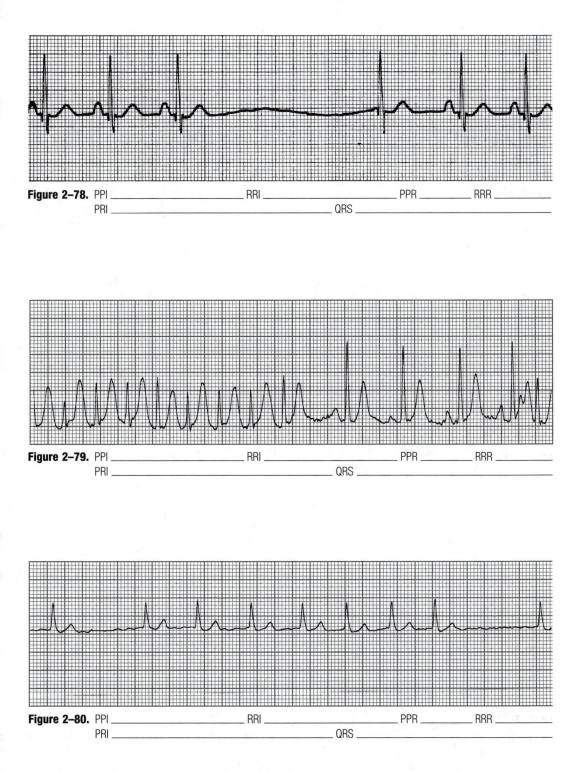

Figure 2–78. PPI _____ RRI _____ PPR _____ RRR _____
PRI _____ QRS _____

Figure 2–79. PPI _____ RRI _____ PPR _____ RRR _____
PRI _____ QRS _____

Figure 2–80. PPI _____ RRI _____ PPR _____ RRR _____
PRI _____ QRS _____

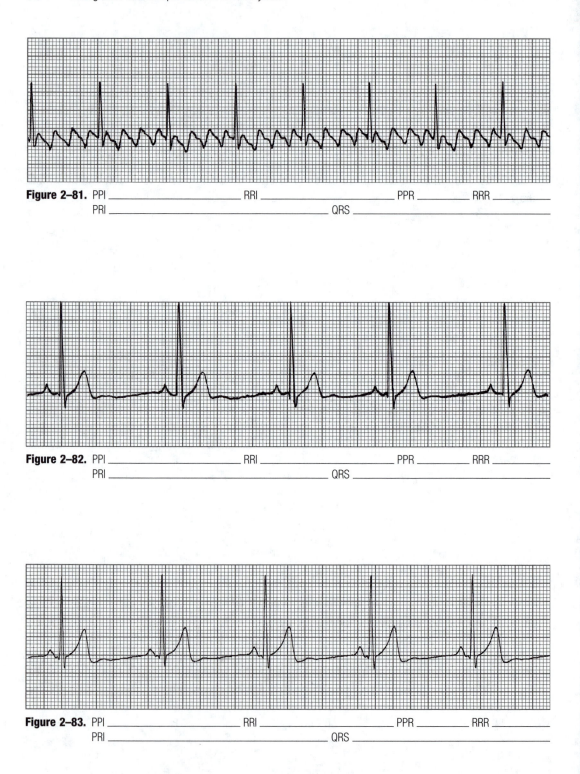

Figure 2–81. PPI _____ RRI _____ PPR _____ RRR _____
PRI _____ QRS _____

Figure 2–82. PPI _____ RRI _____ PPR _____ RRR _____
PRI _____ QRS _____

Figure 2–83. PPI _____ RRI _____ PPR _____ RRR _____
PRI _____ QRS _____

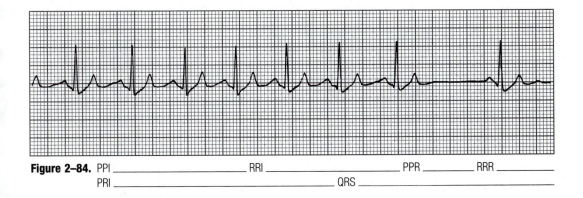

Figure 2–84. PPI _____ RRI _____ PPR _____ RRR _____
          PRI _____ QRS _____

Junctional Dysrhythmias

I. Premature Junctional Complex (PJC)

A. ECG features

1. *PP interval:* regular except for early complex
2. *RR interval:* regular except for early complex
3. *PP rate:* usually 60–100/min
4. *RR rate:* usually 60–100/min
5. *P wave:* pacemaker site is the junctional tissue; therefore, in Lead II the P wave may be
   a. Inverted before QRS
   b. Buried in QRS
   c. Inverted behind QRS
6. *PRI:* 0.12 second or less
7. *QRS interval:* less than (<) 0.12 second (Figs. 3–1 and 3–2)

B. Common etiology

1. Ischemia or insult to atrioventricular (A-V) junction
2. Hypoxemia
3. Valvular disease
4. Digitalis toxicity
5. Normal variant

C. Clinical signs and symptoms

1. Seldom produces symptoms
2. Patient may have an irregular pulse
3. Serious only if occurs frequently
4. May be a warning of a more serious junctional dysrhythmia

II. Junctional Rhythm

A. ECG features

1. *PP interval:* regular or absent
2. *RR interval:* regular
3. *PP rate:* 40–60/min
4. *RR rate:* 40–60/min

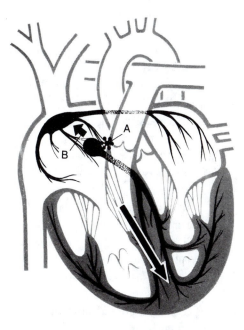

Figure 3–1. Premature junctional complex: **A.** Irritable focus in junction initiates impulse early. **B.** Retrograde conduction through the atria causes an inverted P wave in Lead II.

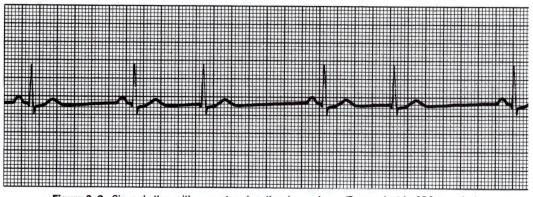

Figure 3–2. Sinus rhythm with premature junctional complexes (P wave lost in QRS complex).

5. *P wave:* pacemaker site is the junctional tissue; therefore, in Lead II the P wave may be
   a. Inverted before QRS
   b. Buried in QRS
   c. Inverted behind QRS
6. *PRI:* 0.12 second or less
7. *QRS interval:* less than (<) 0.12 second (Figs: 3–3, 3–4, and 3–5)

B. Common etiology
   1. Insult to S-A node
   2. Increased vagal tone on the S-A node
   3. Hypoxemia
   4. Digitalis toxicity

C. Clinical signs and symptoms
   1. Slow, regular pulse
   2. Often a temporary dysrhythmia; S-A node may regain control
   3. If rate dramatically decreases, cardiac output may drop
   4. Because of slow rate, ventricular escape or irritability may occur

III. Accelerated Junctional Rhythm

A. ECG features
   1. *PP interval:* regular or absent
   2. *RR interval:* regular
   3. *PP rate:* 61–100/min
   4. *RR rate:* 61–100/min
   5. *P wave:* pacemaker site is the junctional tissue; therefore, in Lead II the P wave may be
      a. Inverted before QRS

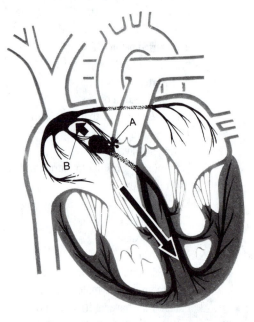

Figure 3–3. Junctional rhythm. **A.** Junction initiates impulse at 40–60/min. **B.** Retrograde conduction through the atria causes an inverted P wave in Lead II.

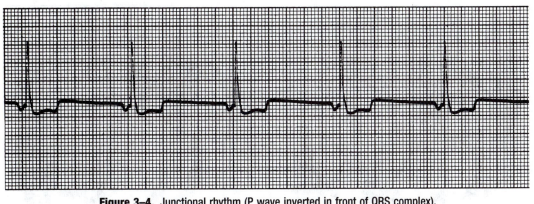

Figure 3–4. Junctional rhythm (P wave inverted in front of QRS complex).

b. Buried in QRS

c. Inverted behind QRS

6. *PRI:* 0.12 second or less

7. *QRS interval:* less than (<) 0.12 second (Figs. 3–6 and 3–7)

B. Common etiology

1. Insult to A-V junction

2. Digitalis toxicity

3. Acute MI

C. Clinical signs and symptoms

1. Usually benign

2. May deteriorate into junctional tachycardia

IV. Junctional Tachycardia

A. ECG features

1. *PP interval:* regular or absent

2. *RR interval:* regular

3. *PP rate:* 101–140/min (may be as high as 240/min and unable to detect P waves)

4. *RR rate:* 101–140/min

5. *P wave:* pacemaker site is the junctional tissue; therefore, in Lead II the P wave may be

a. Inverted before QRS

b. Buried in QRS

c. Inverted behind QRS

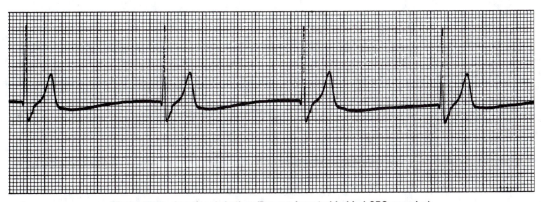

Figure 3–5. Junctional rhythm (P wave inverted behind QRS complex).

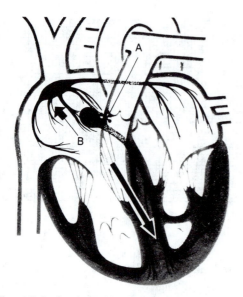

Figure 3–6. Accelerated junctional rhythm: **A.** Junction initiates impulse at 61–100/min. **B.** Retrograde conduction through the atria causes an inverted P wave in Lead II.

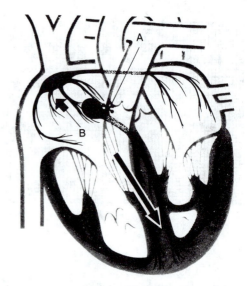

Figure 3–8. Junctional tachycardia: **A.** Junction initiates impulse at 101–140/min. **B.** Retrograde conduction through the atria causes an inverted P wave in Lead II.

6. *PRI:* 0.12 second or less
7. *QRS interval:* less than (<) 0.12 second
  (Figs. 3–8 and 3–9)
*Note: If unable to detect P waves, called SVT
  B. Common etiology

1. Insult to A-V junction
2. Digitalis toxicity
3. Acute MI
C. Clinical signs and symptoms
  1. May decrease cardiac output

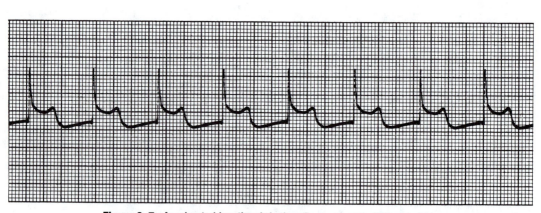

Figure 3–7. Accelerated junctional rhythm (P wave lost in QRS complex).

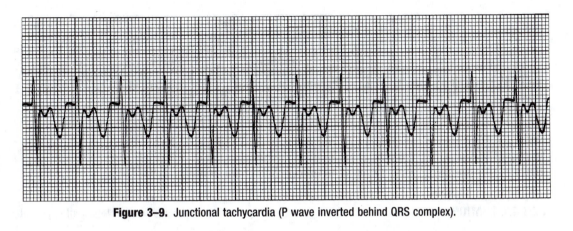

Figure 3–9. Junctional tachycardia (P wave inverted behind QRS complex).

2. May be paroxysmal
3. May deteriorate into ventricular tachycardia or ventricular fibrillation
4. If heart rate rapid, signs/symptoms same as atrial tachycardia

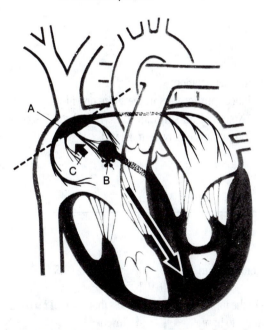

Figure 3–10. Junctional escape complex: **A.** S-A node fails to fire intermittently. **B.** Junctional escape complex comes in as a protective mechanism. **C.** Retrograde conduction through the atria causes an inverted P wave in Lead II.

V. Junctional Escape Complex

A. ECG features
1. *PP interval:* depends upon underlying dysrhythmia
2. *RR interval:* depends upon underlying dysrhythmia; escape complexes occur late in the cardiac cycle
3. *PP rate:* depends upon underlying dysrhythmia, usually 60–100/min (may be bradycardic)
4. *RR rate:* depends upon underlying dysrhythmia; usually 60–100/min (may be bradycardic)
5. *P wave:* on escape complexes may be
   a. Inverted before QRS
   b. Buried in QRS
   c. Inverted behind QRS
6. *PRI:* if present on escape complex, 0.12 second or less
7. *QRS interval:* less than (<) 0.12 second (Figs. 3–10 and 3–11)
B. Common etiology
1. Failure of a higher center in the conduction system to fire
2. Protective mechanism
C. Clinical signs and symptoms
1. Patient may be asymptomatic
2. May feel skipped beats

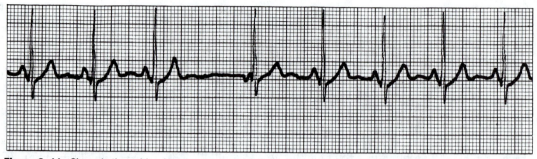

Figure 3–11. Sinus rhythm with a junctional escape complex (P wave inverted in front of QRS complex).

SELF-EVALUATION

Directions

Answer keys for the Self-Evaluation section begin on page 287.

1. **Matching.** Place the letter of the appropriate item(s) before each numbered statement. Some answers are used more than once, and not all answers will be used.
2. **ECG practice strips.** For simplicity and practicality, all rates have been calculated by using Method 3 (Fig. 1–14). Keep in mind that your measurements for PRIs and QRS complexes may vary slightly and still be correct. Use the systematic approach shown in Chapter 1 to interpret the ECG

strips. It is important that you follow all steps and not take shortcuts.
For the following ECG strips:
1. Determine if the PPI and RRI are regular or irregular.
2. Calculate rates using the appropriate method:
   a. PPR
   b. RRR
3. Measure:
   a. PRI
   b. QRS
4. Interpretation
Place your answers in the space provided.
*Note that all strips are Lead II and are 6 seconds long unless otherwise indicated.

MATCHING

_____ 1. Part of the conduction system in which a junctional rhythm originates

_____ 2. In a Lead II, the shape of a P wave originating in the junction

_____ 3. The type of conduction causing junctional rhythms to have inverted P waves

_____ 4. Three possible places to find a P wave in a junctional rhythm

_____ 5. Where in the cardiac cycle a PJC occurs

_____ 6. Where in the cardiac cycle a junctional escape complex occurs

a. behind the QRS
b. early
c. less than (<) 0.12 second
d. inverted
e. on time
f. junctional tissue
g. retrograde
h. 101–140/min

_____ 7. The measurement of the PR interval in a junctional rhythm
_____ 8. The RRI of a junctional rhythm
_____ 9. Inherent rate of the junction
_____ 10. RRR of an accelerated junctional rhythm
_____ 11. RRR of a junctional tachycardia

i. in the QRS
j. late
k. 0.12–0.20 second
l. regular
m. bundle of His
n. 61–100/min
o. upright
p. before the QRS
q. slightly irregular
r. 40–60/min
s. grossly irregular

ECG PRACTICE STRIPS

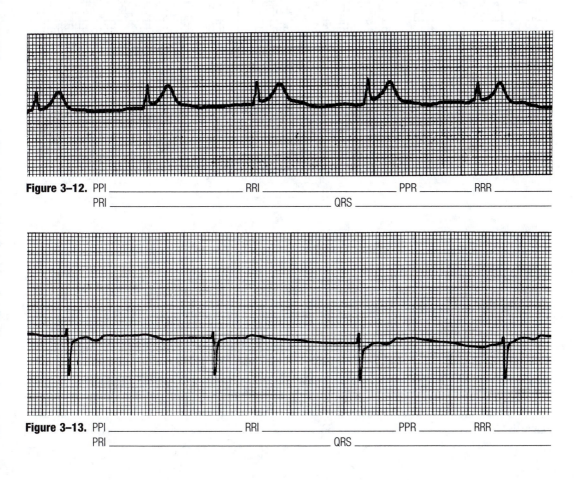

Figure 3–12. PPI _____ RRI _____ PPR _____ RRR _____
PRI _____ QRS _____

Figure 3–13. PPI _____ RRI _____ PPR _____ RRR _____
PRI _____ QRS _____

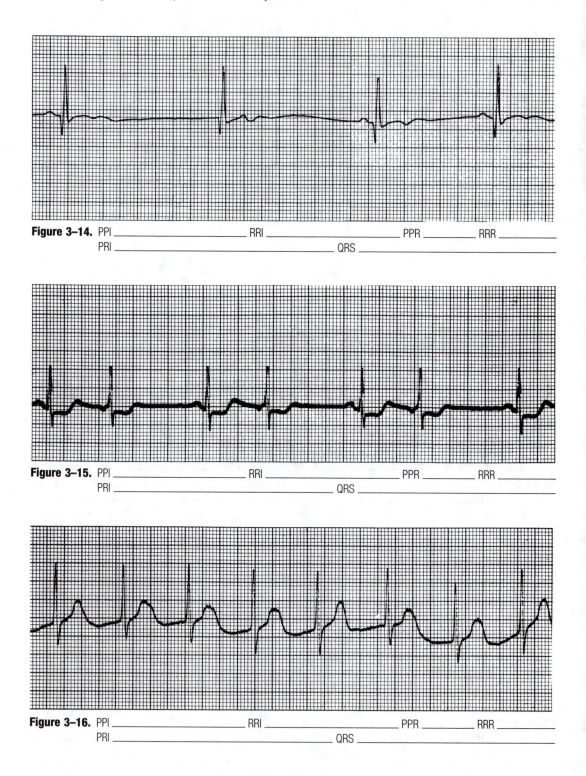

Figure 3–14. PPI _____ RRI _____ PPR _____ RRR _____
PRI _____ QRS _____

Figure 3–15. PPI _____ RRI _____ PPR _____ RRR _____
PRI _____ QRS _____

Figure 3–16. PPI _____ RRI _____ PPR _____ RRR _____
PRI _____ QRS _____

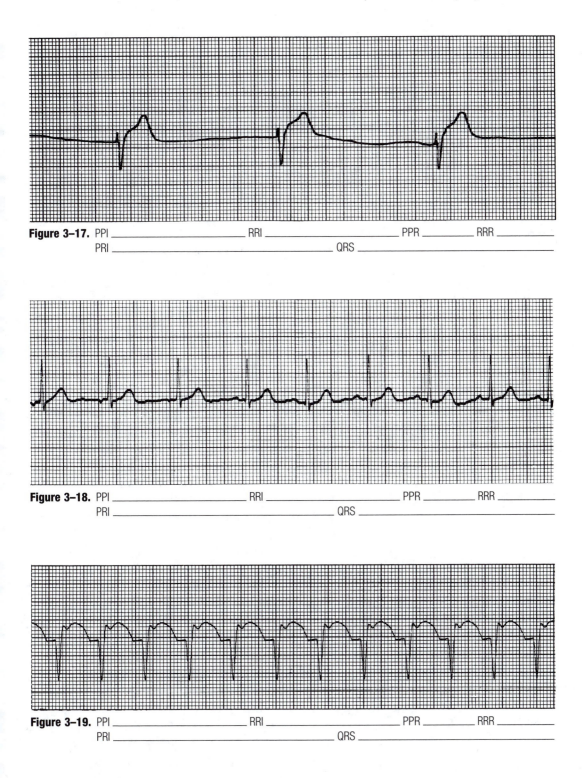

Figure 3–17. PPI _____ RRI _____ PPR _____ RRR _____
PRI _____ QRS _____

Figure 3–18. PPI _____ RRI _____ PPR _____ RRR _____
PRI _____ QRS _____

Figure 3–19. PPI _____ RRI _____ PPR _____ RRR _____
PRI _____ QRS _____

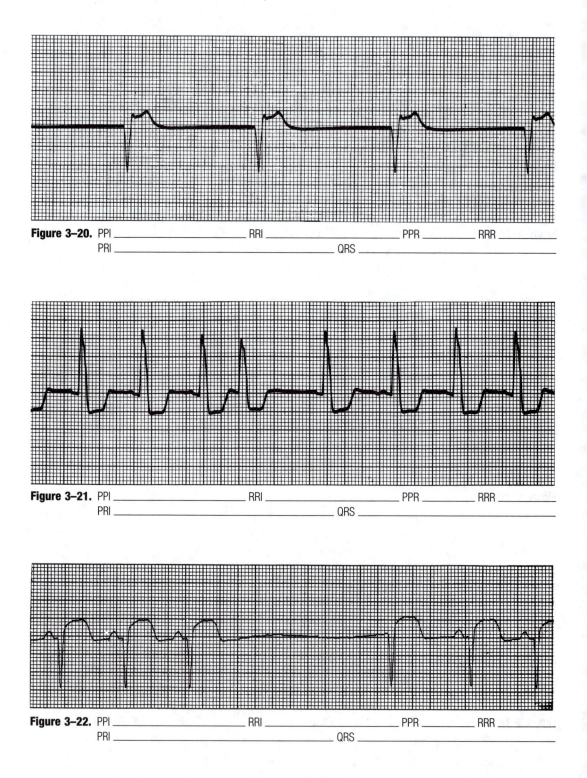

Figure 3–20. PPI _____ RRI _____ PPR _____ RRR _____
PRI _____ QRS _____

Figure 3–21. PPI _____ RRI _____ PPR _____ RRR _____
PRI _____ QRS _____

Figure 3–22. PPI _____ RRI _____ PPR _____ RRR _____
PRI _____ QRS _____

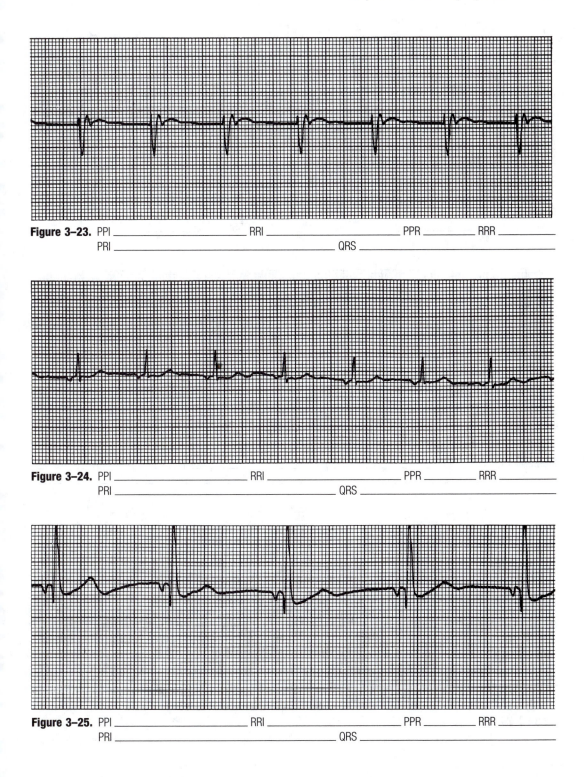

Figure 3–23. PPI _____ RRI _____ PPR _____ RRR _____
PRI _____ QRS _____

Figure 3–24. PPI _____ RRI _____ PPR _____ RRR _____
PRI _____ QRS _____

Figure 3–25. PPI _____ RRI _____ PPR _____ RRR _____
PRI _____ QRS _____

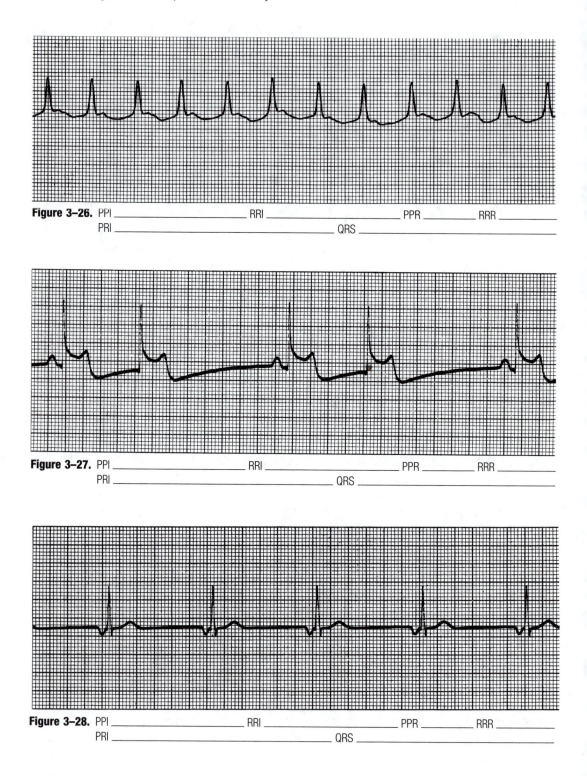

Figure 3–26. PPI _____ RRI _____ PPR _____ RRR _____
PRI _____ QRS _____

Figure 3–27. PPI _____ RRI _____ PPR _____ RRR _____
PRI _____ QRS _____

Figure 3–28. PPI _____ RRI _____ PPR _____ RRR _____
PRI _____ QRS _____

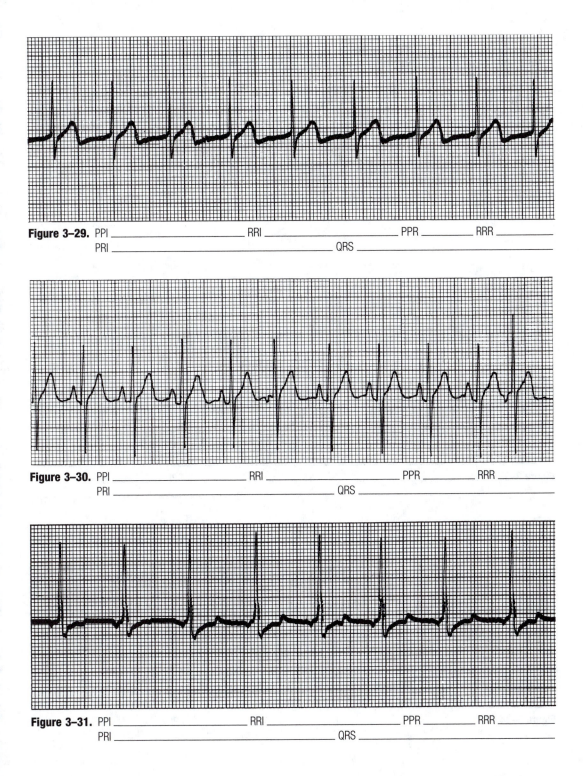

Figure 3–29. PPI _____ RRI _____ PPR _____ RRR _____
PRI _____ QRS _____

Figure 3–30. PPI _____ RRI _____ PPR _____ RRR _____
PRI _____ QRS _____

Figure 3–31. PPI _____ RRI _____ PPR _____ RRR _____
PRI _____ QRS _____

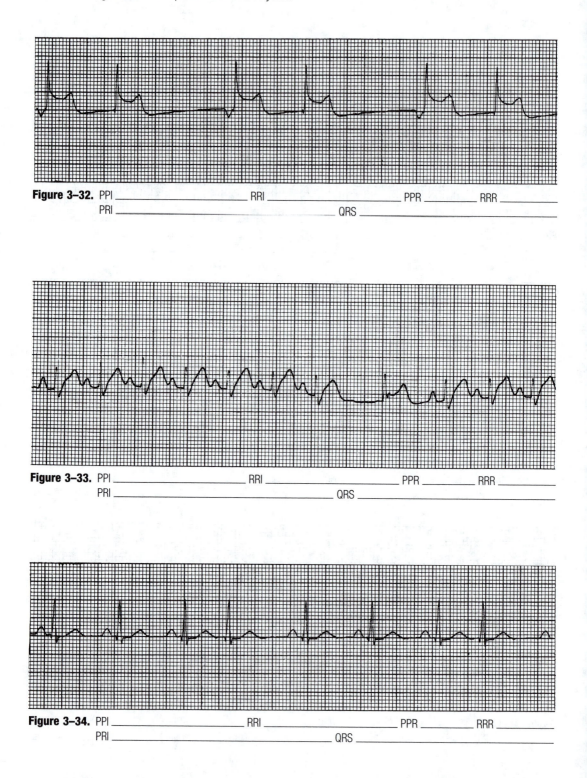

Figure 3–32. PPI _____ RRI _____ PPR _____ RRR _____
PRI _____ QRS _____

Figure 3–33. PPI _____ RRI _____ PPR _____ RRR _____
PRI _____ QRS _____

Figure 3–34. PPI _____ RRI _____ PPR _____ RRR _____
PRI _____ QRS _____

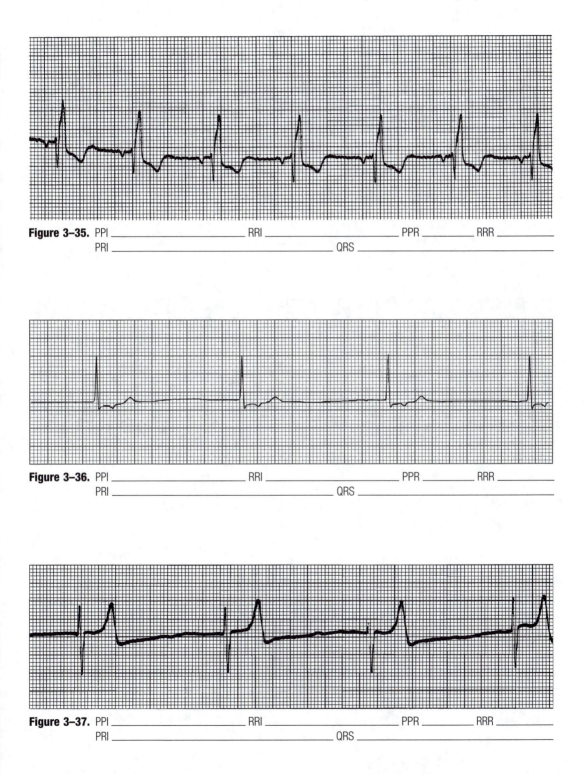

Figure 3–35. PPI _____ RRI _____ PPR _____ RRR _____
PRI _____ QRS _____

Figure 3–36. PPI _____ RRI _____ PPR _____ RRR _____
PRI _____ QRS _____

Figure 3–37. PPI _____ RRI _____ PPR _____ RRR _____
PRI _____ QRS _____

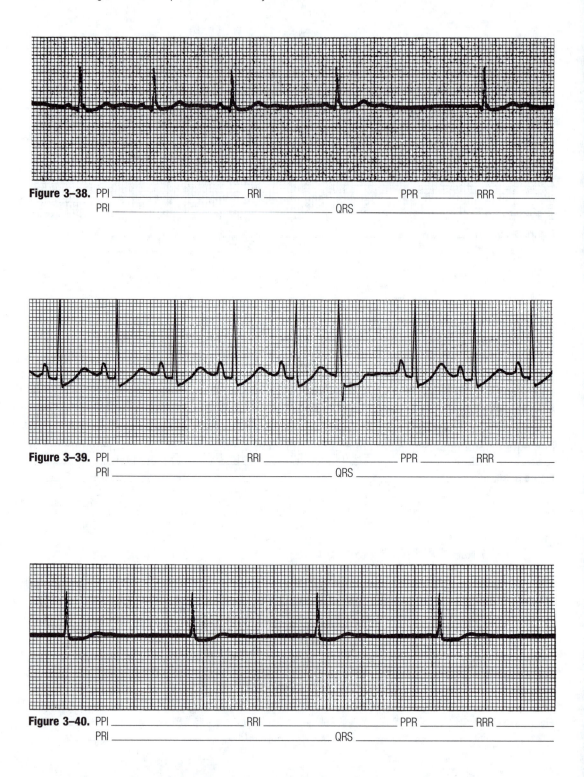

Figure 3–38. PPI _____ RRI _____ PPR _____ RRR _____
PRI _____ QRS _____

Figure 3–39. PPI _____ RRI _____ PPR _____ RRR _____
PRI _____ QRS _____

Figure 3–40. PPI _____ RRI _____ PPR _____ RRR _____
PRI _____ QRS _____

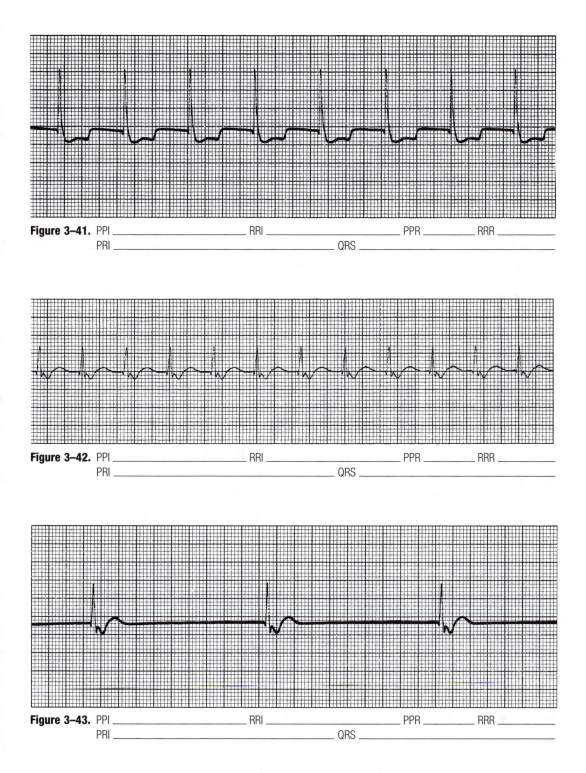

Figure 3–41. PPI _____ RRI _____ PPR _____ RRR _____

PRI _____ QRS _____

Figure 3–42. PPI _____ RRI _____ PPR _____ RRR _____

PRI _____ QRS _____

Figure 3–43. PPI _____ RRI _____ PPR _____ RRR _____

PRI _____ QRS _____

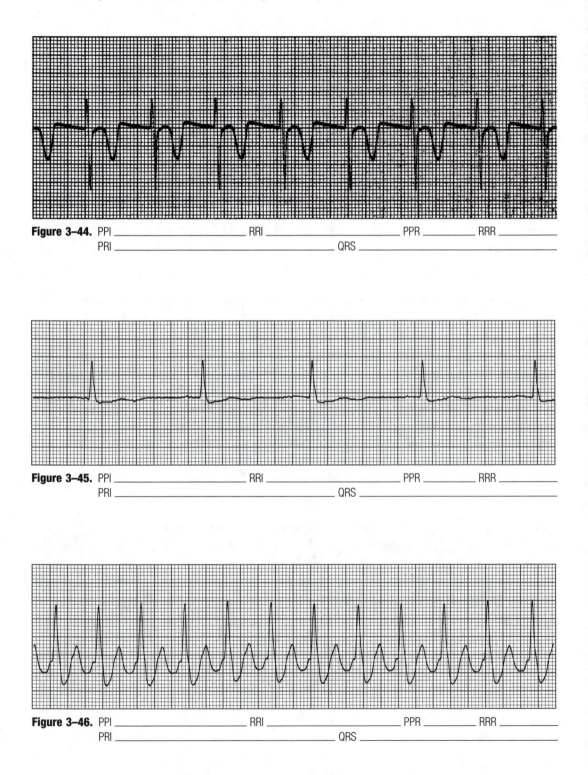

Figure 3–44. PPI _____ RRI _____ PPR _____ RRR _____
PRI _____ QRS _____

Figure 3–45. PPI _____ RRI _____ PPR _____ RRR _____
PRI _____ QRS _____

Figure 3–46. PPI _____ RRI _____ PPR _____ RRR _____
PRI _____ QRS _____

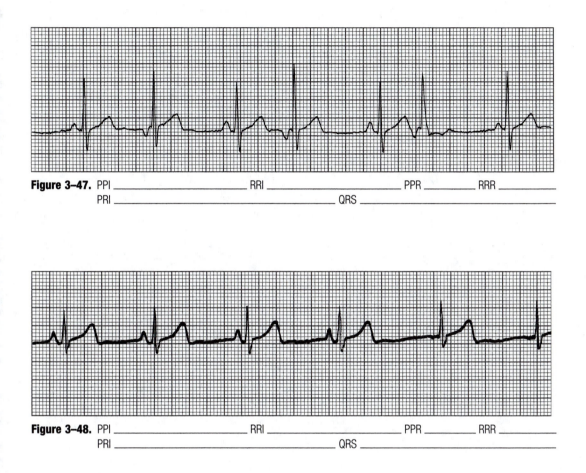

Figure 3–47. PPI _____ RRI _____ PPR _____ RRR _____
PRI _____ QRS _____

Figure 3–48. PPI _____ RRI _____ PPR _____ RRR _____
PRI _____ QRS _____

4

Supraventricular Dysrhythmias—Practice Strips

The following self-evaluation section combines all supraventricular dysrhythmias learned in Chapters 2 and 3: sinus, atrial, and junctional. This practice section will allow you to test your skill in measuring, calculating, and interpreting supraventricular dysrhythmias.

SELF-EVALUATION

Directions

Answer keys for the Self-Evaluation section begin on page 300.

For simplicity and practicality, all rates have been calculated by using Method 3 (Fig. 1–14). Keep in mind that your measurements for PRIs and QRS complexes may vary slightly and still be correct. Use the systematic approach shown in Chapter 1 to interpret the ECG strips. It is important that you follow all steps and not take shortcuts.

For the following ECG strips:

1. Determine if PPI and RRI are regular or irregular
2. Calculate rates using the appropriate method:
   a. PPI
   b. RRI
3. Measure:
   a. PRI
   b. QRS
4. Interpretation

Place your answers in the space provided.

*Note that all strips are Lead II and are 6 seconds long unless otherwise indicated.

ECG PRACTICE STRIPS

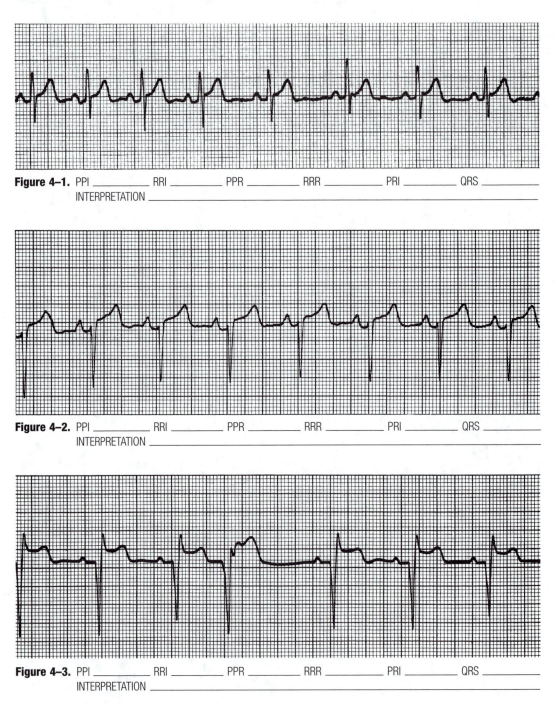

Figure 4–1. PPI _____ RRI _____ PPR _____ RRR _____ PRI _____ QRS _____
INTERPRETATION _____

Figure 4–2. PPI _____ RRI _____ PPR _____ RRR _____ PRI _____ QRS _____
INTERPRETATION _____

Figure 4–3. PPI _____ RRI _____ PPR _____ RRR _____ PRI _____ QRS _____
INTERPRETATION _____

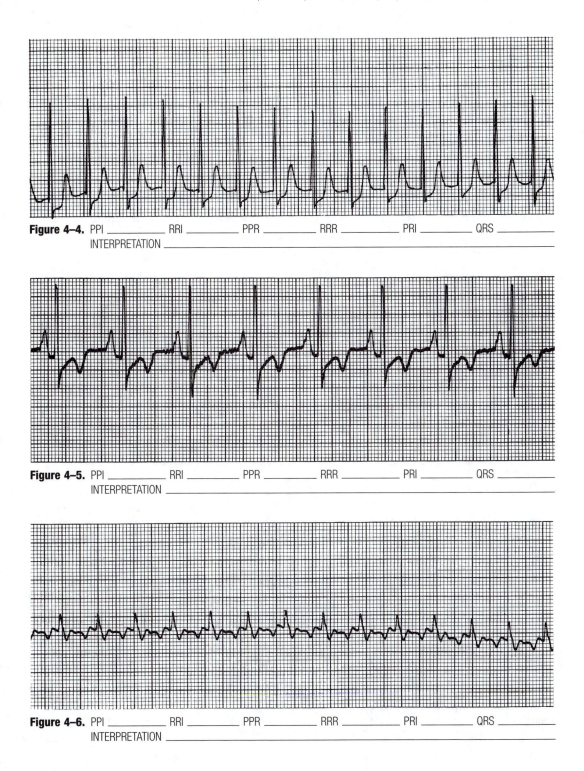

Figure 4–4. PPI _____ RRI _____ PPR _____ RRR _____ PRI _____ QRS _____
INTERPRETATION _____

Figure 4–5. PPI _____ RRI _____ PPR _____ RRR _____ PRI _____ QRS _____
INTERPRETATION _____

Figure 4–6. PPI _____ RRI _____ PPR _____ RRR _____ PRI _____ QRS _____
INTERPRETATION _____

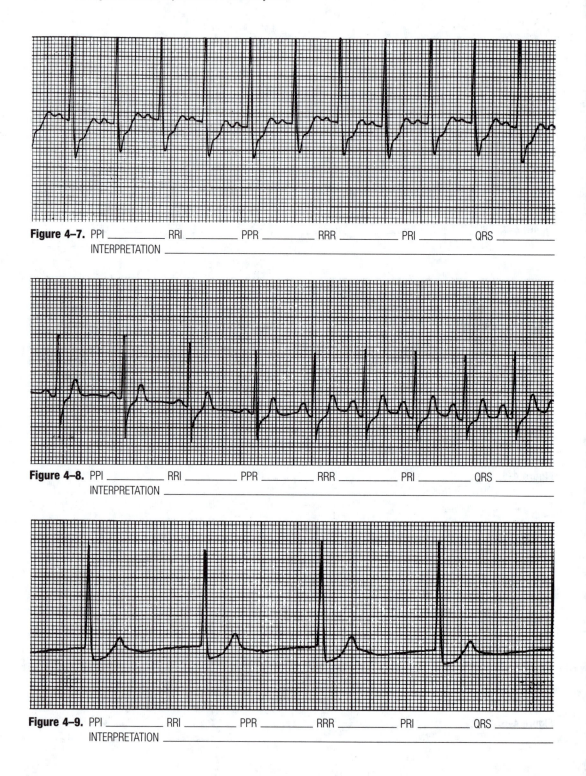

Figure 4–7. PPI _____ RRI _____ PPR _____ RRR _____ PRI _____ QRS _____
INTERPRETATION _____

Figure 4–8. PPI _____ RRI _____ PPR _____ RRR _____ PRI _____ QRS _____
INTERPRETATION _____

Figure 4–9. PPI _____ RRI _____ PPR _____ RRR _____ PRI _____ QRS _____
INTERPRETATION _____

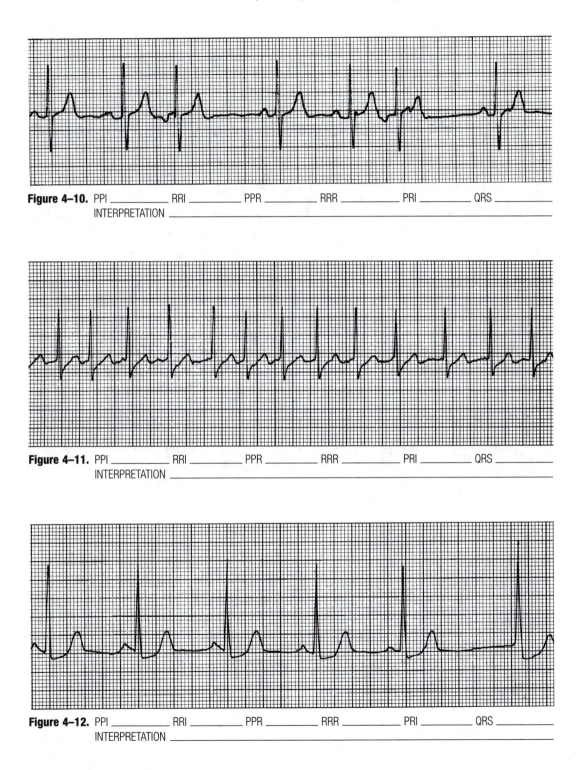

Figure 4–10. PPI _____ RRI _____ PPR _____ RRR _____ PRI _____ QRS _____
INTERPRETATION _____

Figure 4–11. PPI _____ RRI _____ PPR _____ RRR _____ PRI _____ QRS _____
INTERPRETATION _____

Figure 4–12. PPI _____ RRI _____ PPR _____ RRR _____ PRI _____ QRS _____
INTERPRETATION _____

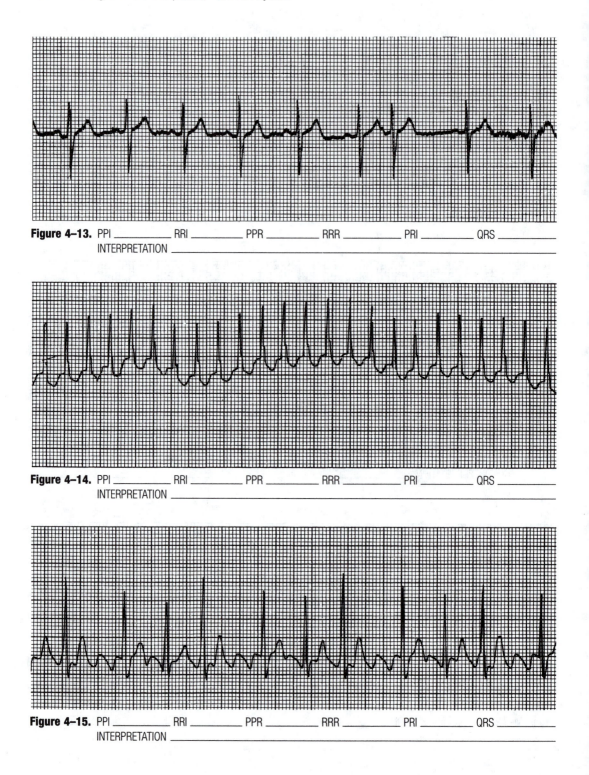

Figure 4–13. PPI _____ RRI _____ PPR _____ RRR _____ PRI _____ QRS _____
INTERPRETATION _____

Figure 4–14. PPI _____ RRI _____ PPR _____ RRR _____ PRI _____ QRS _____
INTERPRETATION _____

Figure 4–15. PPI _____ RRI _____ PPR _____ RRR _____ PRI _____ QRS _____
INTERPRETATION _____

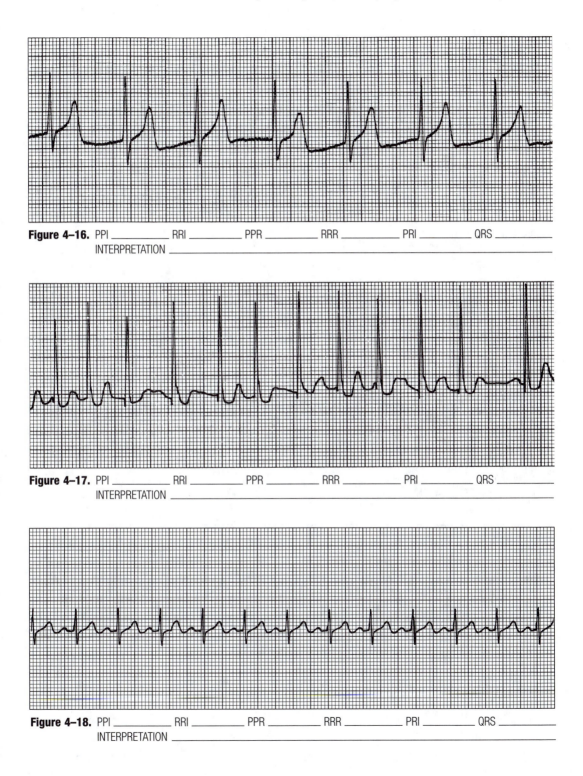

Figure 4–16. PPI _____ RRI _____ PPR _____ RRR _____ PRI _____ QRS _____
INTERPRETATION _____

Figure 4–17. PPI _____ RRI _____ PPR _____ RRR _____ PRI _____ QRS _____
INTERPRETATION _____

Figure 4–18. PPI _____ RRI _____ PPR _____ RRR _____ PRI _____ QRS _____
INTERPRETATION _____

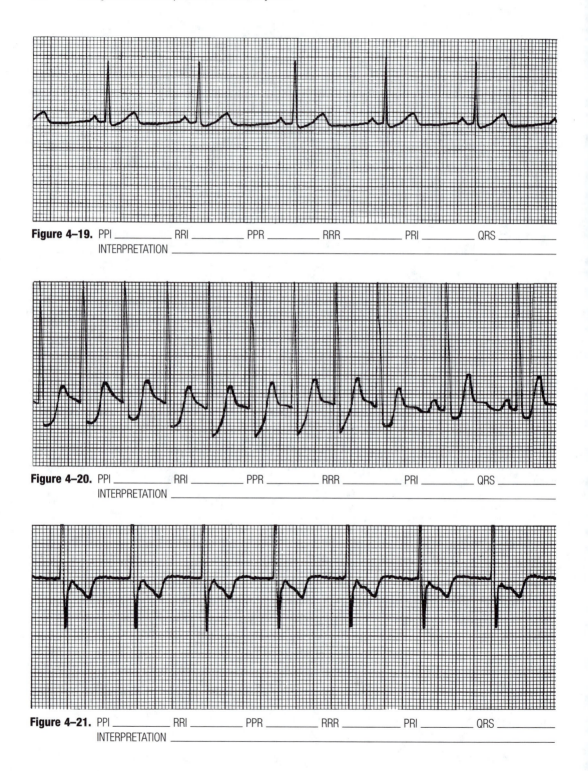

Figure 4–19. PPI _____ RRI _____ PPR _____ RRR _____ PRI _____ QRS _____
INTERPRETATION _____

Figure 4–20. PPI _____ RRI _____ PPR _____ RRR _____ PRI _____ QRS _____
INTERPRETATION _____

Figure 4–21. PPI _____ RRI _____ PPR _____ RRR _____ PRI _____ QRS _____
INTERPRETATION _____

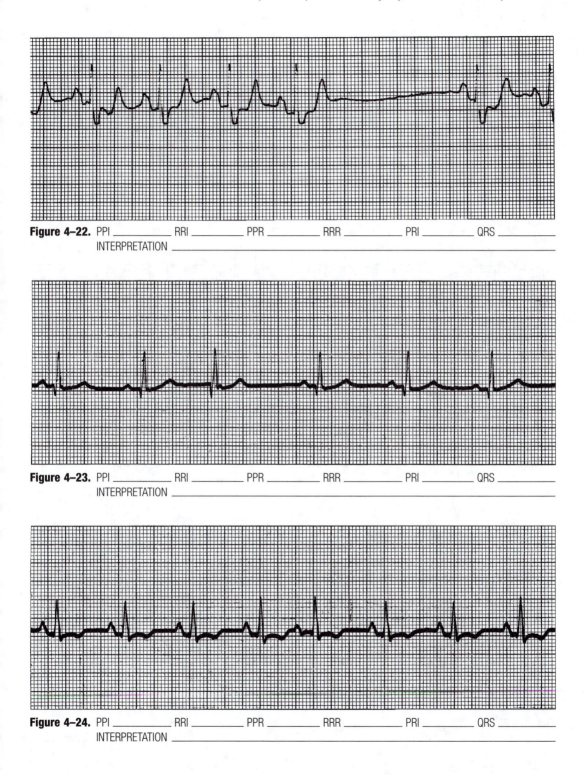

Figure 4–22. PPI _____ RRI _____ PPR _____ RRR _____ PRI _____ QRS _____
INTERPRETATION _____

Figure 4–23. PPI _____ RRI _____ PPR _____ RRR _____ PRI _____ QRS _____
INTERPRETATION _____

Figure 4–24. PPI _____ RRI _____ PPR _____ RRR _____ PRI _____ QRS _____
INTERPRETATION _____

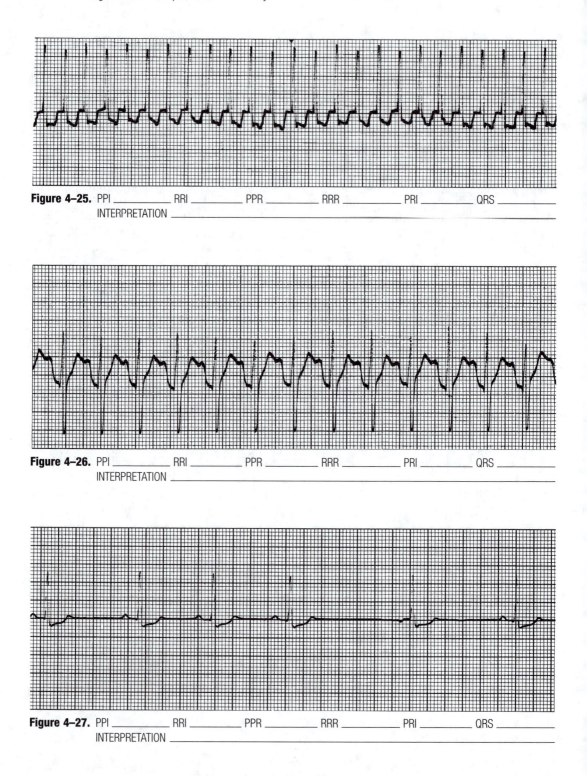

Figure 4–25. PPI _____ RRI _____ PPR _____ RRR _____ PRI _____ QRS _____
INTERPRETATION _____

Figure 4–26. PPI _____ RRI _____ PPR _____ RRR _____ PRI _____ QRS _____
INTERPRETATION _____

Figure 4–27. PPI _____ RRI _____ PPR _____ RRR _____ PRI _____ QRS _____
INTERPRETATION _____

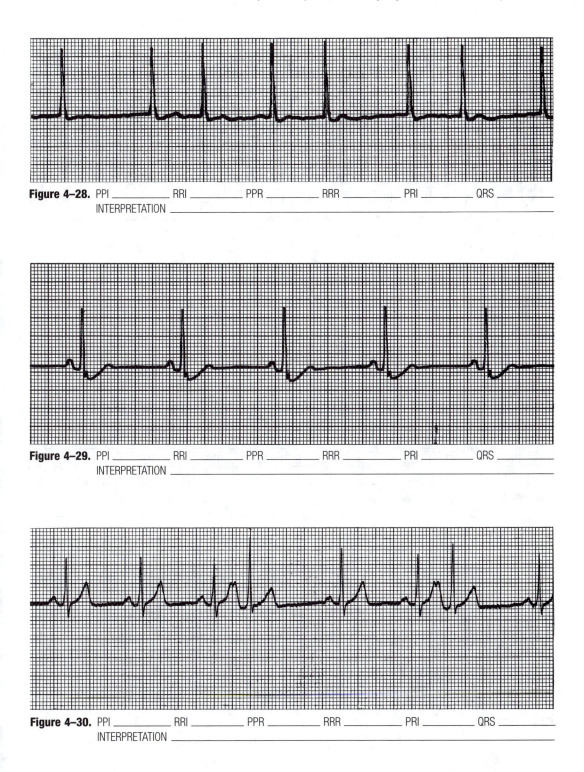

Figure 4–28. PPI _____ RRI _____ PPR _____ RRR _____ PRI _____ QRS _____
INTERPRETATION _____

Figure 4–29. PPI _____ RRI _____ PPR _____ RRR _____ PRI _____ QRS _____
INTERPRETATION _____

Figure 4–30. PPI _____ RRI _____ PPR _____ RRR _____ PRI _____ QRS _____
INTERPRETATION _____

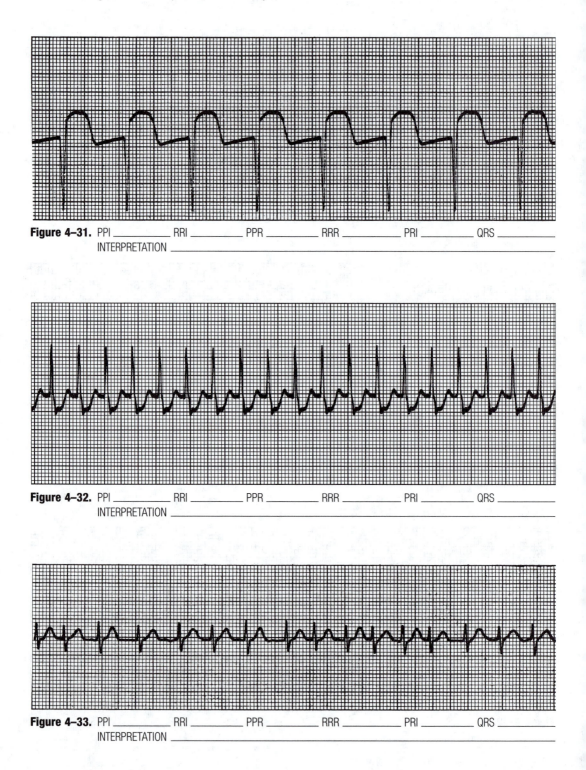

Figure 4–31. PPI _____ RRI _____ PPR _____ RRR _____ PRI _____ QRS _____
INTERPRETATION _____

Figure 4–32. PPI _____ RRI _____ PPR _____ RRR _____ PRI _____ QRS _____
INTERPRETATION _____

Figure 4–33. PPI _____ RRI _____ PPR _____ RRR _____ PRI _____ QRS _____
INTERPRETATION _____

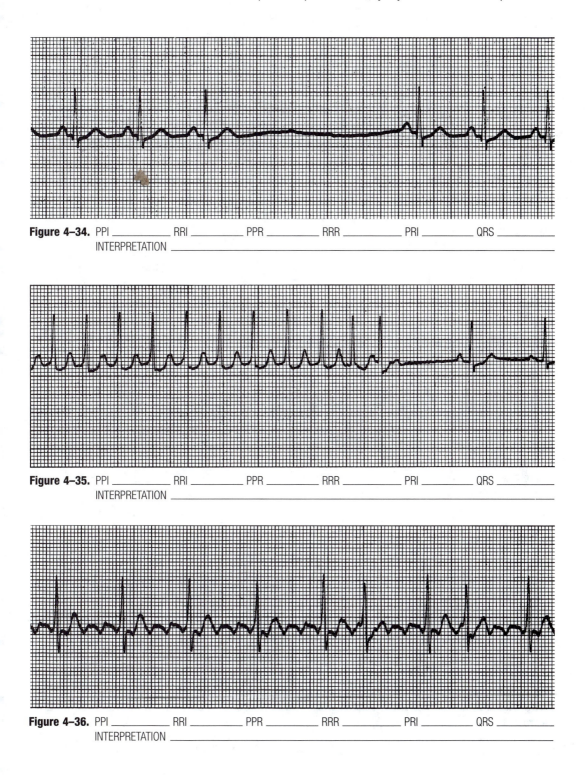

Figure 4–34. PPI _____ RRI _____ PPR _____ RRR _____ PRI _____ QRS _____
INTERPRETATION _____

Figure 4–35. PPI _____ RRI _____ PPR _____ RRR _____ PRI _____ QRS _____
INTERPRETATION _____

Figure 4–36. PPI _____ RRI _____ PPR _____ RRR _____ PRI _____ QRS _____
INTERPRETATION _____

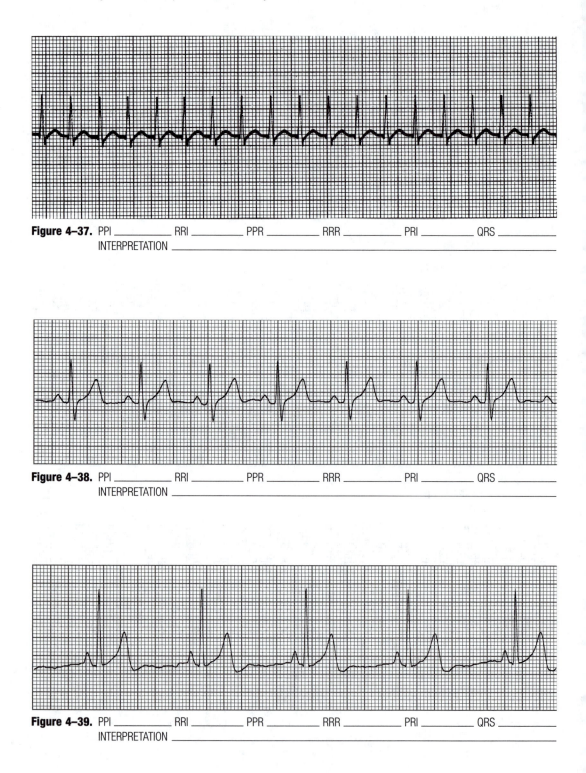

Figure 4–37. PPI _____ RRI _____ PPR _____ RRR _____ PRI _____ QRS _____
INTERPRETATION _____

Figure 4–38. PPI _____ RRI _____ PPR _____ RRR _____ PRI _____ QRS _____
INTERPRETATION _____

Figure 4–39. PPI _____ RRI _____ PPR _____ RRR _____ PRI _____ QRS _____
INTERPRETATION _____

5

A-V Blocks

I. First Degree A-V Block

A. ECG features
1. *PP interval:* regular
2. *RR interval:* regular
3. *PP rate:* usually 60–100/min; may be bradycardic or tachycardic
4. *RR rate:* usually 60–100/min; may be bradycardic or tachycardic
5. *P wave:* upright in Lead II; one P wave for each QRS complex
6. *PRI:* greater than 0.20 second due to a prolonged delay at the A-V node; KEY: PRI IS CONSTANT AND PROLONGED.
7. *QRS interval:* less than (<) 0.12 second (Figs. 5–1 and 5–2)

B. Common etiology
1. Insult to A-V node
2. Hypoxemia
3. Myocardial infarction (MI)
4. Digitalis toxicity
5. Ischemic disease of the conduction system
6. Right coronary artery disease

C. Clinical signs and symptoms
1. None
2. May progress into second or third degree A-V block

II. Second Degree A-V Block (Type I, Wenckebach)

A. ECG features
1. *PP interval:* regular
2. *RR interval:* irregular (grouped beating)
3. *PP rate:* usually 60–100/min
4. *RR rate:* usually 60–100/min; may be bradycardic
5. *P wave:* upright in Lead II; more P waves than QRS complexes

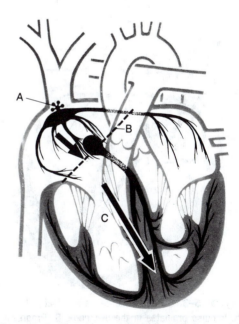

Figure 5–1. First degree A-V block. **A.** Impulse originates in S-A node. **B.** Impulse delayed at A-V node. **C.** Impulse travels normally through ventricles.

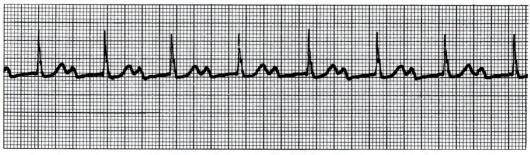

Figure 5–2. Sinus rhythm with first degree A-V block.

6. *PRI:* KEY: BECOMES PROGRESSIVELY LONGER UNTIL A QRS COMPLEX IS DROPPED; P WAVE PRESENT BUT NO QRS.

7. *QRS interval:* less than (<) 0.12 second (Figs. 5–3 and 5–4)

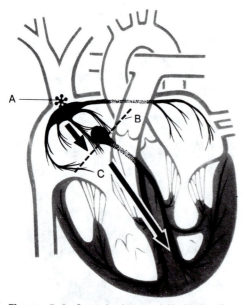

Figure 5–3. Second degree A-V block, Type I. **A.** Impulse orginates in the S-A node. **B.** Progressive delay at A-V node until impulse completely blocked. **C.** Conducted impulses travels normally through the ventricles.

8. In 2:1 conduction, if QRS is of normal duration, probably Type I (second degree A-V block)

B. Common etiology
   1. Insult to the A-V node
   2. Commonly seen in inferior MI
   3. Hypoxemia
   4. Increased vagal tone on the A-V node

C. Clinical signs and symptoms
   1. Usually none
   2. If heart rate dramatically decreases, may produce signs/symptoms of decreased cardiac output
   3. *Usually* does not progress to higher degree heart blocks

III. Second Degree A-V Block (Type II)

A. ECG features
   1. *PP interval:* regular
   2. *RR interval:* regular (may be irregular if conduction has a variable block)
   3. *PP rate:* usually 60–100/min
   4. *RR rate:* usually bradycardic
   5. *P wave:* upright in Lead II; more P waves than QRS complexes
   6. *PRI:* usually 0.12–0.20 second (may be prolonged); KEY: PRI IS CONSTANT ON CONDUCTED COMPLEXES. EVERY SECOND, THIRD, OR FOURTH COMPLEX IS BLOCKED AT THE A-V NODE, RESULTING

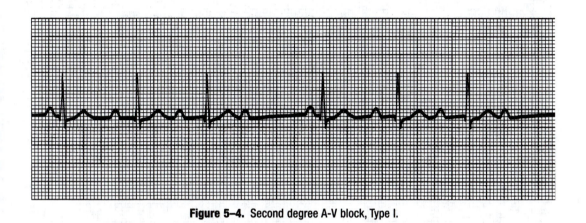

Figure 5–4. Second degree A-V block, Type I.

IN P WAVES WITHOUT QRS COMPLEXES. BLOCK MAY ALSO OCCUR RANDOMLY, WITHOUT A PATTERN.

7. *QRS interval:* usually 0.12 second or greater due to presence of bundle branch block (Figs. 5–5 and 5–6)

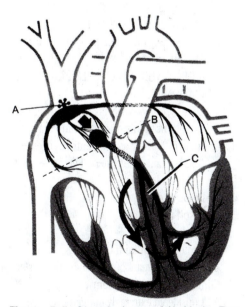

Figure 5–5. Second degree A-V block, Type II. **A.** Impulse originates in S-A node. **B.** Intermittent block at A-V node. **C.** May spread through ventricles abnormally due to presence of bundle branch block.

8. In 2:1 conduction, if QRS is wide, probably Type II (second degree A-V block)

*Note: Authors consider second degree A-V blocks with 2:1 conduction Type I if the QRS is of normal duration (Fig. 5–7) and Type II if the QRS is wide, indicating bundle branch block

B. Common etiology
   1. Insult to A-V node
   2. Myocardial infarction
   3. Hypoxemia
   4. Cardiac drugs
   5. Ischemic disease of the conduction system
C. Clinical signs and symptoms
   1. Slow heart rate may produce signs/symptoms of decreased cardiac output
   2. May suddenly progress to complete A-V block or ventricular standstill

IV. **Third Degree A-V Block (Complete A-V Block; Complete Heart Block—CHB)**
A. ECG features
   1. *PP interval:* regular
   2. *RR interval:* usually regular
   3. *PP rate:* usually 60–100/min
   4. *RR rate:* usually bradycardic; junctional escape dysrhythmia 40–60/min; ventricular escape dysrhythmia 20–40/min
   5. *P wave:* upright in Lead II; more P waves

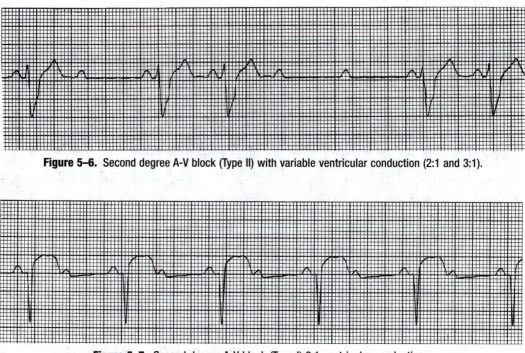

Figure 5–6. Second degree A-V block (Type II) with variable ventricular conduction (2:1 and 3:1).

Figure 5–7. Second degree A-V block (Type I) 2:1 ventricular conduction.

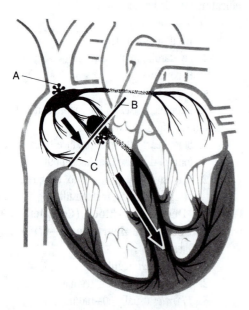

Figure 5–8. Third degree A-V block. **A.** Impulse originates in S-A node. **B.** Total block at A-V node. **C.** Impulse originating in junction paces the heart and travels normally through the ventricles.

than QRS complexes; KEY: P WAVES MAY FALL INSIDE QRS COMPLEX

6. *PRI:* varies; KEY: PRI IS NOT CONSTANT AND BEARS NO CONSISTENT RELATIONSHIP TO THE QRS COMPLEX (A-V DISSOCIATION).

7. *QRS interval:* depends upon origin of escape mechanism: junctional escape-less than (<) 0.12 second; ventricular escape-0.12 second or greater (Figs. 5–8, 5–9, 5–10, and 5–11)

B. Common etiology
   1. Insult to A-V node
   2. Cardiac drugs
   3. Acute myocardial infarction
   4. Ischemic disease of the conduction system

C. Clinical signs and symptoms
   1. Considered extremely dangerous
   2. Rate usually very slow
   3. Dramatic drop in cardiac output
   4. May progress to ventricular standstill

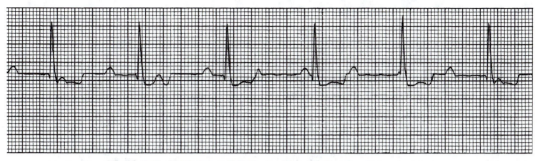

Figure 5–9. Third degree A-V block with a junctional escape response.

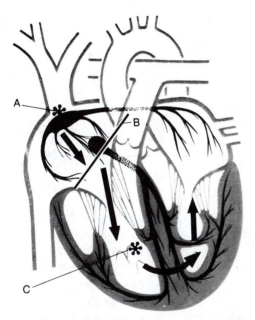

Figure 5–10. Third degree A-V block. **A.** Impulse originates in S-A node. **B.** Total block at A-V node. **C.** Impulse in ventricle paces the heart and travels abnormally through the ventricles.

5. Due to slow rate, ventricular escape or irritability may occur

6. May cause Stokes–Adams attack—syncopal episode caused by cerebral ischemia from a drop in cardiac output due to dysrhythmias

SELF-EVALUATION

Directions

Answer keys for the Self-Evaluation section begin on page 313.

1. **Matching.** Place the letter of the appropriate item(s) before each numbered statement. Some answers are used more than once, and not all answers will be used.

2. **ECG practice strips.** For simplicity and practicality, all rates have been calculated by Method 3 (Fig. 1–14). Keep in mind that your measurements for PRIs and QRS complexes may vary slightly and

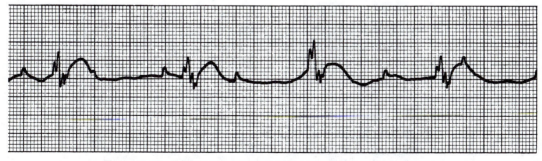

Figure 5–11. Third degree A-V block with a ventricular escape response.

still be correct. Use the systematic approach shown in Chapter 1 to interpret the ECG strips. It is important that you follow all steps and not take shortcuts.

For the following ECG strips:
1. Determine if the PPI and RRI are regular or irregular.
2. Calculate rates using the appropriate method:
   a. PPR

   b. RRR
3. Measure:
   a. PRI
   b. QRS
4. Interpretation

Place your answers in the space provided.
*Note that all strips are Lead II and are six seconds long unless otherwise indicated.

MATCHING

_____ 1. Key to differentiating all types of A-V blocks

_____ 2. Where in the conduction system the impulse originates for A-V blocks

_____ 3. Dysrhythmia that originates in the sinoatrial (S-A) node and has a constant PRI greater than 0.20 second

_____ 4. RRI of first degree A-V block

_____ 5. A type of A-V block in which the PR interval gets progressively longer

_____ 6. In Wenckebach, where in the conduction system atrial impulses are blocked

_____ 7. PPI of Wenckebach

_____ 8. RRI of Wenckebach

_____ 9. An A-V block in which group beating may be present

_____ 10. A-V block that does not usually progress to higher degrees of block

_____ 11. In Wenckebach, number of P waves compared to QRS complexes

_____ 12. A-V block that has more than one P wave for each QRS and constant PR intervals (on conducted beats)

_____ 13. A-V blocks with a constant PR interval

a. QRS interval
b. S-A node
c. second degree A-V block (Type I, Wenckebach)
d. second degree A-V block (Type II)
e. first degree A-V block
f. third degree A-V block
g. irregular
h. more
i. PR interval
j. A-V node
k. regular
l. less

_____ 14. A-V block that *always* has an irregular RRI

_____ 15. A-V blocks with a regular PPI

_____ 16. Type of second degree A-V block that may suddenly progress to third degree

_____ 17. A-V blocks with variable PR intervals

_____ 18. A-V block that is a form of A-V dissociation

_____ 19. In third degree A-V block, where in the conduction system *all* atrial impulses are blocked

_____ 20. In third degree A-V block, where the atrial impulse originates

_____ 21. In third degree A-V block, where the ventricular impulse originates

_____ 22. In third degree A-V block, if the QRS measures less than 0.12 second, where the impulse would originate

_____ 23. In third degree A-V block, if the QRS measures 0.12 second, or greater, where the impulse would originate

_____ 24. In this A-V block, P waves march through the QRS complex

a. first degree A-V block

b. second degree A-V block (Type I, Wenckebach)

c. second degree A-V block (Type II)

d. third degree A-V block

e. 0.12 second or greater

f. less than 0.12 second

g. S-A node

h. A-V node

i. atrium

j. junction

k. His–Purkinje system

ECG PRACTICE STRIPS

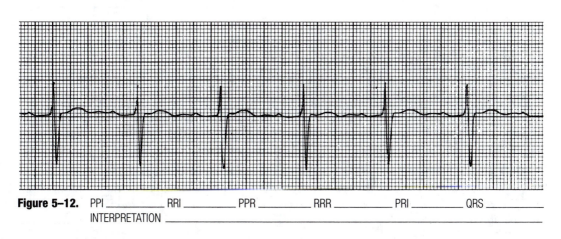

Figure 5–12. PPI _____ RRI _____ PPR _____ RRR _____ PRI _____ QRS _____
INTERPRETATION _____

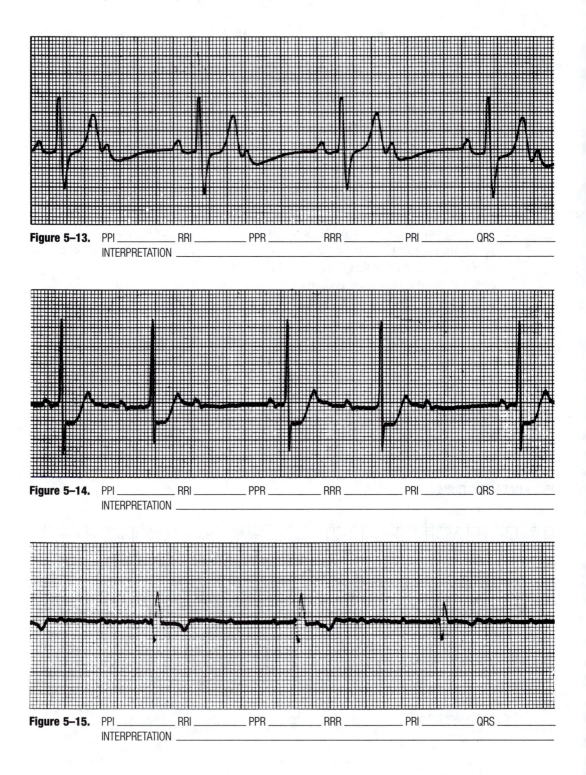

Figure 5–13. PPI _____ RRI _____ PPR _____ RRR _____ PRI _____ QRS _____
INTERPRETATION _____

Figure 5–14. PPI _____ RRI _____ PPR _____ RRR _____ PRI _____ QRS _____
INTERPRETATION _____

Figure 5–15. PPI _____ RRI _____ PPR _____ RRR _____ PRI _____ QRS _____
INTERPRETATION _____

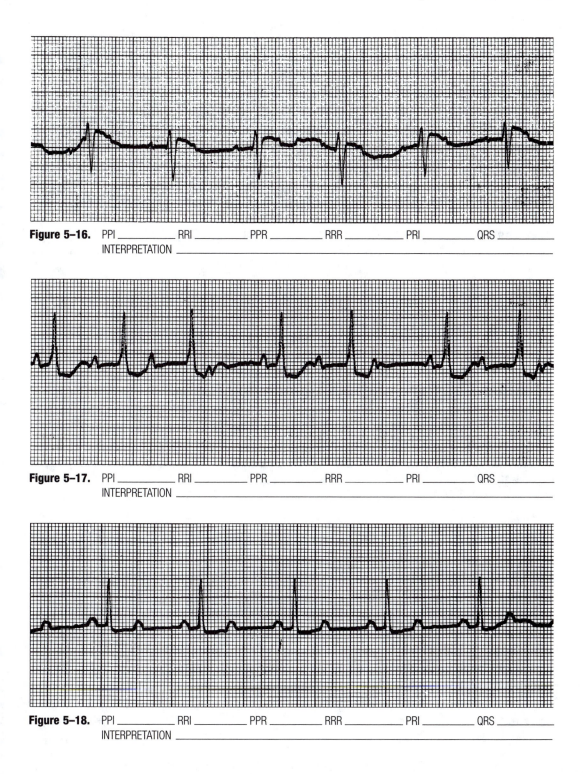

Figure 5–16. PPI _____ RRI _____ PPR _____ RRR _____ PRI _____ QRS _____
INTERPRETATION _____

Figure 5–17. PPI _____ RRI _____ PPR _____ RRR _____ PRI _____ QRS _____
INTERPRETATION _____

Figure 5–18. PPI _____ RRI _____ PPR _____ RRR _____ PRI _____ QRS _____
INTERPRETATION _____

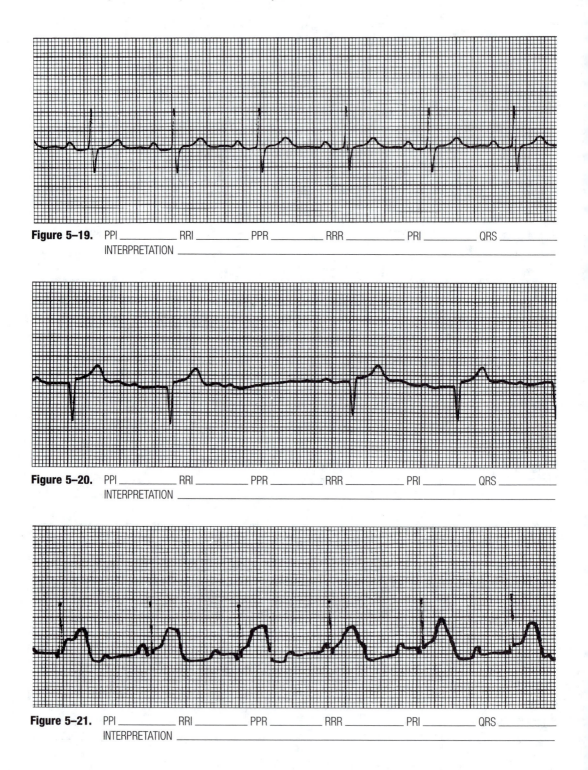

Figure 5–19. PPI _____ RRI _____ PPR _____ RRR _____ PRI _____ QRS _____
INTERPRETATION _____

Figure 5–20. PPI _____ RRI _____ PPR _____ RRR _____ PRI _____ QRS _____
INTERPRETATION _____

Figure 5–21. PPI _____ RRI _____ PPR _____ RRR _____ PRI _____ QRS _____
INTERPRETATION _____

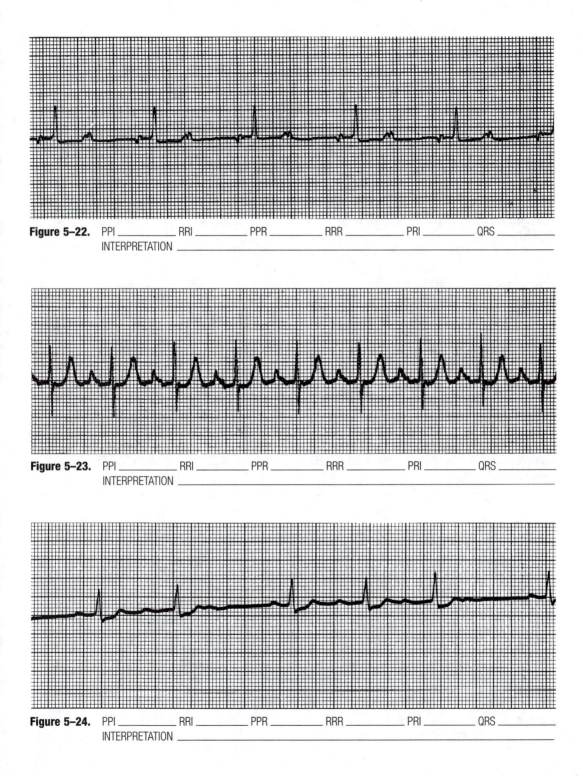

Figure 5–22. PPI _____ RRI _____ PPR _____ RRR _____ PRI _____ QRS _____
INTERPRETATION _____

Figure 5–23. PPI _____ RRI _____ PPR _____ RRR _____ PRI _____ QRS _____
INTERPRETATION _____

Figure 5–24. PPI _____ RRI _____ PPR _____ RRR _____ PRI _____ QRS _____
INTERPRETATION _____

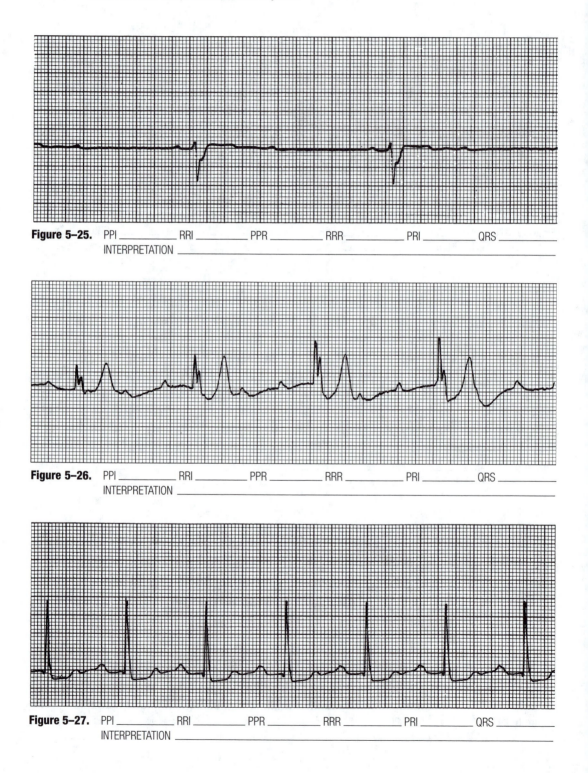

Figure 5–25.   PPI _____ RRI _____ PPR _____ RRR _____ PRI _____ QRS _____
INTERPRETATION _____

Figure 5–26.   PPI _____ RRI _____ PPR _____ RRR _____ PRI _____ QRS _____
INTERPRETATION _____

Figure 5–27.   PPI _____ RRI _____ PPR _____ RRR _____ PRI _____ QRS _____
INTERPRETATION _____

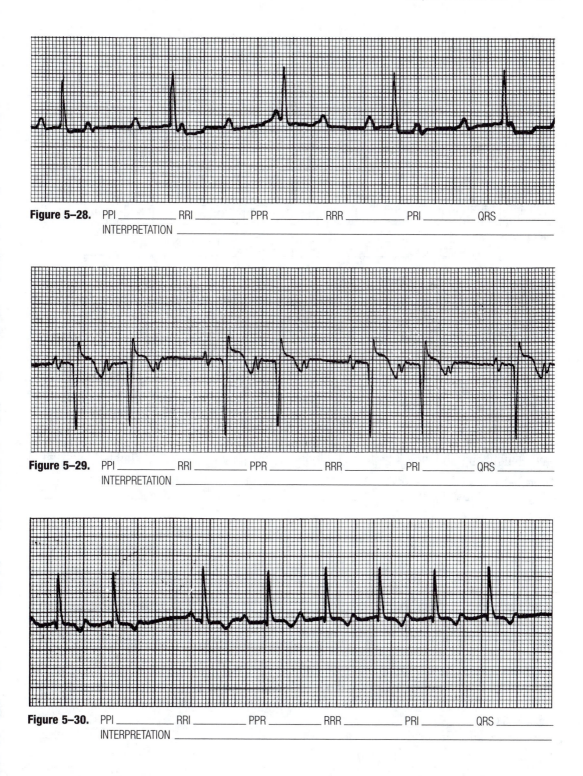

Figure 5–28. PPI _____ RRI _____ PPR _____ RRR _____ PRI _____ QRS _____
INTERPRETATION _____

Figure 5–29. PPI _____ RRI _____ PPR _____ RRR _____ PRI _____ QRS _____
INTERPRETATION _____

Figure 5–30. PPI _____ RRI _____ PPR _____ RRR _____ PRI _____ QRS _____
INTERPRETATION _____

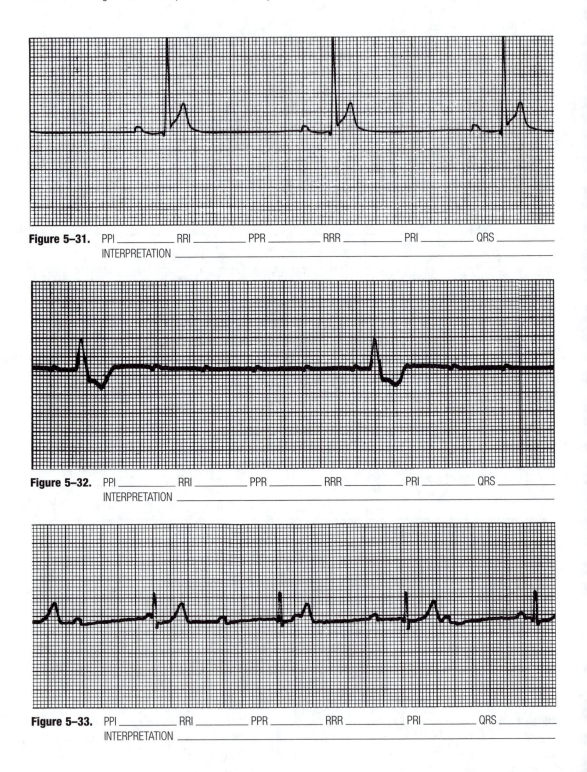

Figure 5–31.   PPI _____ RRI _____ PPR _____ RRR _____ PRI _____ QRS _____
INTERPRETATION _____

Figure 5–32.   PPI _____ RRI _____ PPR _____ RRR _____ PRI _____ QRS _____
INTERPRETATION _____

Figure 5–33.   PPI _____ RRI _____ PPR _____ RRR _____ PRI _____ QRS _____
INTERPRETATION _____

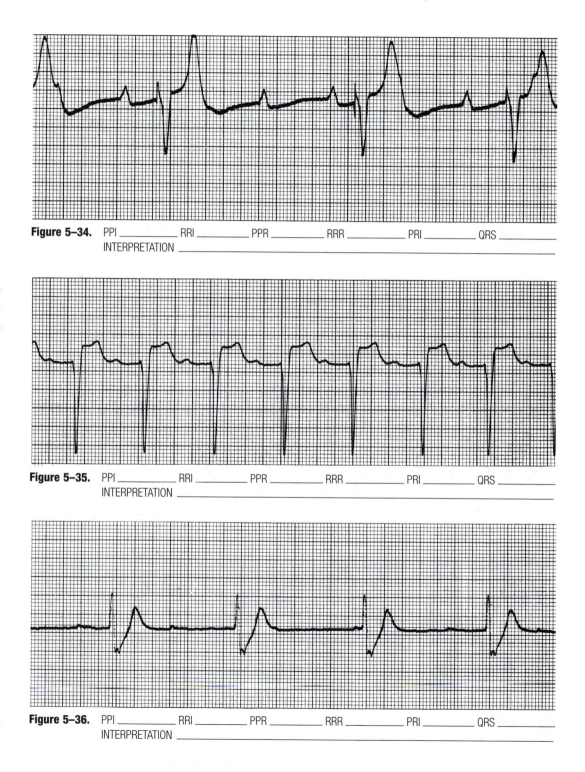

Figure 5–34.   PPI _____ RRI _____ PPR _____ RRR _____ PRI _____ QRS _____
INTERPRETATION _____

Figure 5–35.   PPI _____ RRI _____ PPR _____ RRR _____ PRI _____ QRS _____
INTERPRETATION _____

Figure 5–36.   PPI _____ RRI _____ PPR _____ RRR _____ PRI _____ QRS _____
INTERPRETATION _____

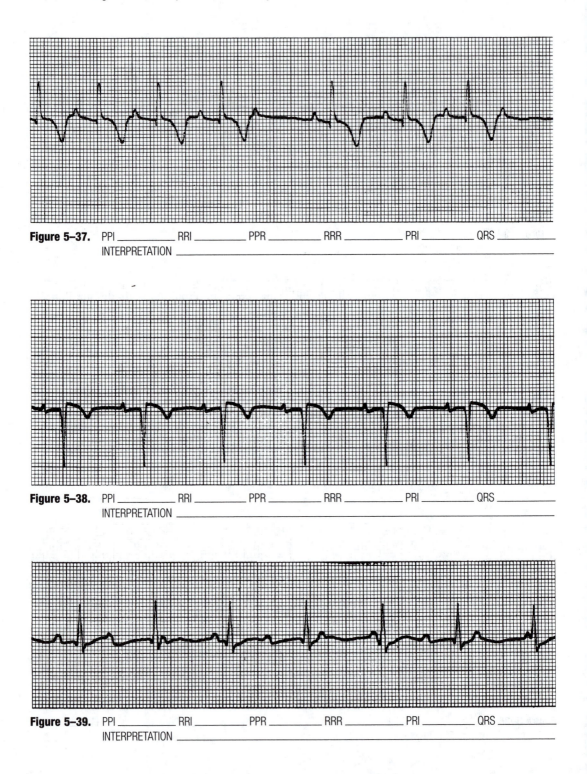

Figure 5–37. PPI _____ RRI _____ PPR _____ RRR _____ PRI _____ QRS _____
INTERPRETATION _____

Figure 5–38. PPI _____ RRI _____ PPR _____ RRR _____ PRI _____ QRS _____
INTERPRETATION _____

Figure 5–39. PPI _____ RRI _____ PPR _____ RRR _____ PRI _____ QRS _____
INTERPRETATION _____

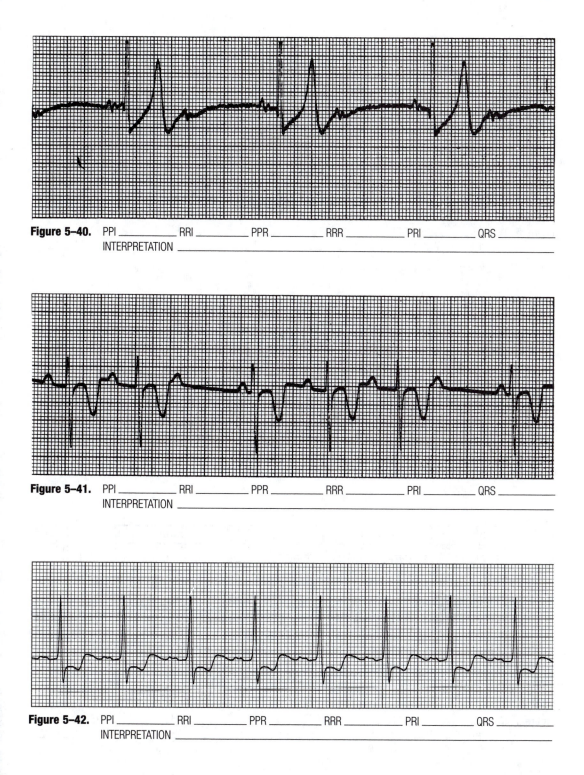

Figure 5–40. PPI _____ RRI _____ PPR _____ RRR _____ PRI _____ QRS _____
INTERPRETATION _____

Figure 5–41. PPI _____ RRI _____ PPR _____ RRR _____ PRI _____ QRS _____
INTERPRETATION _____

Figure 5–42. PPI _____ RRI _____ PPR _____ RRR _____ PRI _____ QRS _____
INTERPRETATION _____

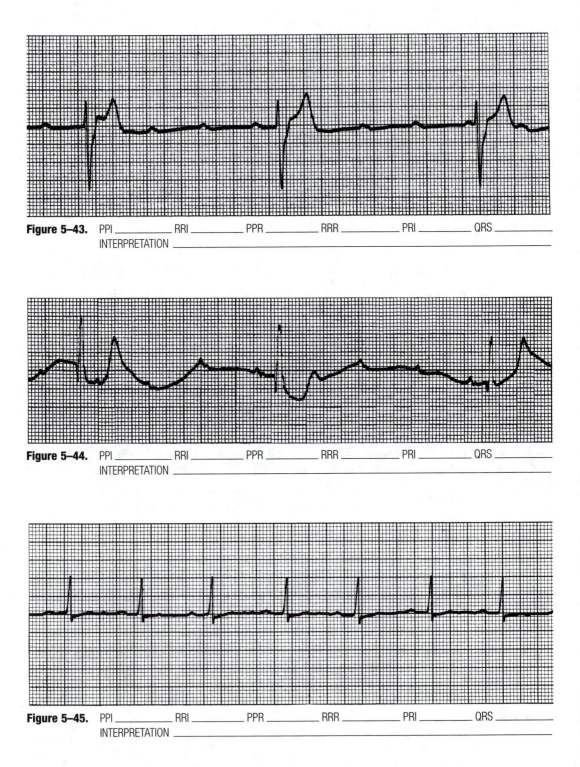

Figure 5–43. PPI _____ RRI _____ PPR _____ RRR _____ PRI _____ QRS _____
INTERPRETATION _____

Figure 5–44. PPI _____ RRI _____ PPR _____ RRR _____ PRI _____ QRS _____
INTERPRETATION _____

Figure 5–45. PPI _____ RRI _____ PPR _____ RRR _____ PRI _____ QRS _____
INTERPRETATION _____

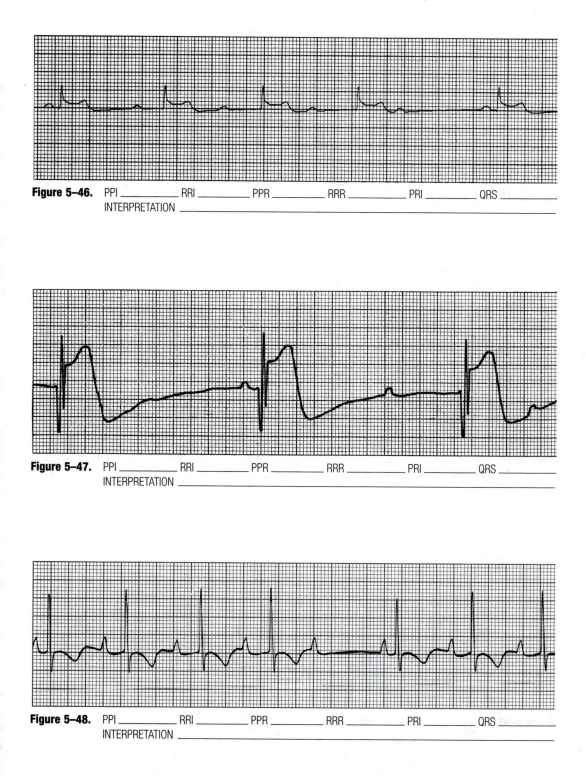

Figure 5–46.   PPI _____ RRI _____ PPR _____ RRR _____ PRI _____ QRS _____
INTERPRETATION _____

Figure 5–47.   PPI _____ RRI _____ PPR _____ RRR _____ PRI _____ QRS _____
INTERPRETATION _____

Figure 5–48.   PPI _____ RRI _____ PPR _____ RRR _____ PRI _____ QRS _____
INTERPRETATION _____

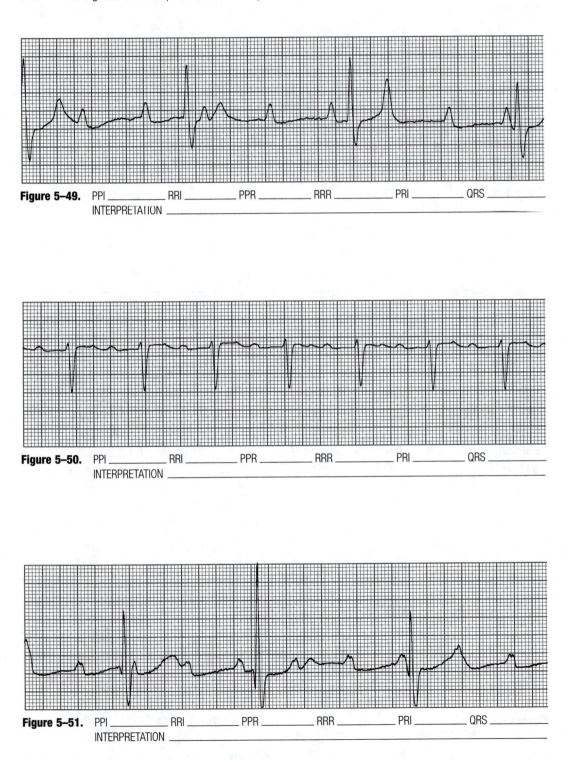

Figure 5–49.   PPI _____ RRI _____ PPR _____ RRR _____ PRI _____ QRS _____
INTERPRETATION _____

Figure 5–50.   PPI _____ RRI _____ PPR _____ RRR _____ PRI _____ QRS _____
INTERPRETATION _____

Figure 5–51.   PPI _____ RRI _____ PPR _____ RRR _____ PRI _____ QRS _____
INTERPRETATION _____

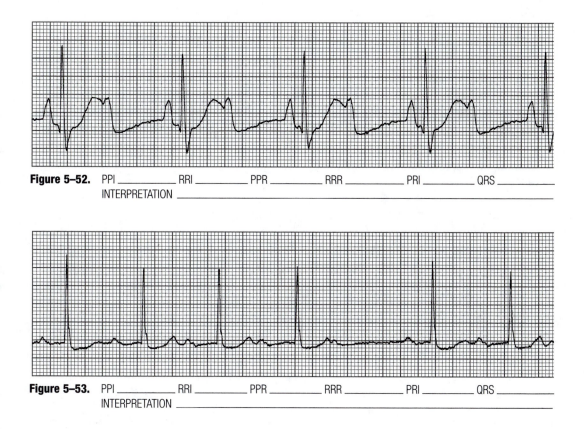

Figure 5–52.   PPI _____ RRI _____ PPR _____ RRR _____ PRI _____ QRS _____
INTERPRETATION _____

Figure 5–53.   PPI _____ RRI _____ PPR _____ RRR _____ PRI _____ QRS _____
INTERPRETATION _____

Ventricular Dysrhythmias

I. Premature Ventricular Complex (PVC)

  A. ECG features

    1. *PP interval:* depends upon underlying rhythm

    2. *RR interval:* depends upon underlying rhythm. PVC occurs prematurely in the cardiac cycle (prior to the next expected beat)

    3. *PP rate:* varies

    4. *RR rate:* varies

    5. *P wave:* PVC may be followed by an inverted P wave in Lead II (retrograde conduction) or P wave may be lost in QRS complex or may be seen before a PVC (if present, PPI is usually regular)

    6. *PRI:* depends upon underlying rhythm

    7. *QRS interval:* usually 0.12 second or greater (different from the QRS complex in the underlying rhythm; Figs. 6–1, 6–2, 6–3, and 6–4)

*Notes: PVCs may be seen in any rhythm. T wave of PVC is usually in opposite direction of the QRS complex. Usually followed by a full compensatory pause. The compensatory pause is a result of the P wave not being conducted due to the refractoriness of the ventricles following the PVC.

    Considered dangerous if (a) frequent (greater than 6 PVCs/min); (b) bigeminy or trigeminy (every other or every third beat is a PVC); (c) paired (couplets) or runs; (d) multiformed (PVCs from more than one focus and look different from each other); (e) R on T phenomenon (PVC falls on preceding T wave); (f) in the presence of acute myocardial infarction (MI)

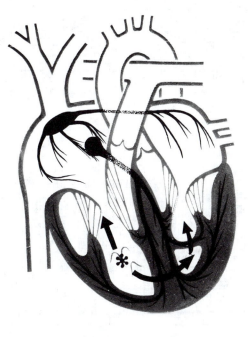

Figure 6–1. Premature ventricular complex. Irritable focus in ventricle initiates impulse early.

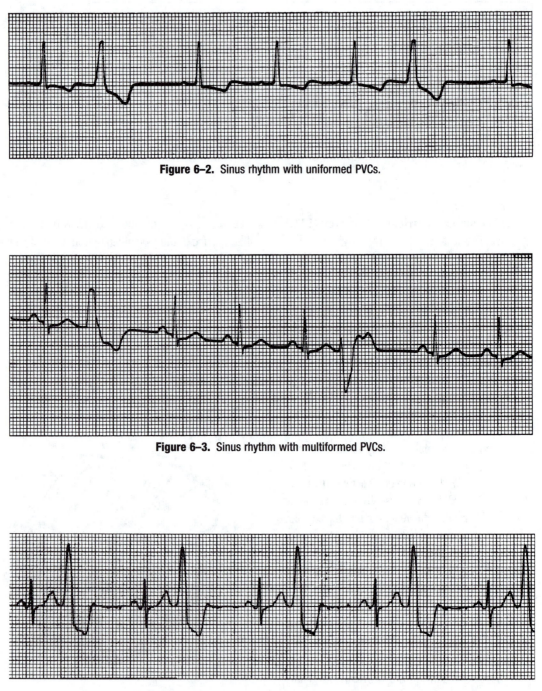

Figure 6–2. Sinus rhythm with uniformed PVCs.

Figure 6–3. Sinus rhythm with multiformed PVCs.

Figure 6–4. Sinus rhythm with bigeminy of uniformed PVCs.

B. Common etiology
   1. Ischemia
   2. Insult to His–Purkinje system or ventricle (MI)
   3. Acidosis
   4. Low potassium level
   5. Drugs (digitalis and catecholamines)
C. Clinical signs and symptoms
   1. Patient may complain of palpitations
   2. Patient may complain of skipped beats
   3. Pulse will have pause followed by a strong beat
   4. May lead to ventricular tachycardia or ventricular fibrillation

II. Ventricular Tachycardia (VT)
A. ECG features
   1. *PP interval:* unable to determine
   2. *RR interval:* usually regular
   3. *PP rate:* unable to determine
   4. *RR rate:* usually 150–250/min (may be as slow as 101)
   5. *P wave:* if present, has no relationship to QRS complex (A-V dissociation)
   6. *PRI:* unable to measure
   7. *QRS interval:* usually 0.12 second or greater; wide and bizarre (Figs. 6–5, 6–6, and 6–7)

*Note: Three or more PVCs in a row are defined as VT.

B. Common etiology
   1. Insult to the His–Purkinje system or ventricle (MI)
   2. Hypoxemia
   3. Acidosis
   4. Low potassium level
   5. Drugs (digitalis and catecholamines)
C. Clinical signs and symptoms
   1. Most patients are immediately aware of this dysrhythmia

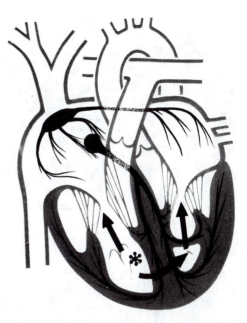

Figure 6–5. Ventricular tachycardia. Irritable focus in ventricle paces the heart at 150–250 beats/min.

   2. Decreased level of consciousness
   3. Patient may complain of palpitations, dyspnea, dizziness, anxiety, diaphoresis, and/or angina
   4. Decreased blood pressure
   5. If short bursts, may be asymptomatic
   6. Patient may have a seizure due to cerebral ischemia
   7. May have no cardiac output—pulseless ventricular tachycardia

III. Ventricular Fibrillation (VF)
A. ECG features
   1. *PP interval:* no discernible P waves
   2. *RR interval:* no discernible R waves
   3. *PP rate:* unable to determine
   4. *RR rate:* unable to determine
   5. *P wave:* no discernible P wave
   6. *PRI:* unable to measure

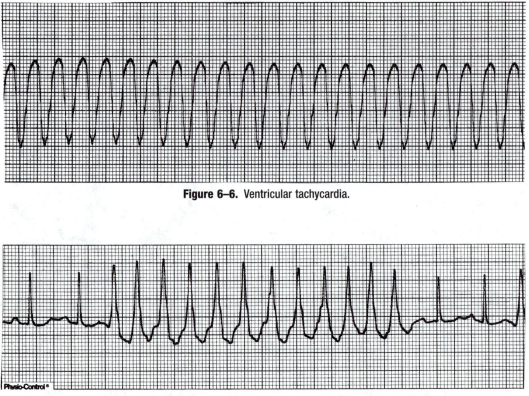

Figure 6–6. Ventricular tachycardia.

Figure 6–7. Sinus tachycardia with a burst of ventricular tachycardia.

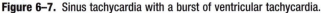

7. *QRS interval:* repetitive series of chaotic waves (Figs. 6–8 and 6–9)

*Note: No discernible PQRST complexes

B. Common etiology
   1. Exact mechanism unknown but usually preceded by ventricular irritability or a PVC on a T wave (R on T phenomenon)
   2. Insult to the His–Purkinje system or ventricle (MI)
   3. Hypoxemia
   4. Electrolyte disturbances
   5. Electrical shock
   6. Drugs (digitalis and catecholamines)

C. Clinical signs and symptoms
   1. Loss of consciousness

   2. No pulse, respirations, or blood pressure
   3. Possible seizure activity
   4. Cyanosis
   5. Clinical death

IV. Idioventricular Rhythm

A. ECG features
   1. *PP interval:* most often absent but usually regular if present
   2. *RR interval:* usually regular
   3. *PP rate:* usually regular if present
   4. *RR rate:* 40/min or less
   5. *P wave:* if present, normal and upright in Lead II
   6. *PRI:* if present, varies (no relationship to QRS complex—A-V dissociation)

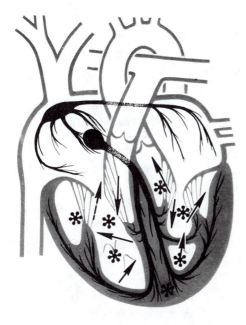

Figure 6–8. Ventricular fibrillation. Multiple foci initiate impulses in ventricles.

7. *QRS interval:* 0.12 second or greater; wide and bizarre (Figs. 6–10 and 6–11)

*Note: If ventricular rate is 41–100/min, it is interpreted as *accelerated idioventricular rhythm* (Fig. 6–12).

B. Common etiology
   1. Protective mechanism (an escape rhythm)
   2. Failure of normal conduction system
   3. Dying heart
C. Clinical signs and symptoms
   1. Slow heart rate
   2. May have no pulse or blood pressure present (pulseless electrical activity)
   3. Decreased cardiac output
   4. Syncopal episode

V. Ventricular Standstill
A. ECG features
   1. *PP interval:* usually regular
   2. *RR interval:* absent
   3. *PP rate:* varies
   4. *RR rate:* absent
   5. *P wave:* upright and normal in Lead II
   6. *PRI:* absent
   7. *QRS interval:* absent (Figs. 6–13 and 6–14)
B. Common etiology
   1. Failure of the conduction system to transmit impulse
   2. Insult to heart muscle
C. Clinical signs and symptoms
   1. Same as ventricular fibrillation (clinically dead)

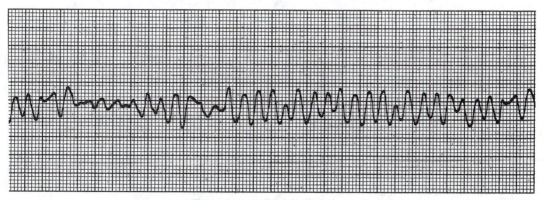

Figure 6–9. Ventricular fibrillation.

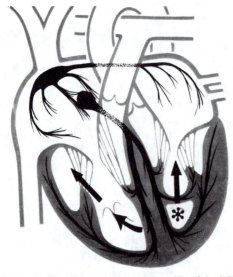

Figure 6–10. Idioventricular rhythm. Ventricle initiates impulse at 20–40/min.

2. Can be distinguished from ventricular fibrillation only by an ECG

VI. **Asystole**

  A. ECG features

    1. *PP interval:* absent

    2. *RR interval:* absent

    3. *PP rate:* absent

    4. *RR rate:* absent

    5. *P wave:* absent

    6. *PRI:* absent

    7. *QRS interval:* absent (Figs. 6–15 and 6–16)

*Note: Straight line on monitor (no PQRST complexes)

  B. Common etiology

    1. Failure of the conduction system to fire

    2. Insult to heart muscle

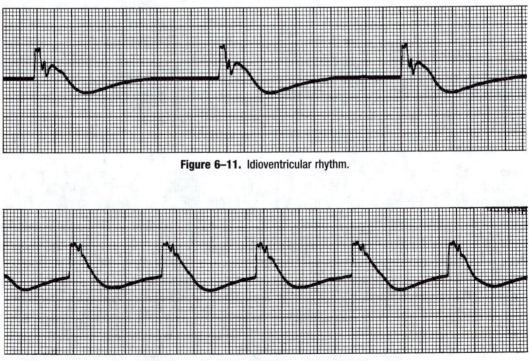

Figure 6–11. Idioventricular rhythm.

Figure 6–12. Accelerated idioventricular rhythm.

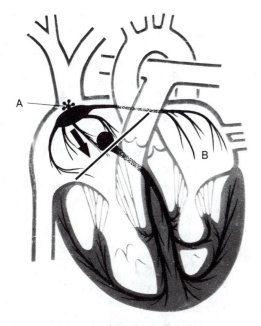

Figure 6–13. Ventricular standstill. **A.** S-A node initiates impulse. **B.** Complete block at A-V node. **C.** Ventricular tissue fails to fire.

C. Clinical signs and symptoms
   1. Same as ventricular fibrillation (clinically dead)
   2. Can be distinguished from ventricular fib-

rillation or ventricular standstill only by an ECG

VII. Pulseless Electrical Activity

A. ECG features
   1. May show any rhythm on the ECG, but patient has no pulse or blood pressure
   2. Commonly seen in
      a. Bradycardias with a ventricular response less than 40/min
      b. Idioventricular rhythm
      c. Tachycardia (suggestive of hypovolemia, cardiac tamponade, tension pneumothorax, or ventricular rupture)
B. Common etiology
   1. Poor pumping action of the heart muscle
   2. Massive MI
   3. Pulmonary embolism
   4. Hypovolemia
   5. Cardiac tamponade
   6. Tension pneumothorax
   7. Ventricular rupture
   8. Acidosis
C. Clinical signs and symptoms
   1. No palpable pulses
   2. No obtainable blood pressure
   3. No respirations

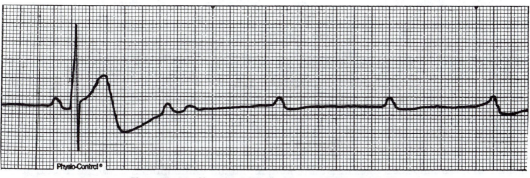

Figure 6–14. Sinus beat followed by ventricular standstill.

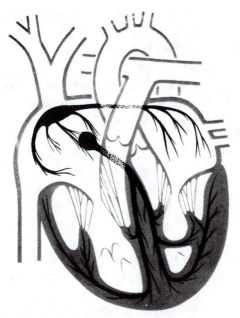

Figure 6–15. Asystole. No electrical activity.

4. Unconsciousness
5. Cyanosis
6. Clinically dead

VIII. Ventricular Escape Complex

A. ECG features

1. *PP interval:* depends upon underlying rhythm
2. *RR interval:* depends upon underlying rhythm; a ventricular escape complex occurs late in the cardiac cycle
3. *PP rate:* depends upon underlying rhythm
4. *RR rate:* depends upon underlying rhythm
5. *P wave:* absent prior to ventricular escape complex
6. *PRI:* absent on ventricular escape complex
7. *QRS interval:* usually 0.12 second or greater; wide and bizarre on escape complex (Figs. 6–17 and 6–18)

B. Common etiology
1. Failure of a higher center in the conduction system to fire
2. A protective mechanism

C. Clinical signs and symptoms
1. Depend on ventricular rate
2. Patient may be asymptomatic
3. If heart rate decreases dramatically, signs/symptoms of decreased cardiac output may occur

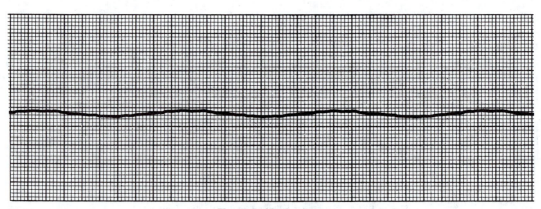

Figure 6–16. Asystole.

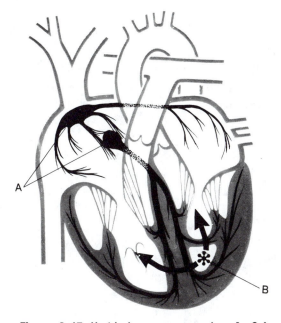

Figure 6–17. Ventricular escape complex. **A.** S-A node and junctional tissue fail to fire. **B.** Ventricular escape complex comes in as a protective mechanism.

SELF-EVALUATION

Directions

Answer keys for the Self-Evaluation section begin on page 327.

1. **Matching.** Place the letter of the appropriate item(s) before each numbered statement. Some answers are used more than once, and not all answers will be used.
2. **ECG practice strips.** For simplicity and practicality, all rates have been calculated by using Method 3 (Fig. 1–14). Keep in mind that your measurements for PRIs and QRS complexes may vary slightly and still be correct. Use the systematic approach shown in Chapter 1 to interpret the ECG strips. It is important that you follow all steps and not take shortcuts.

For the following ECG strips:

1. Determine if the PPI and RRI are regular or irregular
2. Calculate rates using the appropriate method:
   a. PPR
   b. RRR
3. Measure:
   a. PRI
   b. QRS
4. Interpretation
   Place your answers in the space provided.
*Note that all strips are Lead II and are 6 seconds long unless otherwise indicated.

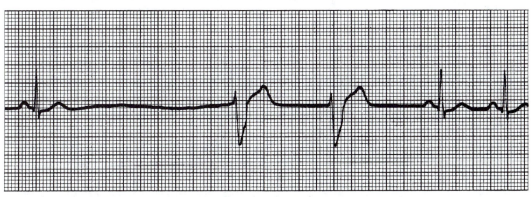

Figure 6–18. Sinus rhythm followed by sinus arrest and two ventricular escape complexes.

MATCHING

_____ 1. Early complex that indicates ventricular irritability

_____ 2. Dysrhythmias characterized by wide and bizarre QRS complexes

_____ 3. The usual direction of the T wave in a negative (downward) PVC

_____ 4. The usual direction of the T wave in a positive (upright) PVC

_____ 5. Three or more PVCs in a row

_____ 6. The width of the QRS complex in a PVC

_____ 7. Part of the PQRST complex that is considered the vulnerable period of the cardiac cycle

_____ 8. Location of the retrograde P waves of a PVC

_____ 9. How ventricular dysrhythmias alter cardiac output

Indicate if the following types of PVCs are dangerous or benign:

_____ 10. R on T phenomenon

_____ 11. Less than three per minute

_____ 12. In presence of chest pain

_____ 13. A young person with no chest pain

_____ 14. Trigeminy

a. positive (upright)
b. usually 0.12 second or greater
c. ventricular fibrillation
d. P wave
e. PVC
f. inverted
g. before the QRS complex
h. ventricular tachycardia
i. decrease
j. S wave
k. negative (downward)
l. after the QRS complex
m. T wave
n. increase
o. benign
p. dangerous
q. supraventricular
r. ventricular

Indicate if the following types of PVCs are dangerous or benign:

_____ 15. Multiformed

_____ 16. Runs of PVCs

_____ 17. Paired

_____ 18. Bigeminy

_____ 19. Frequent (more than six per minute)

_____ 20. Uniformed

_____ 21. PVCs dangerous because they can lead to these two dysrhythmias

_____ 22. Dysrhythmia associated with patients complaining of feeling skipped beats

_____ 23. A repetitive pattern of one sinus beat followed by one PVC

_____ 24. A repetitive pattern of two sinus beats followed by one PVC

_____ 25. Common causes of PVCs

_____ 26. A dysrhythmia in which you see P waves but no QRS complexes

_____ 27. A dysrhythmia characterized by a repetitive series of chaotic waves

_____ 28. Usual rate of idioventricular rhythm

_____ 29. Rate of an accelerated idioventricular rhythm

a. PVCs
b. ventricular standstill
c. bigeminy
d. dangerous
e. asystole
f. 20–40/min
g. trigeminy
h. benign
i. 40–60/min
j. 60–100/min
k. hypoxemia/ischemia
l. ventricular fibrillation
m. ventricular tachycardia
n. ventricular escape complexes
o. quadrigeminy
p. idioventricular rhythm
q. 41–100/min

_____ 30. RRI of an idioventricular rhythm

_____ 31. Width of QRS complexes in an idioventricular rhythm

_____ 32. RRR of ventricular tachycardia

_____ 33. RRI of ventricular tachycardia

_____ 34. Width of QRS complexes in ventricular tachycardia

_____ 35. A dysrhythmia characterized by continued electrical activity but cessation of mechanical activity

_____ 36. P waves are present but have no relation to the QRS complexes

_____ 37. A dysrhythmia characterized by no mechanical activity or PQRST complexes

_____ 38. Dysrhythmias associated with a patient experiencing seizure activity

_____ 39. Ventricular complexes that come late in the cardiac cycle

_____ 40. Ventricular complex considered a protective mechanism

_____ 41. Effect of ventricular fibrillation on cardiac output

_____ 42. Dysrhythmias associated with a patient who presents clinically dead

a. less than (<) 0.12 second

b. 100–150/min

c. 250–350/min

d. regular

e. pulseless electrical activity

f. 150–250/min

g. asystole

h. ventricular tachycardia

i. 0.12 second or greater

j. A-V dissociation

k. escape

l. decreased

m. ventricular fibrillation

n. irregular

o. premature

p. increased

ECG PRACTICE STRIPS

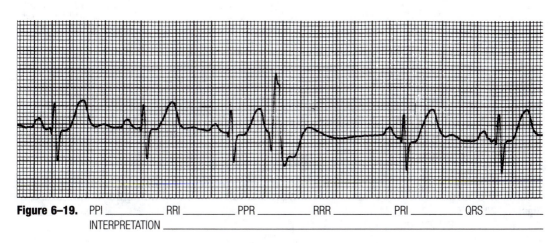

Figure 6–19. PPI _____ RRI _____ PPR _____ RRR _____ PRI _____ QRS _____

INTERPRETATION _____

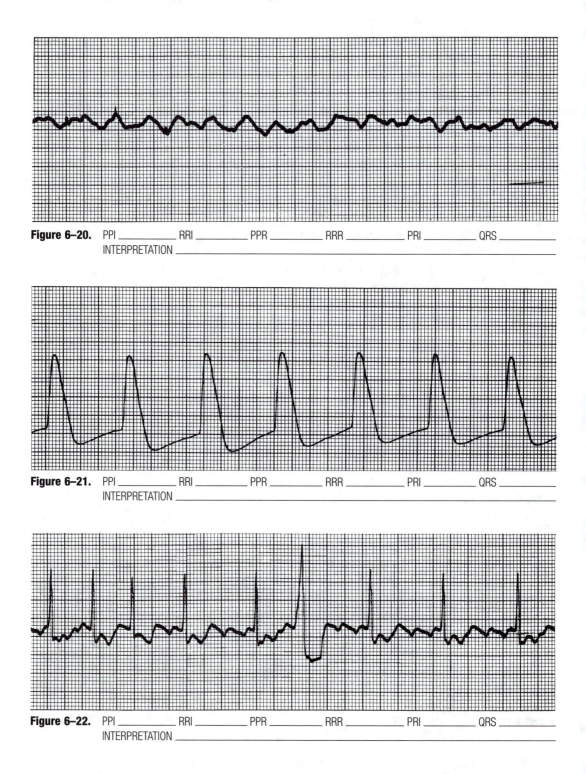

Figure 6–20. PPI _____ RRI _____ PPR _____ RRR _____ PRI _____ QRS _____
INTERPRETATION _____

Figure 6–21. PPI _____ RRI _____ PPR _____ RRR _____ PRI _____ QRS _____
INTERPRETATION _____

Figure 6–22. PPI _____ RRI _____ PPR _____ RRR _____ PRI _____ QRS _____
INTERPRETATION _____

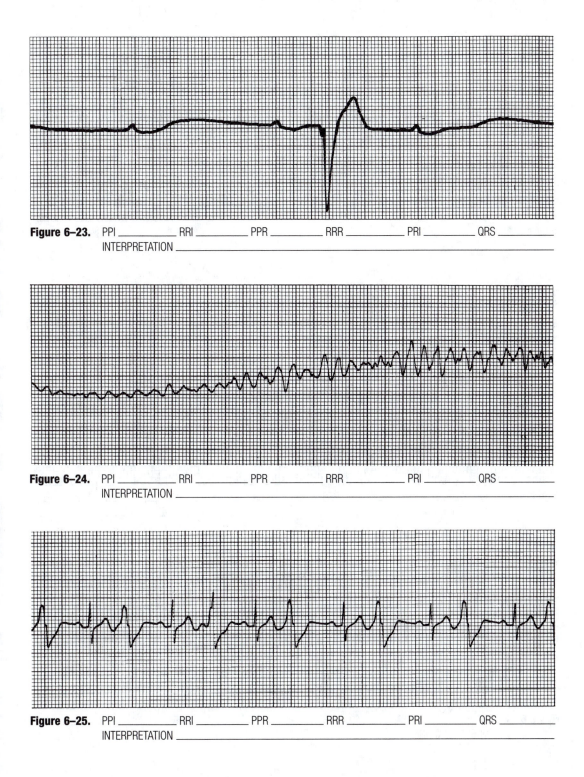

Figure 6–23. PPI _____ RRI _____ PPR _____ RRR _____ PRI _____ QRS _____
INTERPRETATION _____

Figure 6–24. PPI _____ RRI _____ PPR _____ RRR _____ PRI _____ QRS _____
INTERPRETATION _____

Figure 6–25. PPI _____ RRI _____ PPR _____ RRR _____ PRI _____ QRS _____
INTERPRETATION _____

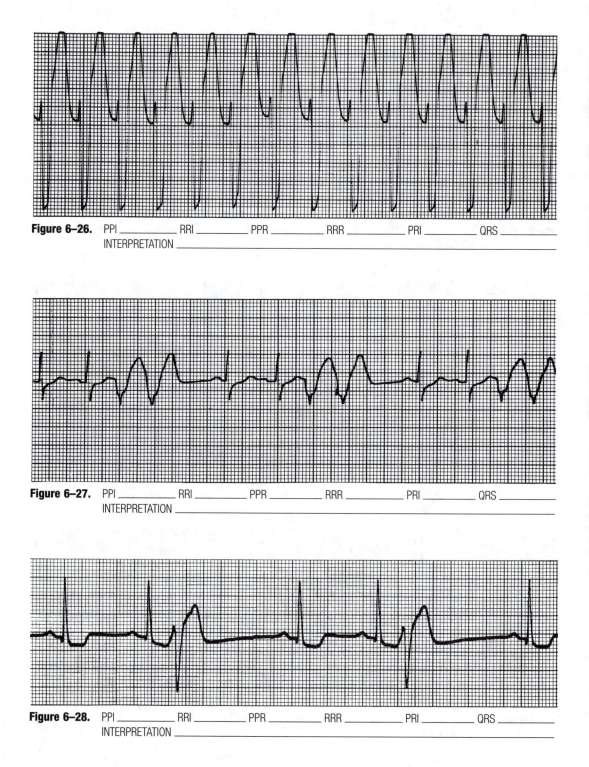

Figure 6–26. PPI _____ RRI _____ PPR _____ RRR _____ PRI _____ QRS _____
INTERPRETATION _____

Figure 6–27. PPI _____ RRI _____ PPR _____ RRR _____ PRI _____ QRS _____
INTERPRETATION _____

Figure 6–28. PPI _____ RRI _____ PPR _____ RRR _____ PRI _____ QRS _____
INTERPRETATION _____

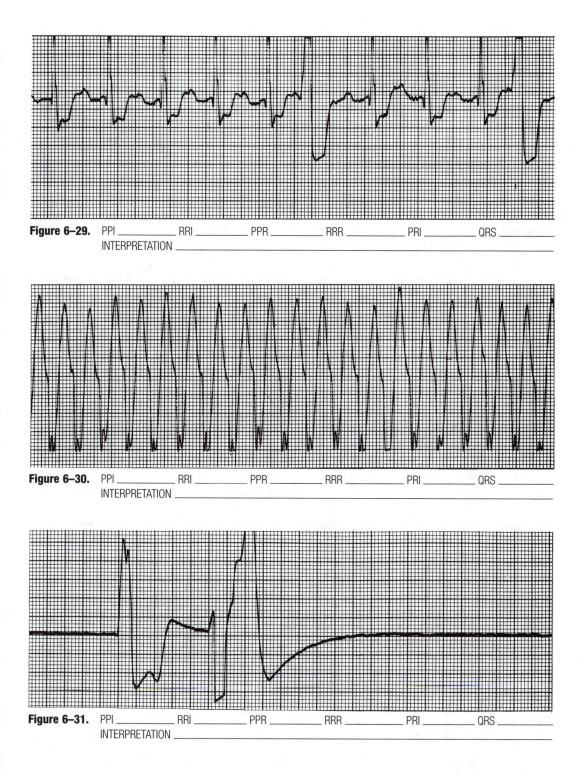

Figure 6–29. PPI _____ RRI _____ PPR _____ RRR _____ PRI _____ QRS _____
INTERPRETATION _____

Figure 6–30. PPI _____ RRI _____ PPR _____ RRR _____ PRI _____ QRS _____
INTERPRETATION _____

Figure 6–31. PPI _____ RRI _____ PPR _____ RRR _____ PRI _____ QRS _____
INTERPRETATION _____

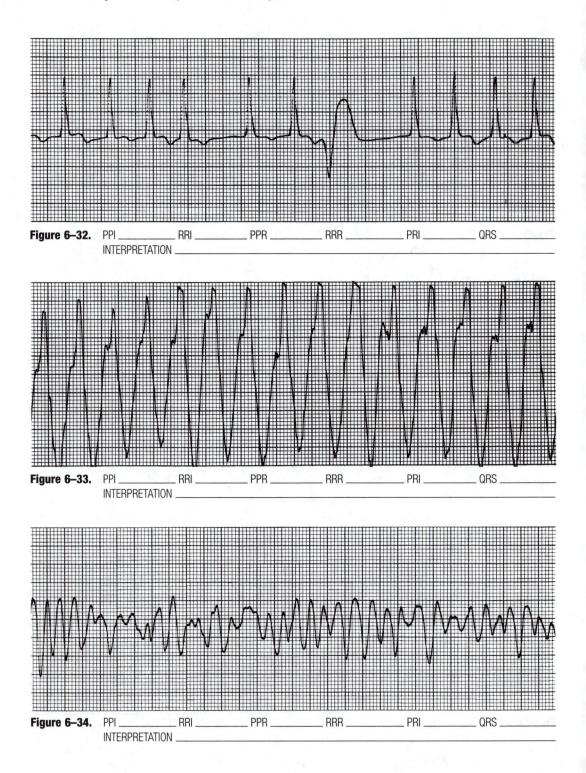

Figure 6–32. PPI _____ RRI _____ PPR _____ RRR _____ PRI _____ QRS _____
INTERPRETATION _____

Figure 6–33. PPI _____ RRI _____ PPR _____ RRR _____ PRI _____ QRS _____
INTERPRETATION _____

Figure 6–34. PPI _____ RRI _____ PPR _____ RRR _____ PRI _____ QRS _____
INTERPRETATION _____

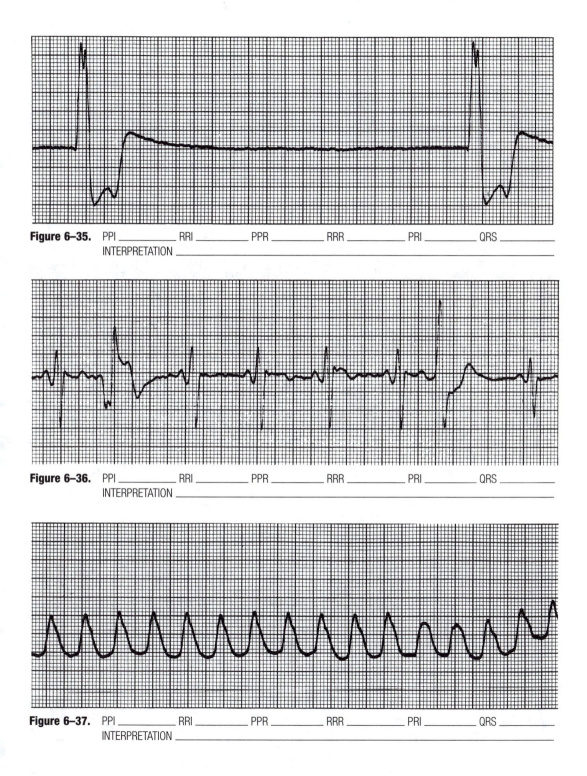

Figure 6–35. PPI _____ RRI _____ PPR _____ RRR _____ PRI _____ QRS _____

INTERPRETATION _____

Figure 6–36. PPI _____ RRI _____ PPR _____ RRR _____ PRI _____ QRS _____

INTERPRETATION _____

Figure 6–37. PPI _____ RRI _____ PPR _____ RRR _____ PRI _____ QRS _____

INTERPRETATION _____

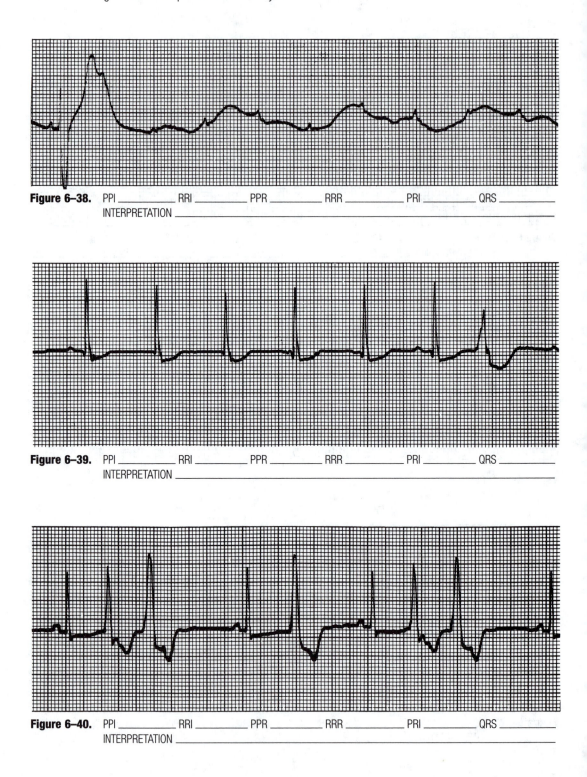

Figure 6–38. PPI _____ RRI _____ PPR _____ RRR _____ PRI _____ QRS _____

INTERPRETATION _____

Figure 6–39. PPI _____ RRI _____ PPR _____ RRR _____ PRI _____ QRS _____

INTERPRETATION _____

Figure 6–40. PPI _____ RRI _____ PPR _____ RRR _____ PRI _____ QRS _____

INTERPRETATION _____

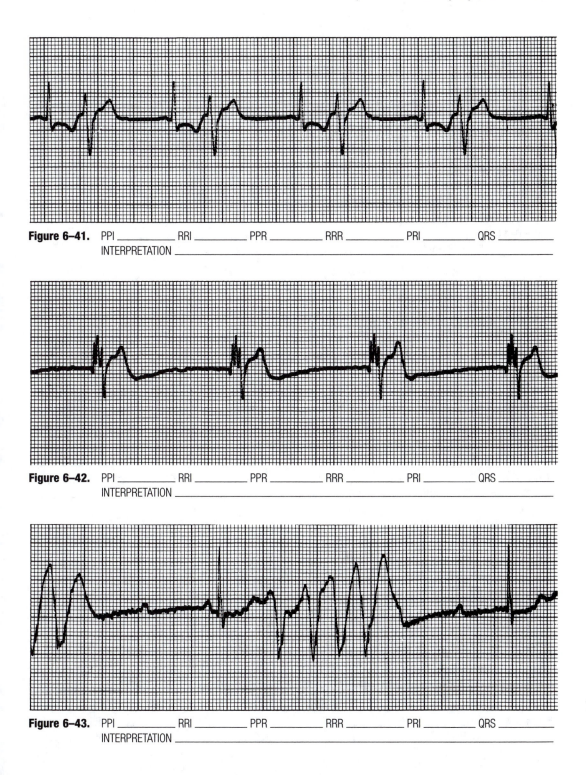

Figure 6–41. PPI _____ RRI _____ PPR _____ RRR _____ PRI _____ QRS _____

INTERPRETATION _____

Figure 6–42. PPI _____ RRI _____ PPR _____ RRR _____ PRI _____ QRS _____

INTERPRETATION _____

Figure 6–43. PPI _____ RRI _____ PPR _____ RRR _____ PRI _____ QRS _____

INTERPRETATION _____

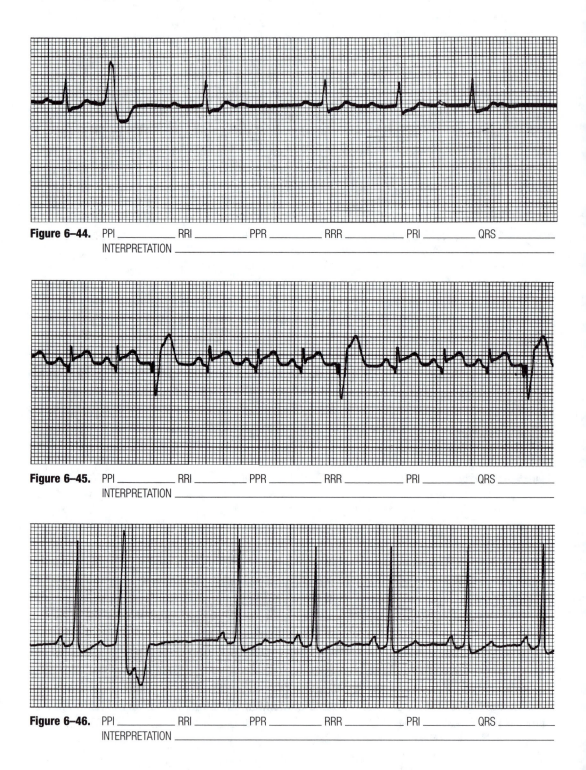

Figure 6–44.   PPI _____ RRI _____ PPR _____ RRR _____ PRI _____ QRS _____
INTERPRETATION _____

Figure 6–45.   PPI _____ RRI _____ PPR _____ RRR _____ PRI _____ QRS _____
INTERPRETATION _____

Figure 6–46.   PPI _____ RRI _____ PPR _____ RRR _____ PRI _____ QRS _____
INTERPRETATION _____

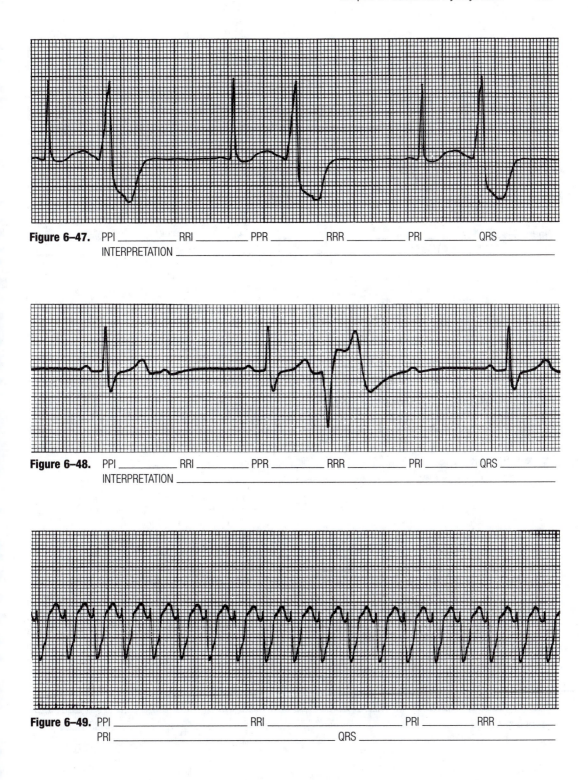

Figure 6–47. PPI _____ RRI _____ PPR _____ RRR _____ PRI _____ QRS _____
INTERPRETATION _____

Figure 6–48. PPI _____ RRI _____ PPR _____ RRR _____ PRI _____ QRS _____
INTERPRETATION _____

Figure 6–49. PPI _____ RRI _____ PRI _____ RRR _____
PRI _____ QRS _____

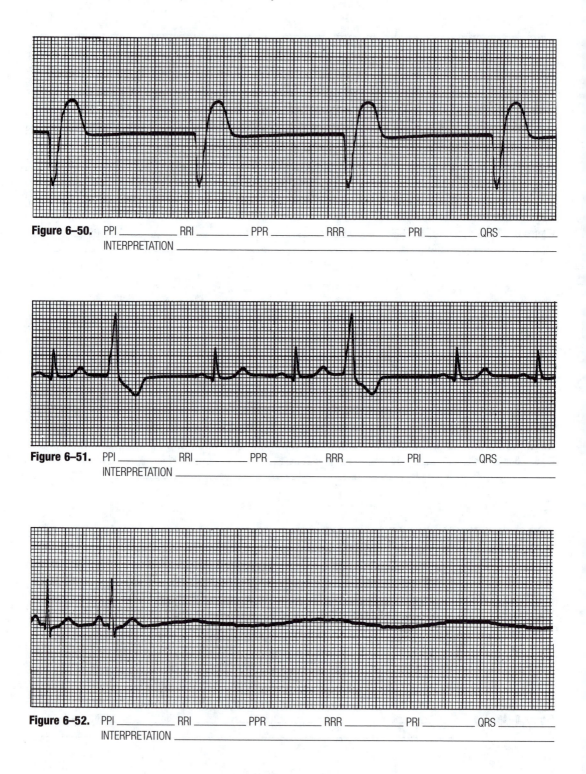

Figure 6–50.   PPI _____ RRI _____ PPR _____ RRR _____ PRI _____ QRS _____
INTERPRETATION _____

Figure 6–51.   PPI _____ RRI _____ PPR _____ RRR _____ PRI _____ QRS _____
INTERPRETATION _____

Figure 6–52.   PPI _____ RRI _____ PPR _____ RRR _____ PRI _____ QRS _____
INTERPRETATION _____

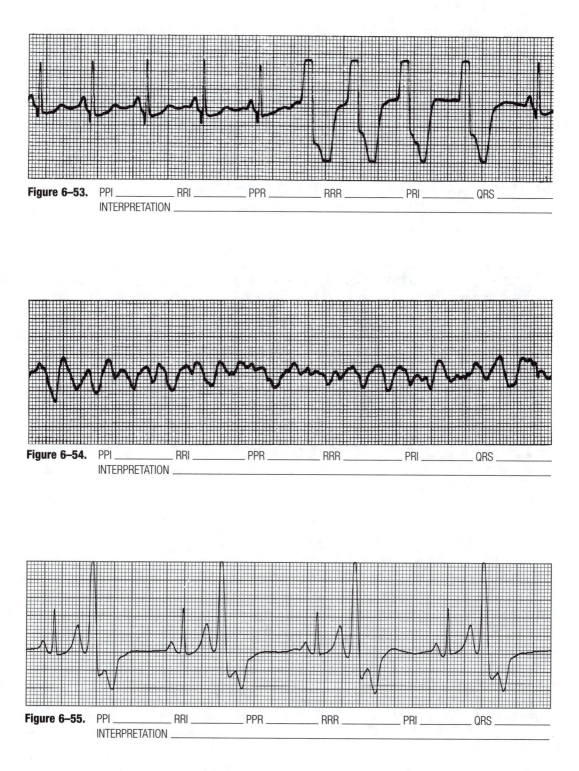

Figure 6–53. PPI _____ RRI _____ PPR _____ RRR _____ PRI _____ QRS _____
INTERPRETATION _____

Figure 6–54. PPI _____ RRI _____ PPR _____ RRR _____ PRI _____ QRS _____
INTERPRETATION _____

Figure 6–55. PPI _____ RRI _____ PPR _____ RRR _____ PRI _____ QRS _____
INTERPRETATION _____

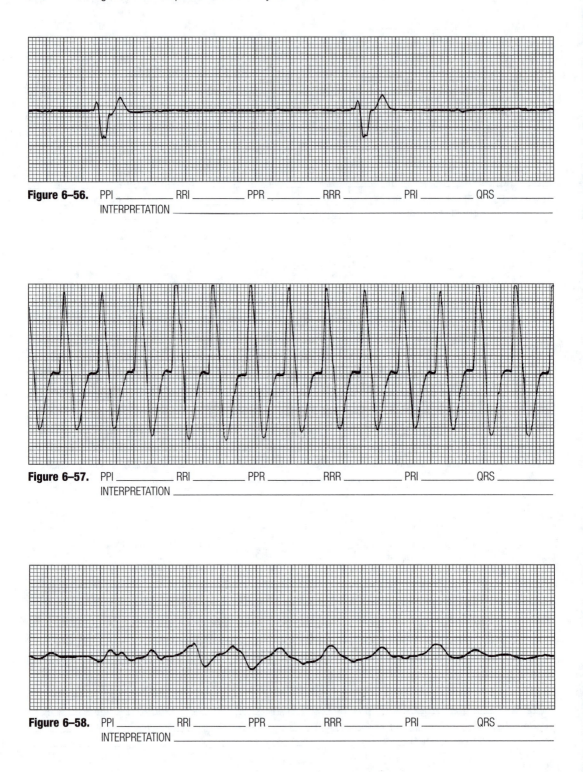

Figure 6–56.   PPI _____ RRI _____ PPR _____ RRR _____ PRI _____ QRS _____
INTERPRETATION _____

Figure 6–57.   PPI _____ RRI _____ PPR _____ RRR _____ PRI _____ QRS _____
INTERPRETATION _____

Figure 6–58.   PPI _____ RRI _____ PPR _____ RRR _____ PRI _____ QRS _____
INTERPRETATION _____

7

Complicating Features

I. **Artificial Pacemakers**
  A. Ventricular pacemaker
    1. ECG features
      a. *PP interval:* usually unable to determine
      b. *RR interval:* usually regular when pacing; when patient's own rhythm is functioning and ventricular pacemaker is on demand, the RR interval may be irregular
      c. *PP rate:* unable to determine
      d. *RR rate:* pacemaker is usually set at a rate of 60–90/min; may be set at a higher rate
      e. *P wave:* if present, has no relationship to QRS complex of paced complex
      f. *PRI:* absent
      g. *QRS interval:* 0.12 second or greater (Figs. 7–1, 7–2, and 7–3)

*Notes: Blip or spike precedes QRS complex. A normally functioning demand pacemaker will not fire unless the patient's own heart rate falls below the preset rate (sensing). Interval between patient's complex and paced complex is constant. Electrical stimulation by the pacemaker should be followed by electrical depolarization of the cardiac cells (capturing). This is demonstrated on the ECG by a blip or spike followed by a QRS complex.

    2. Common indications for ventricular pacemaker
      a. Abnormally slow heart rate
        i. Arteriosclerotic heart disease
        ii. Myocardial infarction
      b. Unreliability or failure of patient's own conduction system
        i. Arteriosclerotic heart disease
        ii. Myocardial infarction
    3. Clinical signs and symptoms

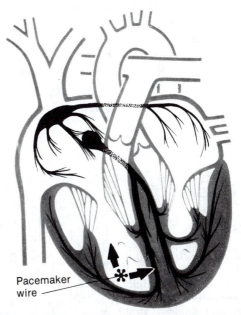

Figure 7–1. Ventricular pacemaker. Pacemaker wire is placed in right ventricle and stimulates conduction.

Pacemaker wire

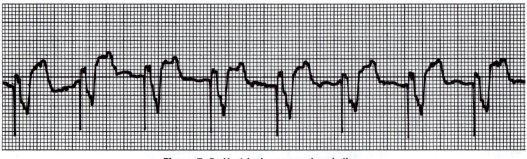

Figure 7–2. Ventricular pacemaker rhythm.

a. None when pacemaker functioning properly

b. If pacemaker is permanent, battery can be seen as a protrusion under the skin (may be very small)

B. Atrioventricular (A-V) synchronous pacemaker

1. ECG features

   a. *PP interval:* usually regular when paced and capturing

   b. *RR interval:* usually regular when paced and capturing

   c. *PP rate:* usually set at a rate of 60–100/min

   d. *RR rate:* usually set at a rate of 60–100/min

   e. *P wave:* if present, all paced P waves look alike

   f. *PRI:* may vary

g. *QRS interval:* less than (<) 0.12 second if captured from atrial stimulus; 0.12 second or greater if paced by ventricular stimulation (Figs. 7–4, 7–5, and 7–6)

*Notes: Two blips or spikes may be present. Patient may have an A-V synchronous pacemaker in which (a) the atria are sensed and/or paced; (b) the ventricle is sensed and/or paced; (c) both the atrium and the ventricle are sensed and paced. Different configurations can be seen on the ECG: (a) spike or blip only before P wave; (b) spike or blip only before QRS complex; spike or blip before both P wave and QRS complex. A-V synchronous pacing is contraindicated in patients with atrial flutter or atrial fibrillation.

2. Common indications for A-V synchronous pacing

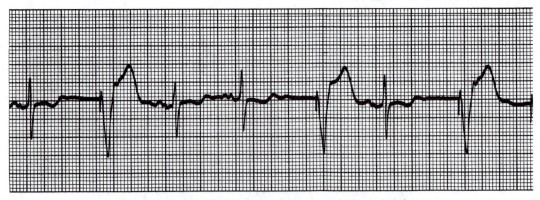

Figure 7–3. Normally functioning demand ventricular pacemaker.

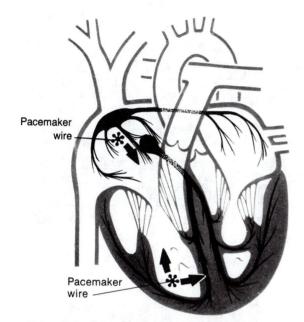

Figure 7–4. Atrioventricular synchronous pacemaker. Pacemaker wires are placed in the right atrium and the right ventricle and are stimulated sequentially.

    a. Abnormally slow heart rate
      i. Arteriosclerotic heart disease
      ii. Myocardial infarction
    b. Unreliability or failure of patient's own conduction system
      i. Arteriosclerotic heart disease
      ii. Myocardial infarction
  3. Clinical signs and symptoms

    a. None when pacemaker functioning properly
    b. If pacemaker is permanent, battery can be seen as a protrusion under the skin (may be very small)
  C. Malfunctioning pacemaker
    1. ECG features
      a. *PP interval:* depends upon underlying rhythm
      b. *RR interval:* depends upon underlying rhythm
      c. *PP rate:* depends upon underlying rhythm; may be absent
      d. *RR rate:* depends upon underlying rhythm
      e. *P wave:* depends upon underlying rhythm
      f. *PRI:* depends upon underlying rhythm
      g. *QRS interval:* depends upon underlying rhythm (Figs. 7–7 and 7–8)

*Notes: In an A-V synchronous pacemaker may see atrial spikes/blips with no P waves or both may be missing. May see ventricular spikes/blips without QRS complexes (represents pacemaker not capturing). May know patient has a pacemaker and see no pacemaker spikes/blips (battery failure). May see spikes/blips falling inside of QRS complexes or on the P or T wave (failure of sensing capability). May cause competition between the pacemaker and the

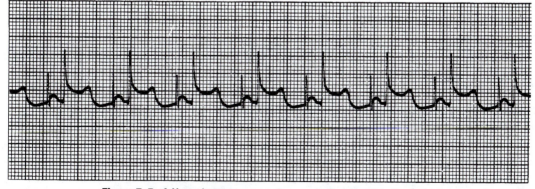

Figure 7–5. A-V synchronous pacemaker responding to atrial stimulation.

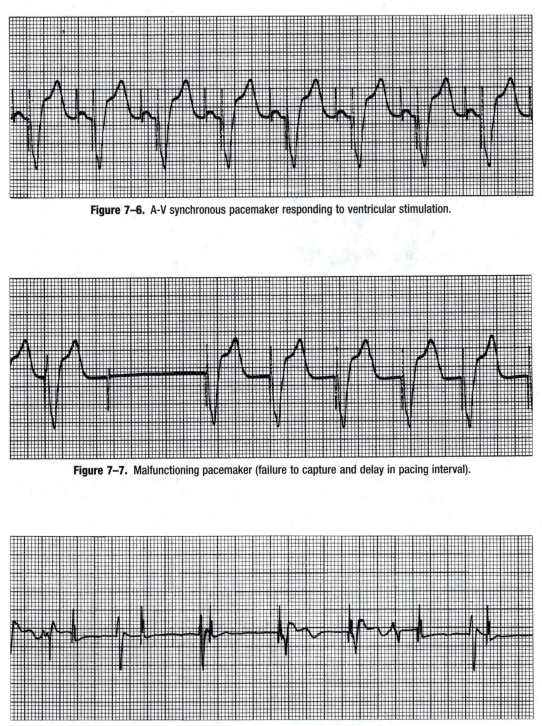

Figure 7–6. A-V synchronous pacemaker responding to ventricular stimulation.

Figure 7–7. Malfunctioning pacemaker (failure to capture and delay in pacing interval).

Figure 7–8. Malfunctioning pacemaker (failure to sense).

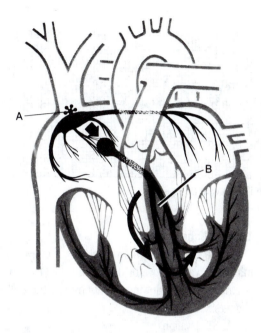

A

B

Figure 7–9. Bundle branch block. **A.** Impulse is initiated normally and spreads through atrium normally. **B.** When impulse reaches bundle branch, it finds one or more branches blocked and takes an alternate route to spread through the ventricles, resulting in a wide QRS.

patient's own heart rhythm. Underlying dysrhythmia will depend on the ability of the patient's own conduction system to function.

    2. Common etiology

        a. Displacement of electrode or pacemaker catheter tip

        b. Low or dead battery

        c. "Runaway" pacemaker (sensing capability fails)

        d. Perforation of atrial or ventricular wall by catheter tip

        e. Broken electrode wire

    3. Clinical signs and symptoms

        a. Depend on patient's underlying rhythm (ability of own conduction system to function)

        b. If ventricular rate extremely slow, may develop decreased cardiac output

        c. If "runaway" pacemaker or competition, may develop ventricular tachycardia or ventricular fibrillation, and/or exhibit palpitations and dyspnea

III. Bundle Branch Block (BBB)

    A. ECG features

        1. *PP interval:* depends upon underlying rhythm

        2. *RR interval:* depends upon underlying rhythm

        3. *PP rate:* depends upon underlying rhythm

        4. *RR rate:* depends upon underlying rhythm

        5. *P wave:* depends upon underlying rhythm

        6. *PRI:* depends upon underlying rhythm

        7. *QRS interval:* 0.12 second or greater (Figs. 7–9, 7–10, and 7–11)

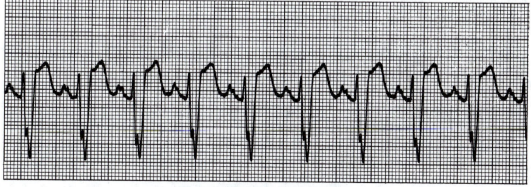

Figure 7–10. Sinus rhythm with BBB.

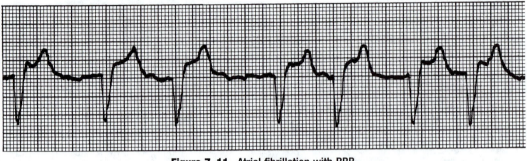

Figure 7–11. Atrial fibrillation with BBB.

*Notes: May be present in any dysrhythmia. RSR′ (notched QRS) may be present in Lead II. In Lead II, if a wide QRS complex is preceded by a P wave, BBB is probably present rather than a ventricular dysrhythmia. To determine right from left BBB, more advanced training in 12-lead ECG interpretation is necessary.

   B. Common etiology
      1. Damage to bundle branch
      2. Usually results from a MI
      3. Fibrotic scarring of the bundle
   C. Clinical signs and symptoms
      1. Usually none
      2. If all three bundle branches become blocked, may result in complete heart block or ventricular standstill

IV. ST Changes

The ST segment is normally isoelectric; however, it may be elevated above or depressed below the isoelectric line. The following conditions may cause ST changes:

   A. ST elevation
      1. MI
      2. Pericarditis
      3. Pericardial tamponade
      4. Cardiac contusion
      5. Ventricular aneurysm (Fig. 7–12)
   B. ST depression
      1. Myocardial ischemia
      2. Tachycardia
      3. Normal effect from digitalis preparations (Fig. 7–13)

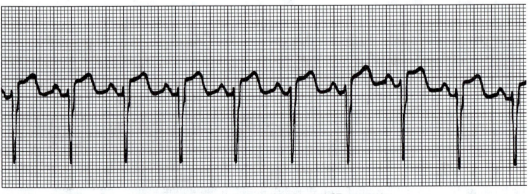

Figure 7–12. Sinus rhythm with elevated ST segments.

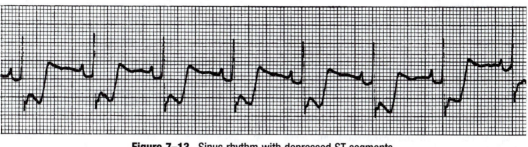

Figure 7-13. Sinus rhythm with depressed ST segments.

V. Pathologic Q Waves

A. Indicative of myocardial death

B. Q wave is one third the height of the QRS complex

C. Q wave is greater than 0.03 second wide

D. Infarction locations are determined by the presence of Q wave

    1. Anterior: Q waves in V1 through V4, I and AVL

    2. Posterior: large R wave in V1 and V2

    3. Inferior: Q wave in II, III, and AV F

    4. Lateral: Q wave in V5 through V6, I and AVL

    5. May have any combination of these; for example, anterolateral MI: Q wave in V1 through V6 and I and AVL

VI. Evolutionary Changes of an MI

ST changes and Q waves are commonly seen in varying stages during the evolutionary process of an MI.

A. ST depression may preceed an MI as well as hyperacute T waves

B. ST depression evolves into ST elevation, and Q waves begin to develop

C. Over a period of hours to days, the T waves will evolve from hyperacute to flattened to inverted

D. Once the evolution is completed, the ST and T waves will return to normal, but the Q wave will deepen and remain permanent (Fig. 7-14)

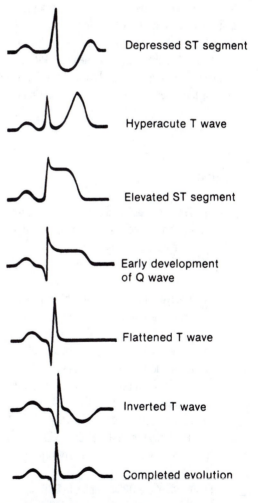

Depressed ST segment

Hyperacute T wave

Elevated ST segment

Early development of Q wave

Flattened T wave

Inverted T wave

Completed evolution

Figure 7-14. Evolutionary changes of an MI. Any of these configurations may indicate the presence of an MI.

SELF-EVALUATION

Directions

Answer keys for the Self-Evaluation section begin on page 341.

1. **Matching.** Place the letter of the appropriate item(s) before each numbered statement. Some answers are used more than once, and not all answers will be used.
2. **ECG practice strips.** For simplicity and practicality, all rates have been calculated by using Method 3 (Fig. 1–14) unless otherwise indicated. Keep in mind that your measurements for PRIs and QRS complexes may vary slightly and still be correct. Use the systematic approach shown in Chapter 1 to interpret the ECG strips. It is important that you follow all steps and not take shortcuts.

For the following ECG strips:
1. Determine if the PPI and RRI are regular or irregular.
2. Calculate rates using the appropriate method:
   a. PPR
   b. RRR
3. Measure:
   a. PRI
   b. QRS
4. Interpretation

Place your answers in the space provided.

Note that all strips are Lead II and are 6 seconds long unless otherwise indicated.

MATCHING

_____ 1. The characteristic feature of a pacemaker rhythm	a. Lead II
_____ 2. Areas of the heart where an implanted pacemaker can generate an impulse	b. malfunctioning pacemaker rhythm
_____ 3. The width of the QRS complex in a ventricular pacemaker rhythm	c. ventricular fibrillation
_____ 4. The type of pacemaker in which spikes/blips may be seen before the P wave and the QRS complex	d. spike/blip
_____ 5. Pacemaker spikes/blips without QRS complexes	e. atrium
_____ 6. A displaced pacemaker catheter result	f. ventricle
_____ 7. A low pacemaker battery result	g. sensing
_____ 8. Result of competition between a pacemaker and the patient's own conduction system	h. ventricular pacemaker
_____ 9. Electrical stimulation by a pacemaker followed by electrical depolarization of the cardiac cells	i. 0.12 second or greater
_____ 10. A pacemaker's ability to fire only if a patient's own heart rate does not exceed a preset rate	j. less than (<) 0.12 second
_____ 11. Width of the QRS complex in BBB	k. complete A-V block
_____ 12. A dysrhythmia that can occur if all three bundle branches are blocked	l. first degree A-V block
	m. asystole
	n. capturing
	o. A-V synchronous pacemaker

_____ 13. ECG change that may indicate pericarditis

_____ 14. ECG change that may indicate myocardial ischemia

_____ 15. ECG change that indicates myocardial death

_____ 16. Seen on the ECG of a patient who takes digitalis

_____ 17. Appearance the QRS complex may have in a BBB

_____ 18. ECG change that might indicate a ventricular aneurysm

_____ 19. Width of pathologic Q wave

_____ 20. ECG change that may indicate cardiac contusion

_____ 21. Shape of T wave that may be an early indication of an MI

a. flattened T wave

b. > 0.03 second

c. ST elevation

d. normal

e. notched

f. pathologic Q waves

g. ST depression

h. S wave

i. 0.12 second or greater

j. hyperacute T wave

ECG PRACTICE STRIPS

Figure 7–15. PPI _____ RRI _____ PPR _____ RRR _____ PRI _____ QRS _____

INTERPRETATION _____

Figure 7–16. PPI _____ RRI _____ PPR _____ RRR _____ PRI _____ QRS _____

INTERPRETATION _____

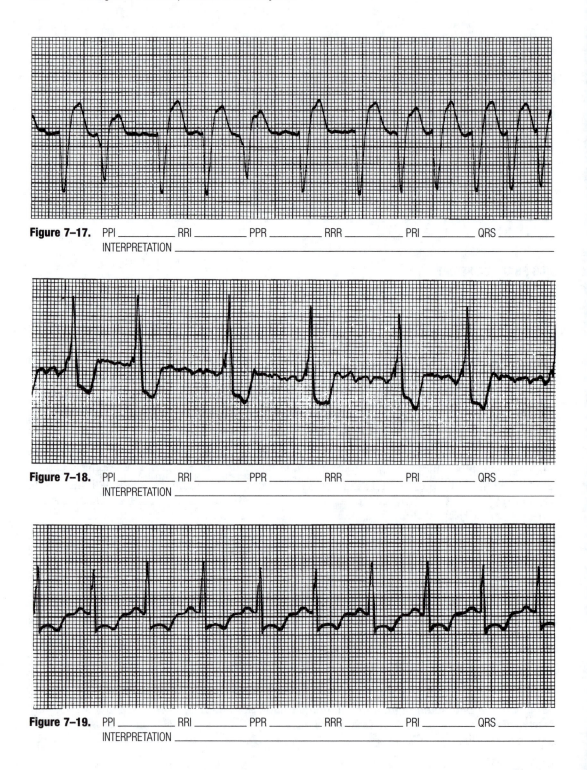

Figure 7–17.   PPI _____ RRI _____ PPR _____ RRR _____ PRI _____ QRS _____
INTERPRETATION _____

Figure 7–18.   PPI _____ RRI _____ PPR _____ RRR _____ PRI _____ QRS _____
INTERPRETATION _____

Figure 7–19.   PPI _____ RRI _____ PPR _____ RRR _____ PRI _____ QRS _____
INTERPRETATION _____

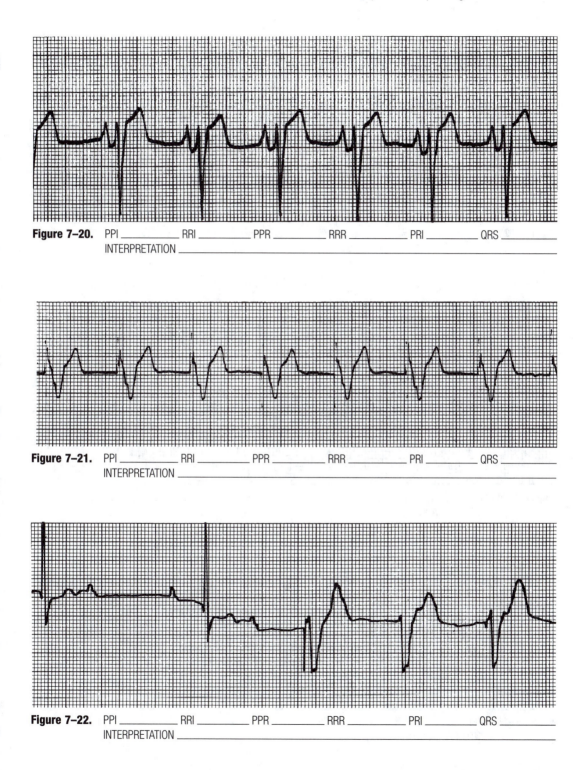

Figure 7–20.   PPI _____ RRI _____ PPR _____ RRR _____ PRI _____ QRS _____
                    INTERPRETATION _____

Figure 7–21.   PPI _____ RRI _____ PPR _____ RRR _____ PRI _____ QRS _____
                    INTERPRETATION _____

Figure 7–22.   PPI _____ RRI _____ PPR _____ RRR _____ PRI _____ QRS _____
                    INTERPRETATION _____

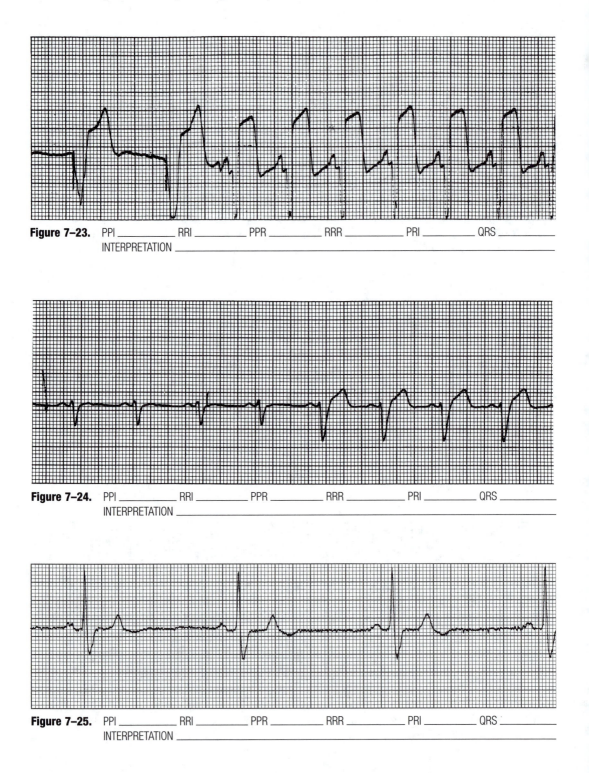

Figure 7–23.   PPI _____ RRI _____ PPR _____ RRR _____ PRI _____ QRS _____
INTERPRETATION _____

Figure 7–24.   PPI _____ RRI _____ PPR _____ RRR _____ PRI _____ QRS _____
INTERPRETATION _____

Figure 7–25.   PPI _____ RRI _____ PPR _____ RRR _____ PRI _____ QRS _____
INTERPRETATION _____

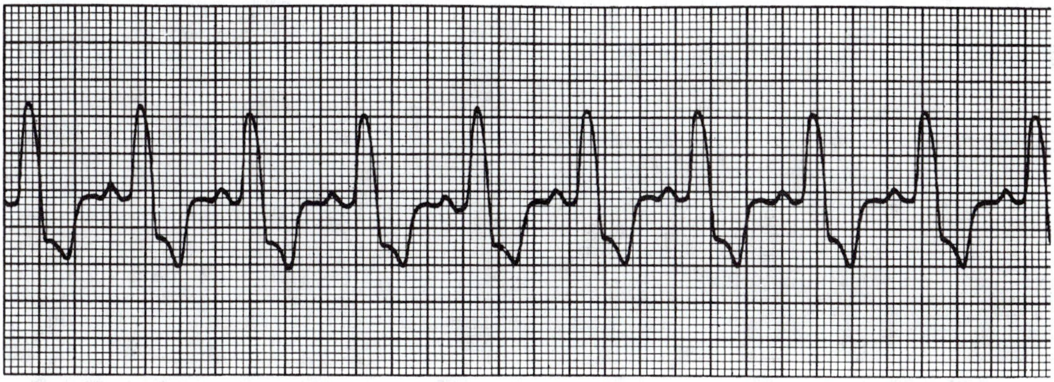

Figure 7–26. PPI ________ RRI ________ PPR ________ RRR ________ PRI ________ QRS ________
INTERPRETATION ____

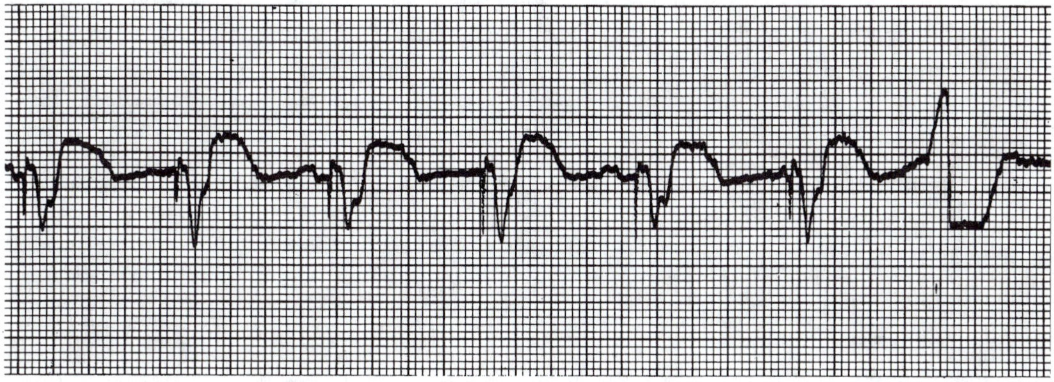

Figure 7–27. PPI ________ RRI ________ PPR ________ RRR ________ PRI ________ QRS ________
INTERPRETATION ____

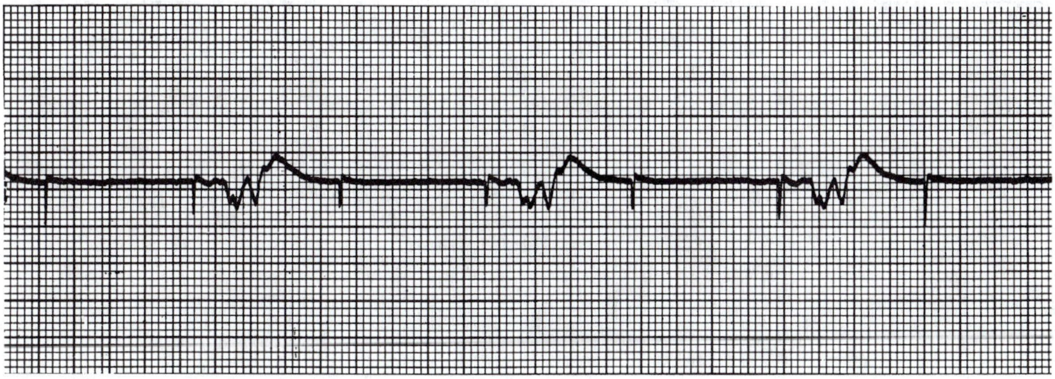

Figure 7–28. PPI ________ RRI ________ PPR ________ RRR ________ PRI ________ QRS ________
INTERPRETATION ____

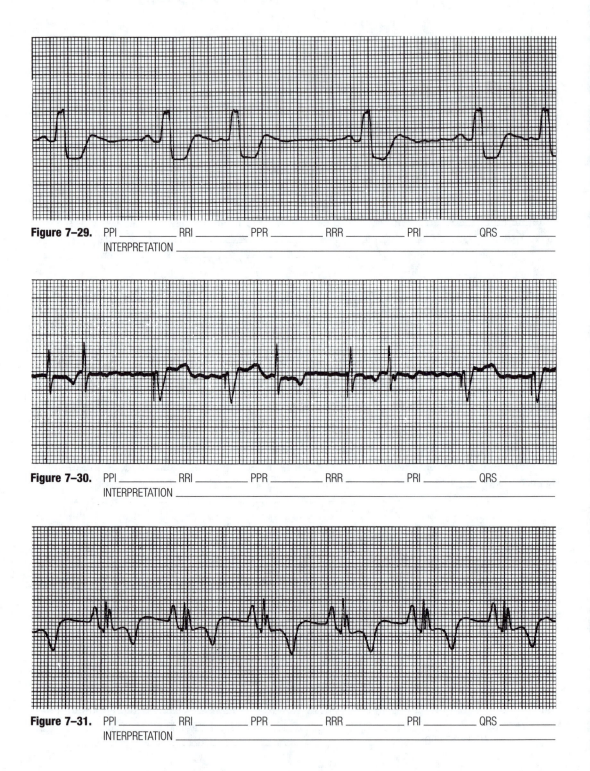

Figure 7–29. PPI _____ RRI _____ PPR _____ RRR _____ PRI _____ QRS _____
INTERPRETATION _____

Figure 7–30. PPI _____ RRI _____ PPR _____ RRR _____ PRI _____ QRS _____
INTERPRETATION _____

Figure 7–31. PPI _____ RRI _____ PPR _____ RRR _____ PRI _____ QRS _____
INTERPRETATION _____

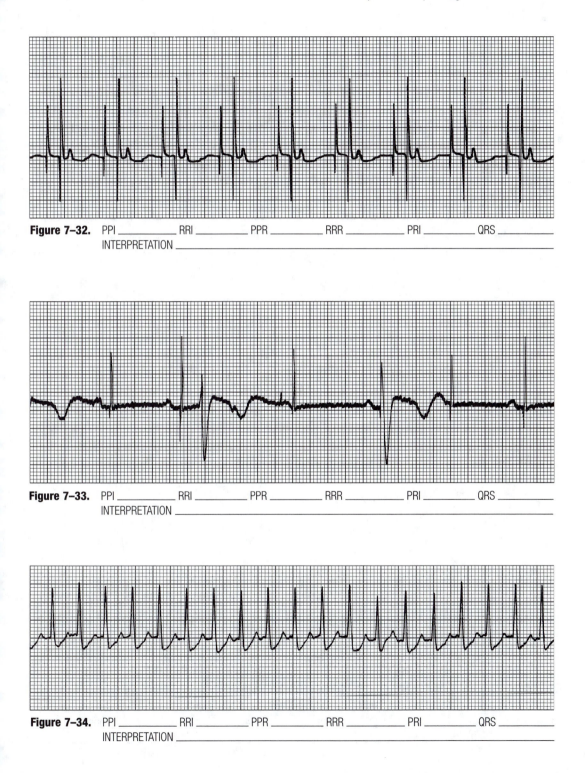

Figure 7–32. PPI _____ RRI _____ PPR _____ RRR _____ PRI _____ QRS _____

INTERPRETATION _____

Figure 7–33. PPI _____ RRI _____ PPR _____ RRR _____ PRI _____ QRS _____

INTERPRETATION _____

Figure 7–34. PPI _____ RRI _____ PPR _____ RRR _____ PRI _____ QRS _____

INTERPRETATION _____

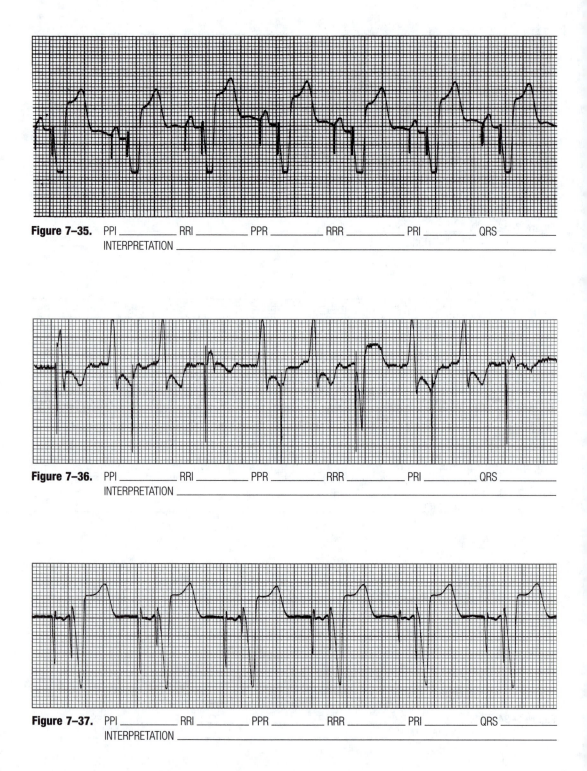

Figure 7–35. PPI _____ RRI _____ PPR _____ RRR _____ PRI _____ QRS _____
INTERPRETATION _____

Figure 7–36. PPI _____ RRI _____ PPR _____ RRR _____ PRI _____ QRS _____
INTERPRETATION _____

Figure 7–37. PPI _____ RRI _____ PPR _____ RRR _____ PRI _____ QRS _____
INTERPRETATION _____

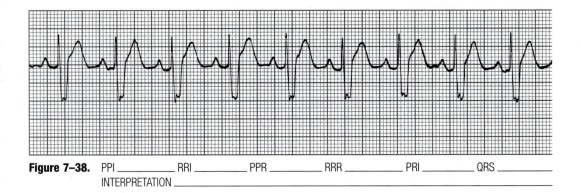

Figure 7–38. PPI _____ RRI _____ PPR _____ RRR _____ PRI _____ QRS _____
INTERPRETATION _____

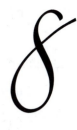

General Review of Dysrhythmias

Chapter 8 is a two-part review of all the dysrhythmias, offering you an opportunity to apply the information learned in the previous chapters.

DIRECTIONS

Answer keys for the Self-Evaluation section begin on page 349.

1. **Review 1.** For simplicity and practicality, all rates have been calculated by using Method 3 (Fig. 1–14) unless otherwise indicated. Keep in mind that your measurements for PRIs and QRS complexes may vary slightly and still be correct. Use the systematic approach shown in Chapter 1 to interpret the ECG strips. It is important that you follow all steps and not take shortcuts.

1. Determine if the PPI and RRI are regular.
2. Calculate rates using the appropriate method:

a. PPR
b. RRR
3. Measure:
a. PRI
b. QRS
4. Interpretation

Place your answer in the space provided.
Note that all strips are Lead II and are 6 seconds long unless otherwise indicated.

2. **Review 2.** At this point you should have become proficient at measuring PRIs and QRSs and at calculating heart rates. Therefore, the ECG strips for Review 2 include space for the interpretation only. However, this does not mean that you should eliminate the other steps in your approach to interpretation.

*Note that all strips are Lead II and are 6 seconds long unless otherwise indicated.

ECG PRACTICE STRIPS—REVIEW 1

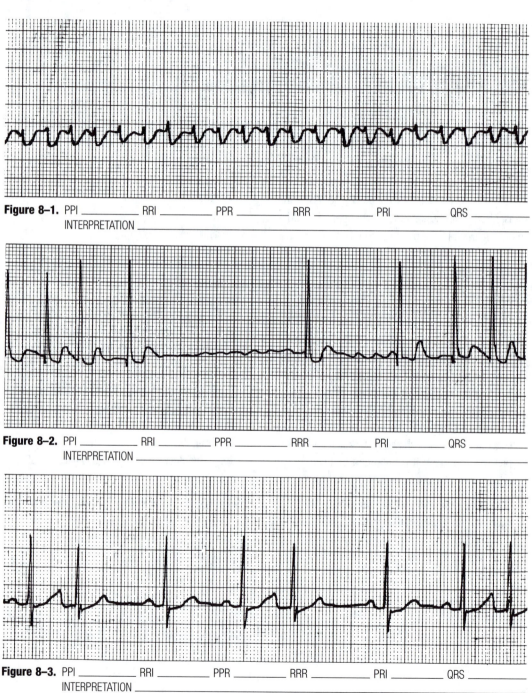

Figure 8–1. PPI _____ RRI _____ PPR _____ RRR _____ PRI _____ QRS _____
INTERPRETATION _____

Figure 8–2. PPI _____ RRI _____ PPR _____ RRR _____ PRI _____ QRS _____
INTERPRETATION _____

Figure 8–3. PPI _____ RRI _____ PPR _____ RRR _____ PRI _____ QRS _____
INTERPRETATION _____

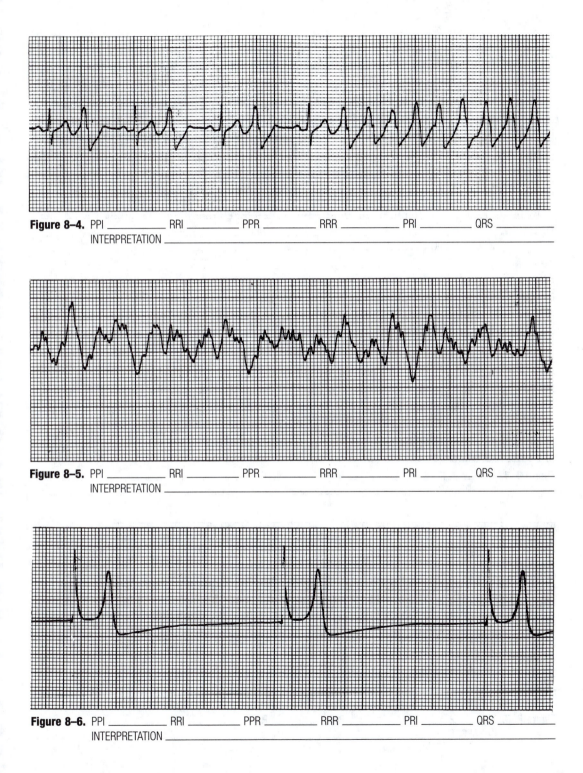

Figure 8–4. PPI _____ RRI _____ PPR _____ RRR _____ PRI _____ QRS _____
INTERPRETATION _____

Figure 8–5. PPI _____ RRI _____ PPR _____ RRR _____ PRI _____ QRS _____
INTERPRETATION _____

Figure 8–6. PPI _____ RRI _____ PPR _____ RRR _____ PRI _____ QRS _____
INTERPRETATION _____

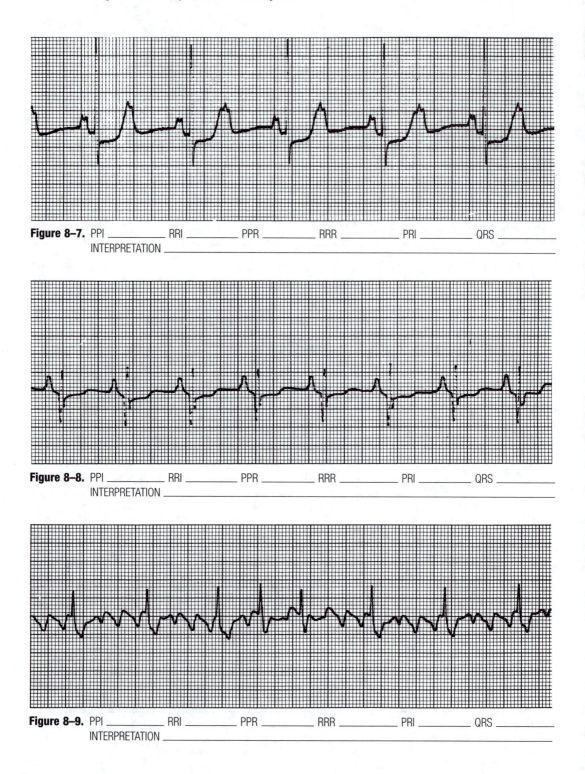

Figure 8–7. PPI _____ RRI _____ PPR _____ RRR _____ PRI _____ QRS _____
INTERPRETATION _____

Figure 8–8. PPI _____ RRI _____ PPR _____ RRR _____ PRI _____ QRS _____
INTERPRETATION _____

Figure 8–9. PPI _____ RRI _____ PPR _____ RRR _____ PRI _____ QRS _____
INTERPRETATION _____

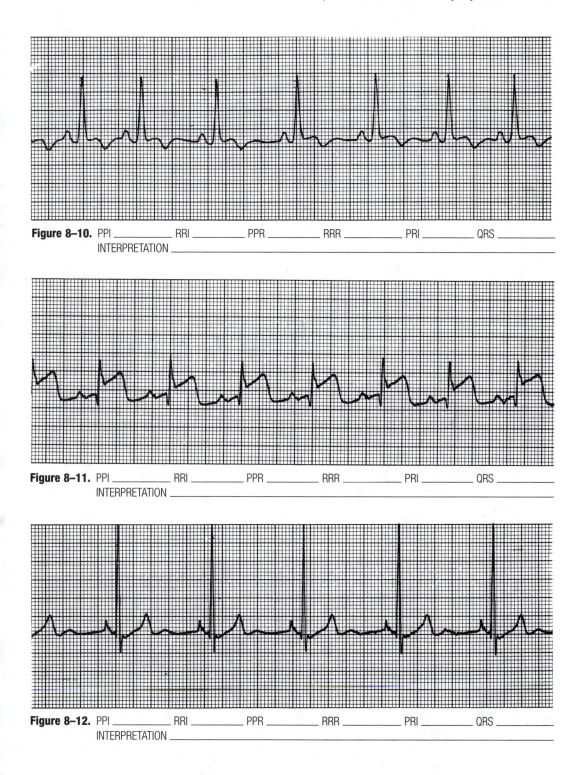

Figure 8–10. PPI _____ RRI _____ PPR _____ RRR _____ PRI _____ QRS _____
INTERPRETATION _____

Figure 8–11. PPI _____ RRI _____ PPR _____ RRR _____ PRI _____ QRS _____
INTERPRETATION _____

Figure 8–12. PPI _____ RRI _____ PPR _____ RRR _____ PRI _____ QRS _____
INTERPRETATION _____

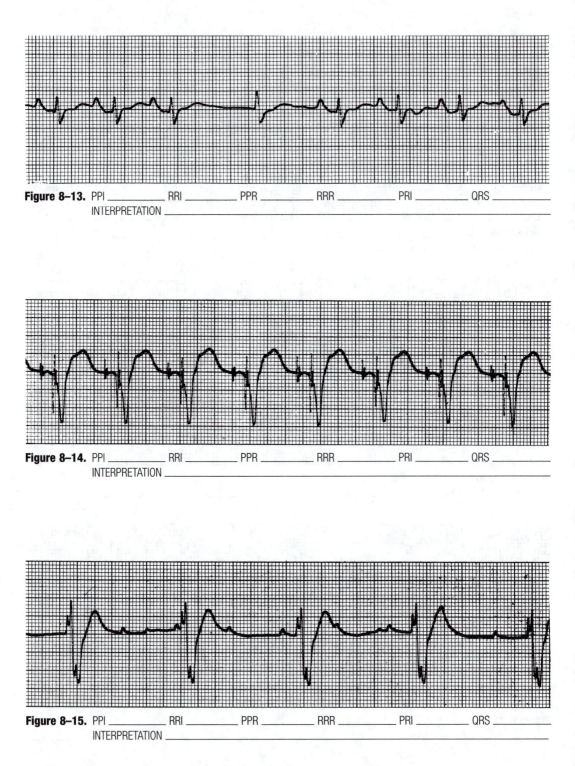

Figure 8–13. PPI _____ RRI _____ PPR _____ RRR _____ PRI _____ QRS _____
INTERPRETATION _____

Figure 8–14. PPI _____ RRI _____ PPR _____ RRR _____ PRI _____ QRS _____
INTERPRETATION _____

Figure 8–15. PPI _____ RRI _____ PPR _____ RRR _____ PRI _____ QRS _____
INTERPRETATION _____

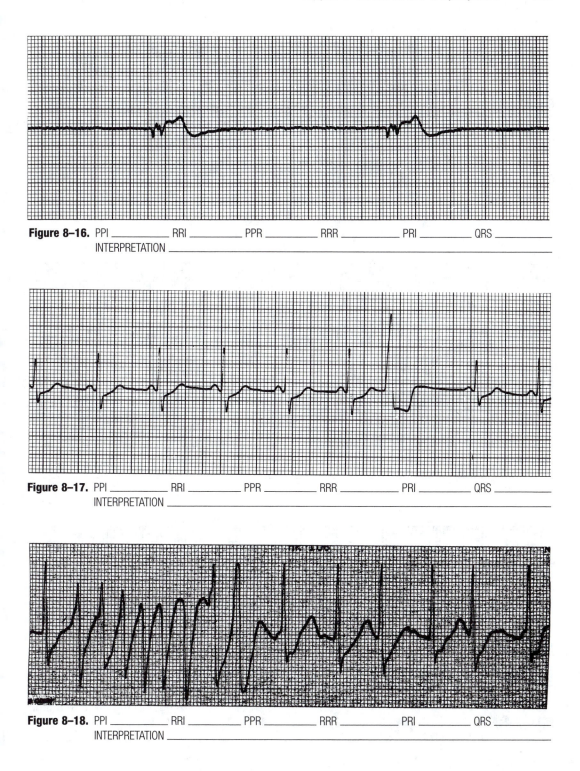

Figure 8–16. PPI _____ RRI _____ PPR _____ RRR _____ PRI _____ QRS _____
INTERPRETATION _____

Figure 8–17. PPI _____ RRI _____ PPR _____ RRR _____ PRI _____ QRS _____
INTERPRETATION _____

Figure 8–18. PPI _____ RRI _____ PPR _____ RRR _____ PRI _____ QRS _____
INTERPRETATION _____

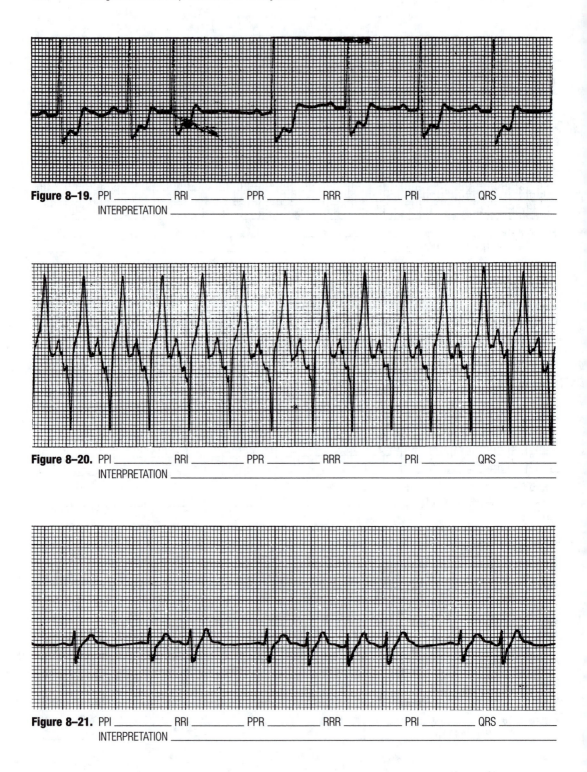

Figure 8–19. PPI _____ RRI _____ PPR _____ RRR _____ PRI _____ QRS _____
INTERPRETATION _____

Figure 8–20. PPI _____ RRI _____ PPR _____ RRR _____ PRI _____ QRS _____
INTERPRETATION _____

Figure 8–21. PPI _____ RRI _____ PPR _____ RRR _____ PRI _____ QRS _____
INTERPRETATION _____

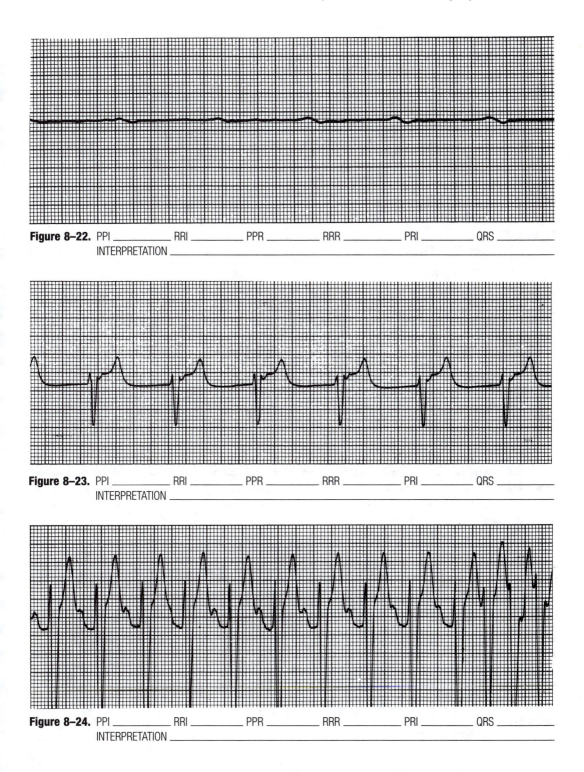

Figure 8–22. PPI _____ RRI _____ PPR _____ RRR _____ PRI _____ QRS _____
INTERPRETATION _____

Figure 8–23. PPI _____ RRI _____ PPR _____ RRR _____ PRI _____ QRS _____
INTERPRETATION _____

Figure 8–24. PPI _____ RRI _____ PPR _____ RRR _____ PRI _____ QRS _____
INTERPRETATION _____

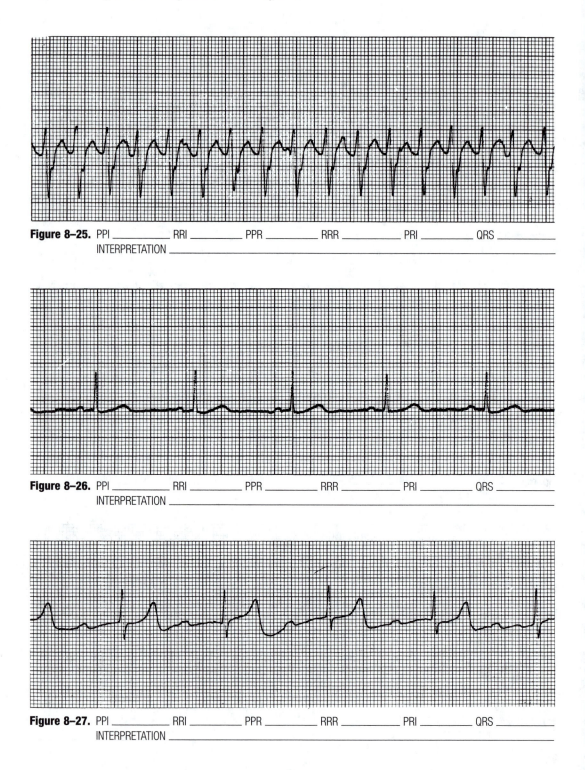

Figure 8–25. PPI _____ RRI _____ PPR _____ RRR _____ PRI _____ QRS _____
INTERPRETATION _____

Figure 8–26. PPI _____ RRI _____ PPR _____ RRR _____ PRI _____ QRS _____
INTERPRETATION _____

Figure 8–27. PPI _____ RRI _____ PPR _____ RRR _____ PRI _____ QRS _____
INTERPRETATION _____

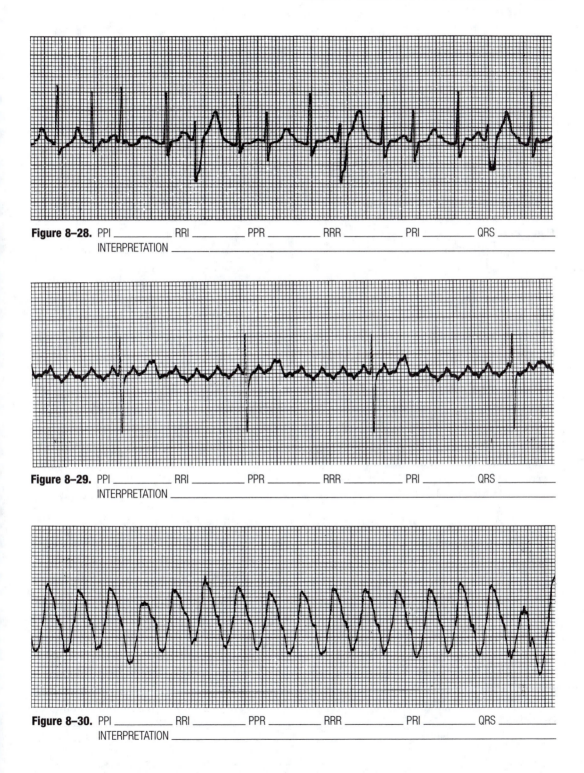

Figure 8–28. PPI _____ RRI _____ PPR _____ RRR _____ PRI _____ QRS _____
INTERPRETATION _____

Figure 8–29. PPI _____ RRI _____ PPR _____ RRR _____ PRI _____ QRS _____
INTERPRETATION _____

Figure 8–30. PPI _____ RRI _____ PPR _____ RRR _____ PRI _____ QRS _____
INTERPRETATION _____

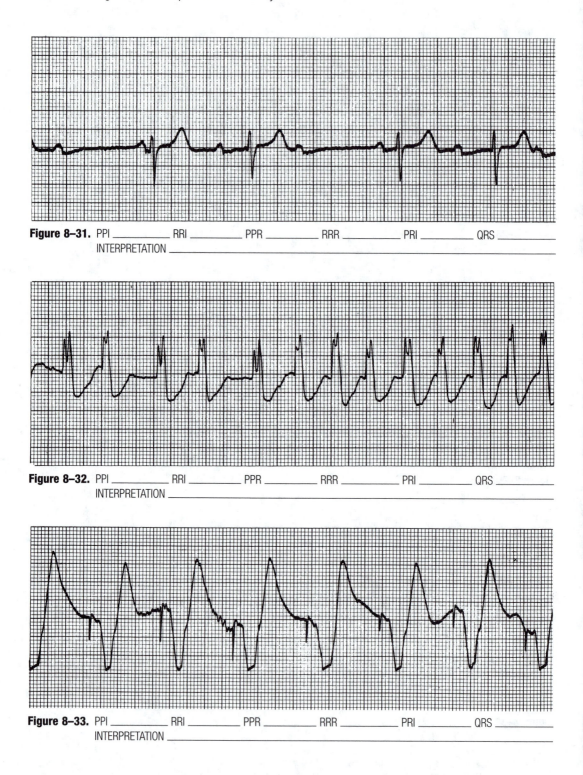

Figure 8–31. PPI _____ RRI _____ PPR _____ RRR _____ PRI _____ QRS _____
INTERPRETATION _____

Figure 8–32. PPI _____ RRI _____ PPR _____ RRR _____ PRI _____ QRS _____
INTERPRETATION _____

Figure 8–33. PPI _____ RRI _____ PPR _____ RRR _____ PRI _____ QRS _____
INTERPRETATION _____

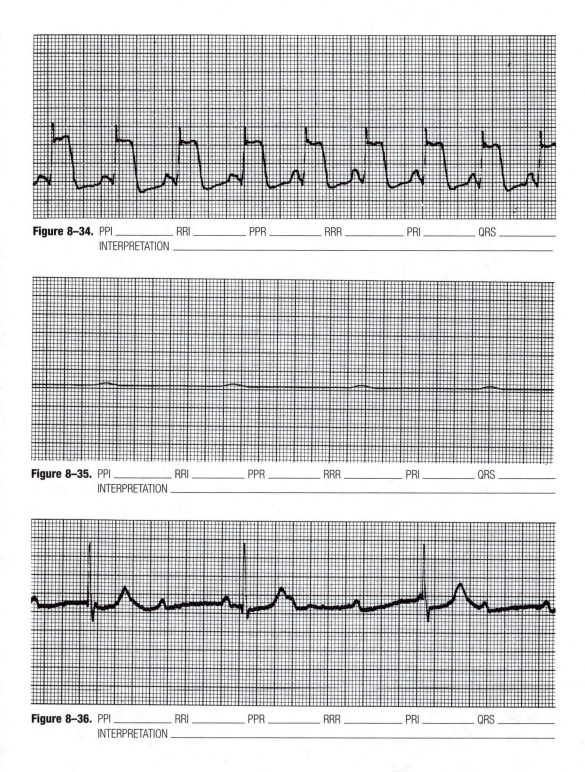

Figure 8–34. PPI _____ RRI _____ PPR _____ RRR _____ PRI _____ QRS _____
INTERPRETATION _____

Figure 8–35. PPI _____ RRI _____ PPR _____ RRR _____ PRI _____ QRS _____
INTERPRETATION _____

Figure 8–36. PPI _____ RRI _____ PPR _____ RRR _____ PRI _____ QRS _____
INTERPRETATION _____

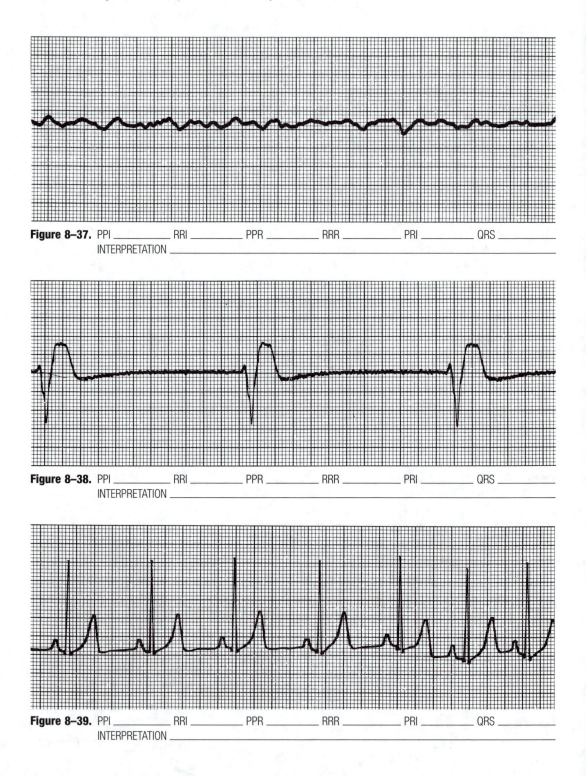

Figure 8–37. PPI _____ RRI _____ PPR _____ RRR _____ PRI _____ QRS _____
INTERPRETATION _____

Figure 8–38. PPI _____ RRI _____ PPR _____ RRR _____ PRI _____ QRS _____
INTERPRETATION _____

Figure 8–39. PPI _____ RRI _____ PPR _____ RRR _____ PRI _____ QRS _____
INTERPRETATION _____

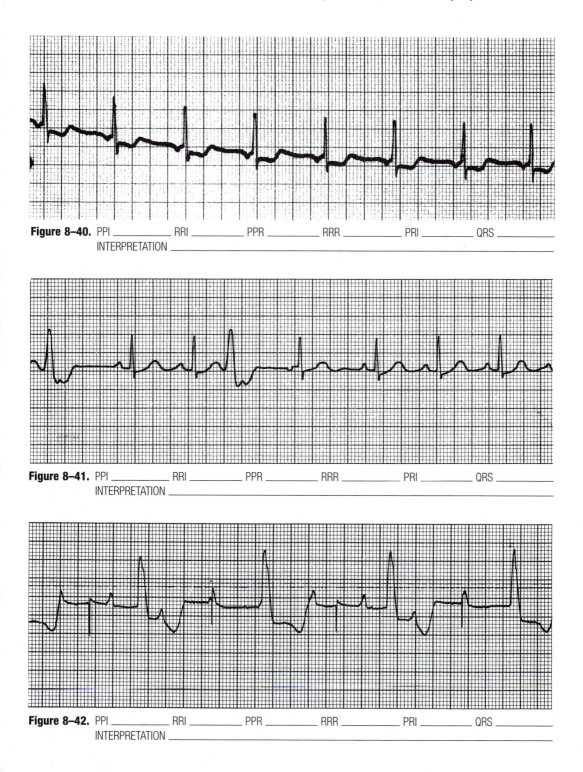

Figure 8–40. PPI _____ RRI _____ PPR _____ RRR _____ PRI _____ QRS _____
INTERPRETATION _____

Figure 8–41. PPI _____ RRI _____ PPR _____ RRR _____ PRI _____ QRS _____
INTERPRETATION _____

Figure 8–42. PPI _____ RRI _____ PPR _____ RRR _____ PRI _____ QRS _____
INTERPRETATION _____

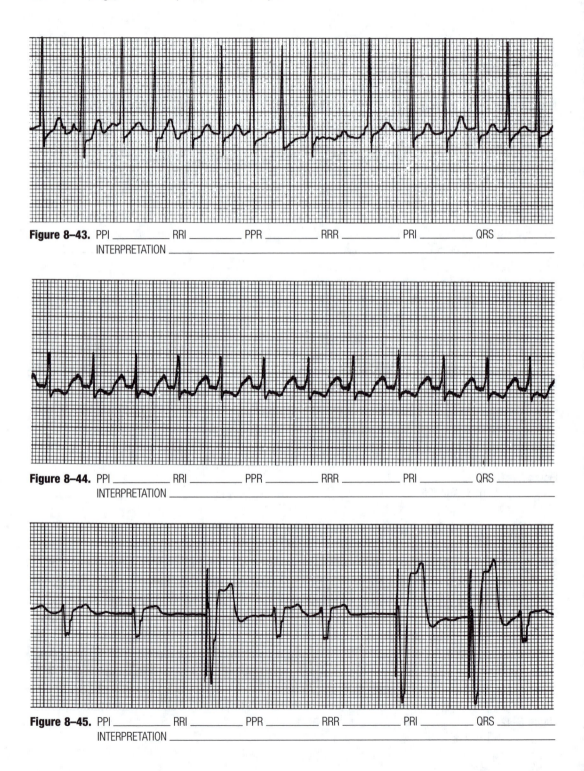

Figure 8–43. PPI _____ RRI _____ PPR _____ RRR _____ PRI _____ QRS _____
INTERPRETATION _____

Figure 8–44. PPI _____ RRI _____ PPR _____ RRR _____ PRI _____ QRS _____
INTERPRETATION _____

Figure 8–45. PPI _____ RRI _____ PPR _____ RRR _____ PRI _____ QRS _____
INTERPRETATION _____

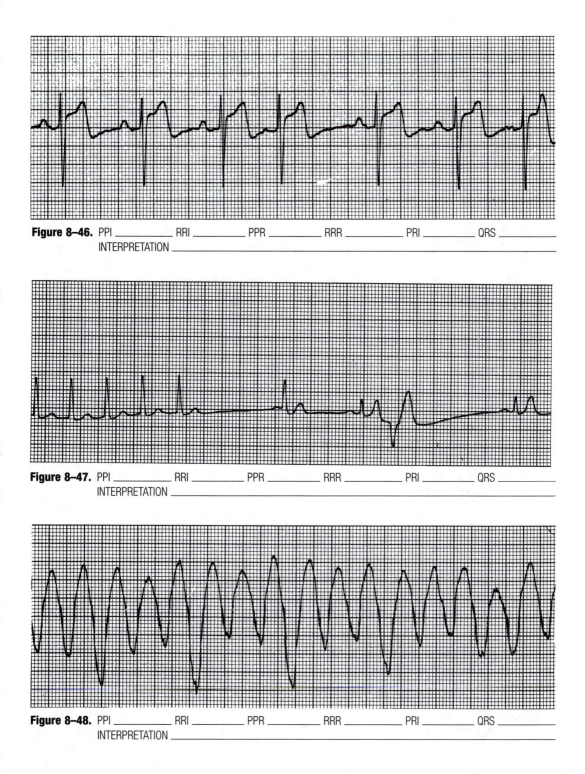

Figure 8–46. PPI _____ RRI _____ PPR _____ RRR _____ PRI _____ QRS _____
INTERPRETATION _____

Figure 8–47. PPI _____ RRI _____ PPR _____ RRR _____ PRI _____ QRS _____
INTERPRETATION _____

Figure 8–48. PPI _____ RRI _____ PPR _____ RRR _____ PRI _____ QRS _____
INTERPRETATION _____

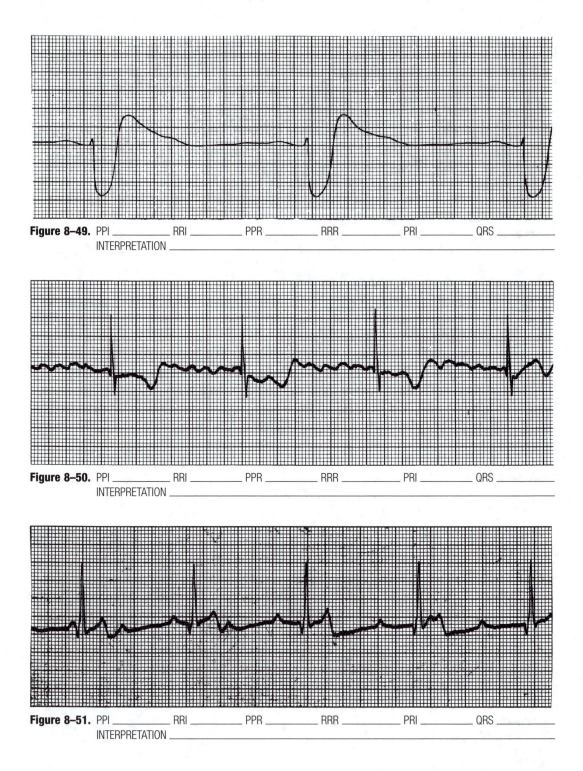

Figure 8–49. PPI _____ RRI _____ PPR _____ RRR _____ PRI _____ QRS _____
INTERPRETATION _____

Figure 8–50. PPI _____ RRI _____ PPR _____ RRR _____ PRI _____ QRS _____
INTERPRETATION _____

Figure 8–51. PPI _____ RRI _____ PPR _____ RRR _____ PRI _____ QRS _____
INTERPRETATION _____

ECG PRACTICE STRIPS—REVIEW 2

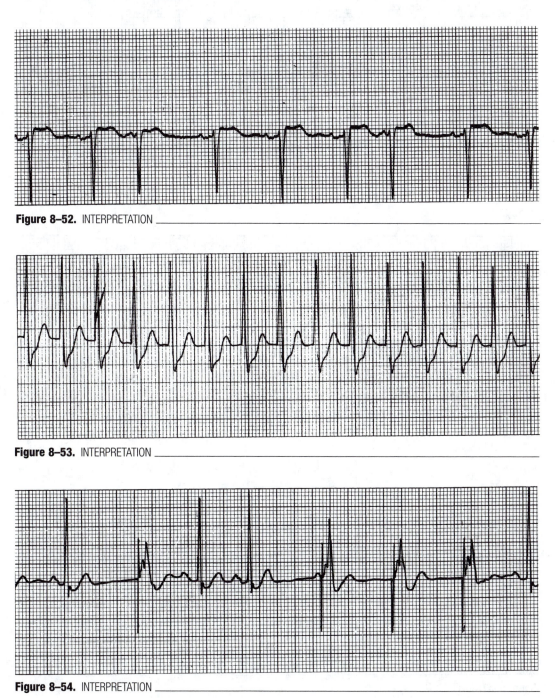

Figure 8–52. INTERPRETATION _____

Figure 8–53. INTERPRETATION _____

Figure 8–54. INTERPRETATION _____

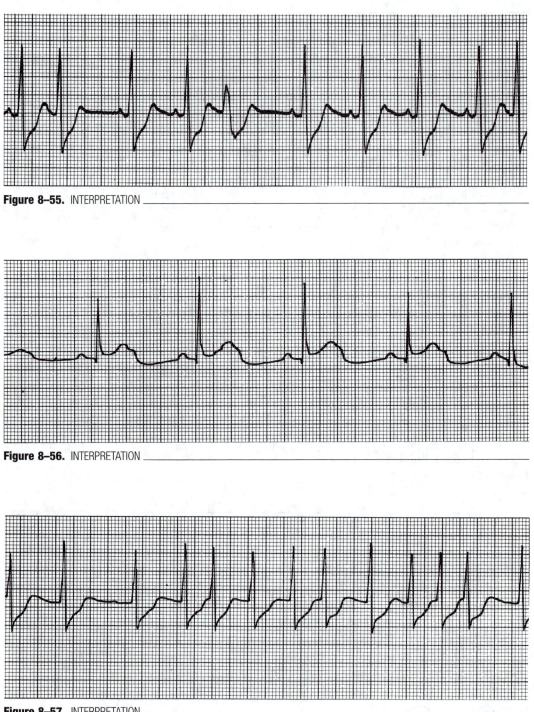

Figure 8–55. INTERPRETATION _____

Figure 8–56. INTERPRETATION _____

Figure 8–57. INTERPRETATION _____

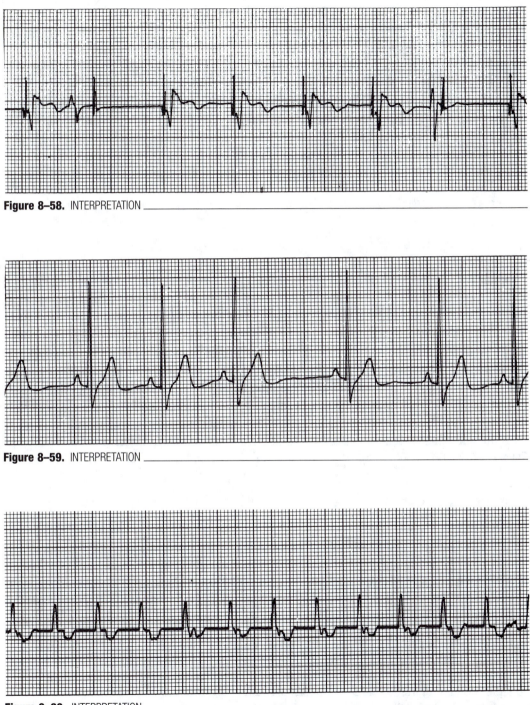

Figure 8–58. INTERPRETATION _____

Figure 8–59. INTERPRETATION _____

Figure 8–60. INTERPRETATION _____

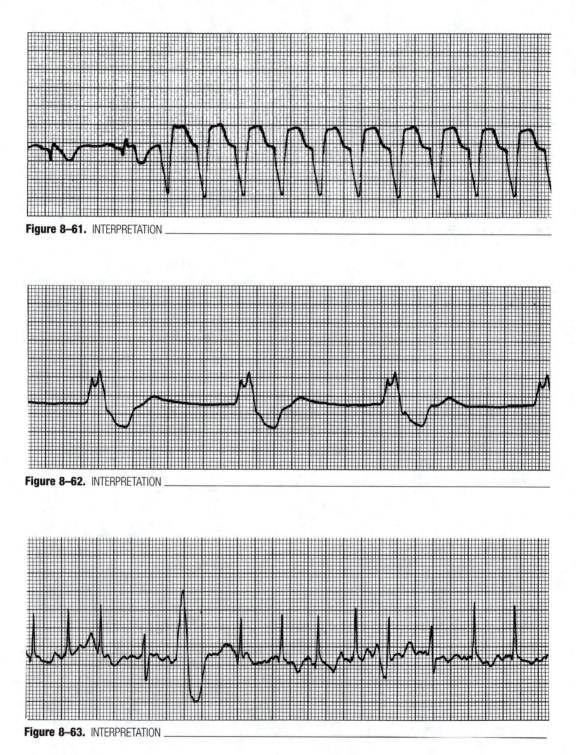

Figure 8–61. INTERPRETATION _____

Figure 8–62. INTERPRETATION _____

Figure 8–63. INTERPRETATION _____

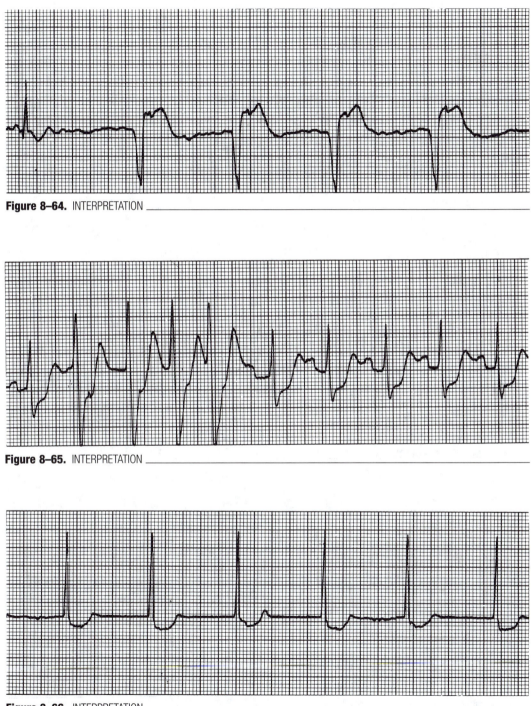

Figure 8–64. INTERPRETATION _____

Figure 8–65. INTERPRETATION _____

Figure 8–66. INTERPRETATION _____

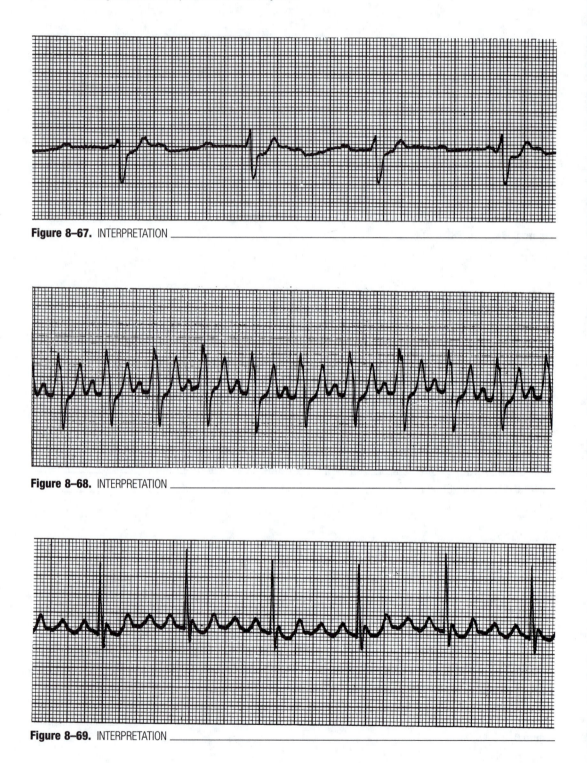

Figure 8–67. INTERPRETATION _____

Figure 8–68. INTERPRETATION _____

Figure 8–69. INTERPRETATION _____

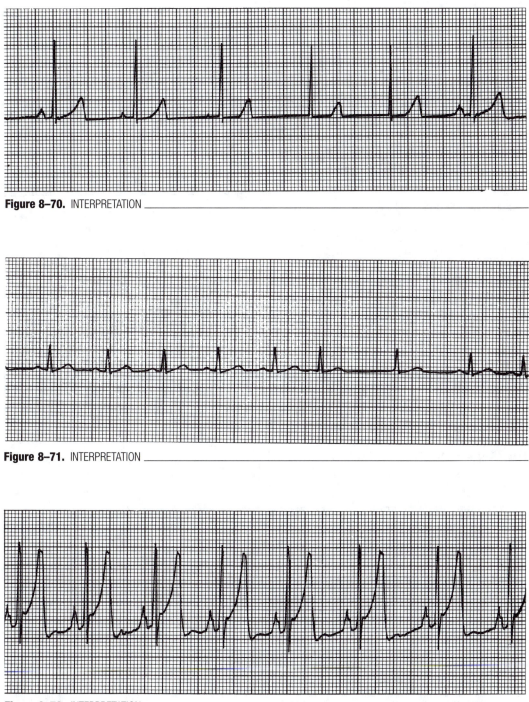

Figure 8–70. INTERPRETATION _____

Figure 8–71. INTERPRETATION _____

Figure 8–72. INTERPRETATION _____

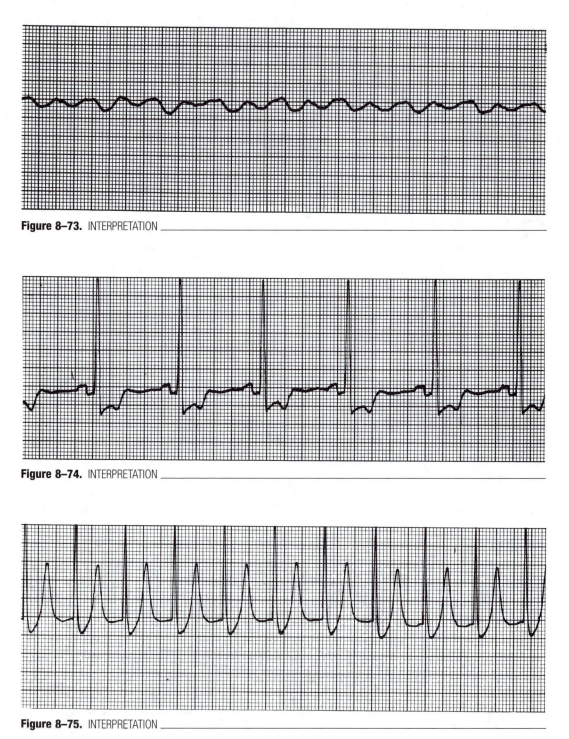

Figure 8–73. INTERPRETATION _____

Figure 8–74. INTERPRETATION _____

Figure 8–75. INTERPRETATION _____

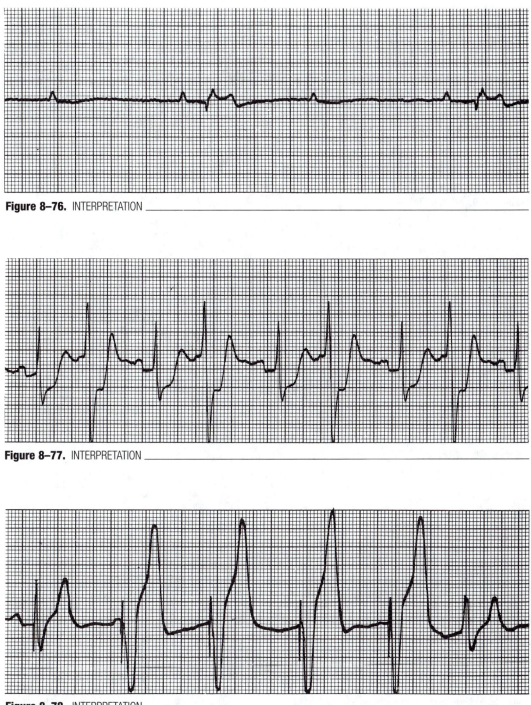

Figure 8–76. INTERPRETATION _____

Figure 8–77. INTERPRETATION _____

Figure 8–78. INTERPRETATION _____

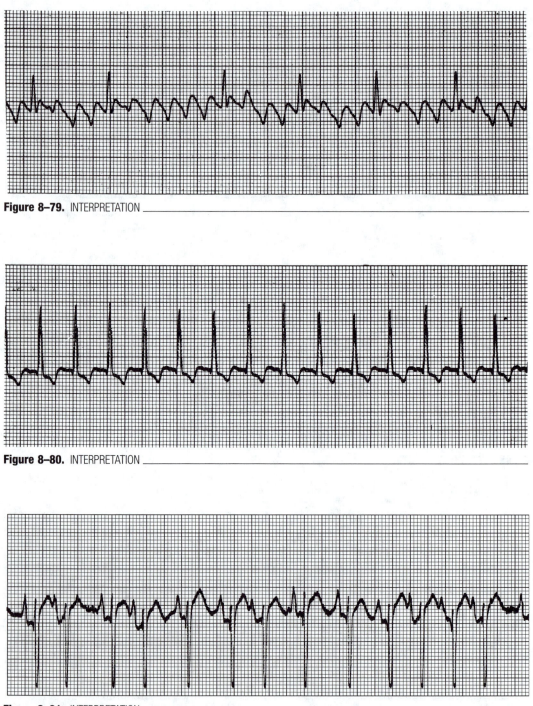

Figure 8–79. INTERPRETATION _____

Figure 8–80. INTERPRETATION _____

Figure 8–81. INTERPRETATION _____

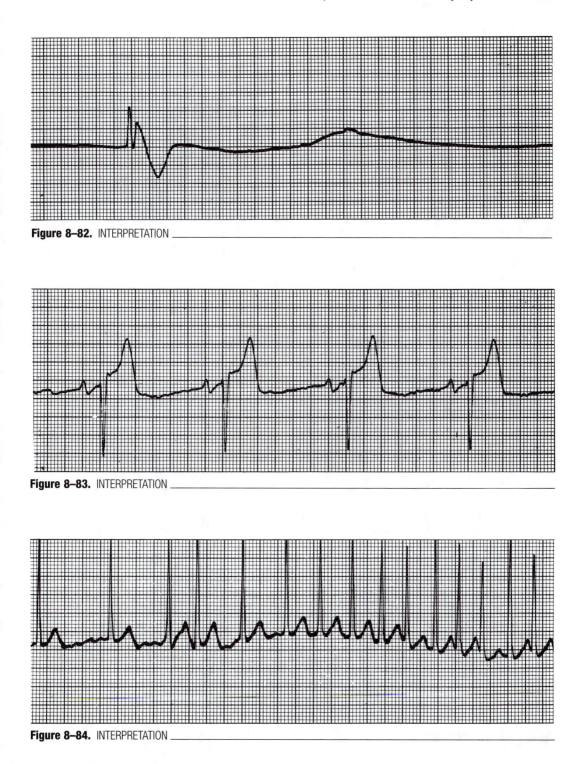

Figure 8–82. INTERPRETATION _____

Figure 8–83. INTERPRETATION _____

Figure 8–84. INTERPRETATION _____

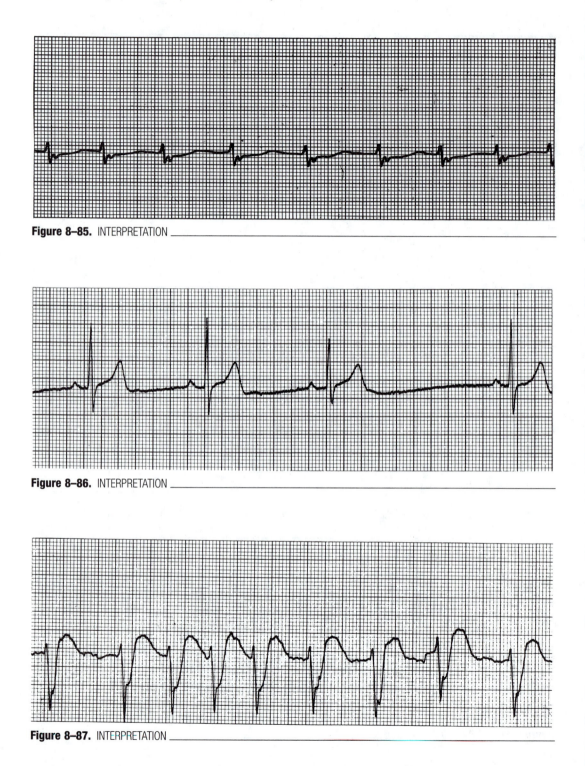

Figure 8–85. INTERPRETATION _____

Figure 8–86. INTERPRETATION _____

Figure 8–87. INTERPRETATION _____

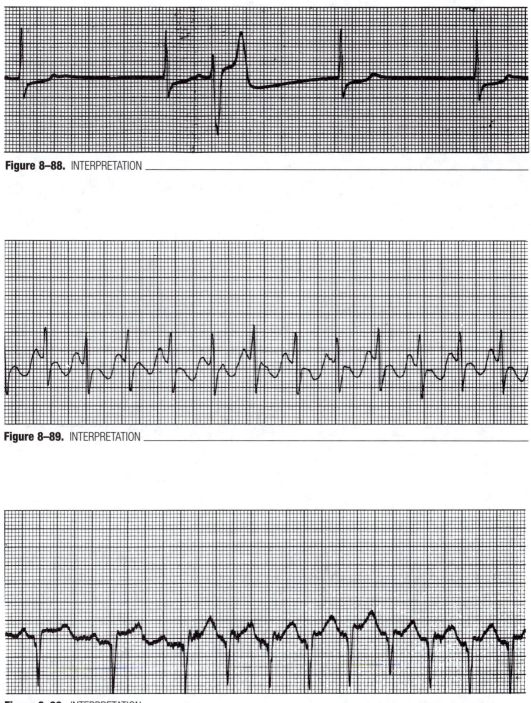

Figure 8–88. INTERPRETATION _____

Figure 8–89. INTERPRETATION _____

Figure 8–90. INTERPRETATION _____

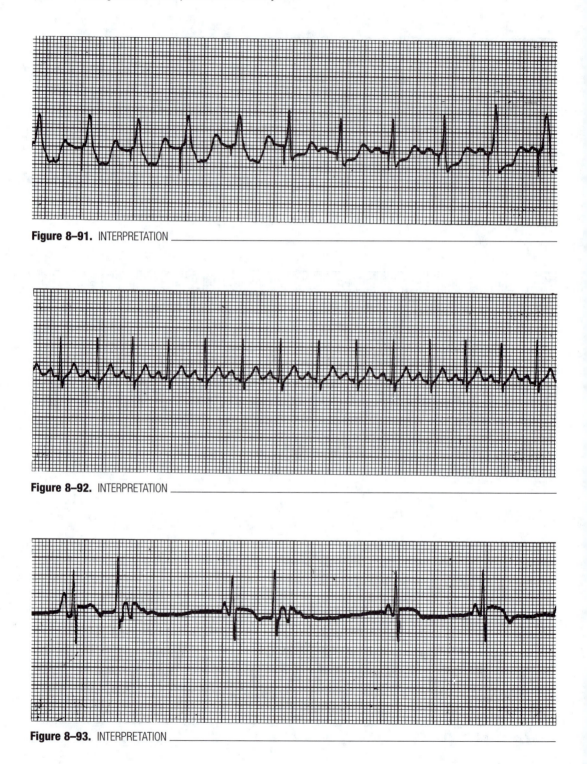

Figure 8–91. INTERPRETATION _____

Figure 8–92. INTERPRETATION _____

Figure 8–93. INTERPRETATION _____

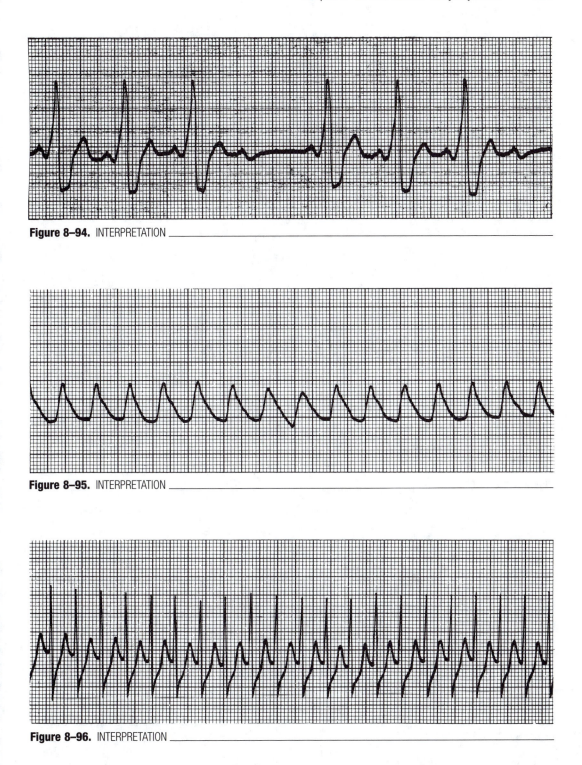

Figure 8–94. INTERPRETATION _____

Figure 8–95. INTERPRETATION _____

Figure 8–96. INTERPRETATION _____

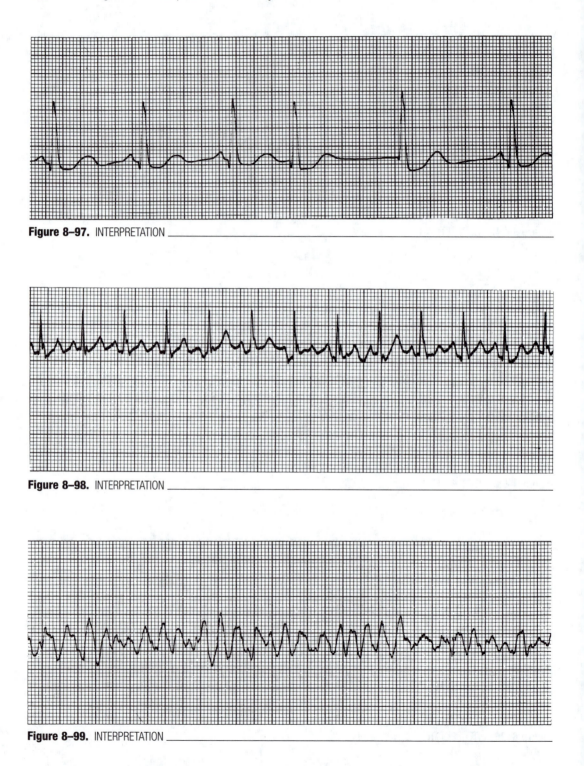

Figure 8–97. INTERPRETATION _____

Figure 8–98. INTERPRETATION _____

Figure 8–99. INTERPRETATION _____

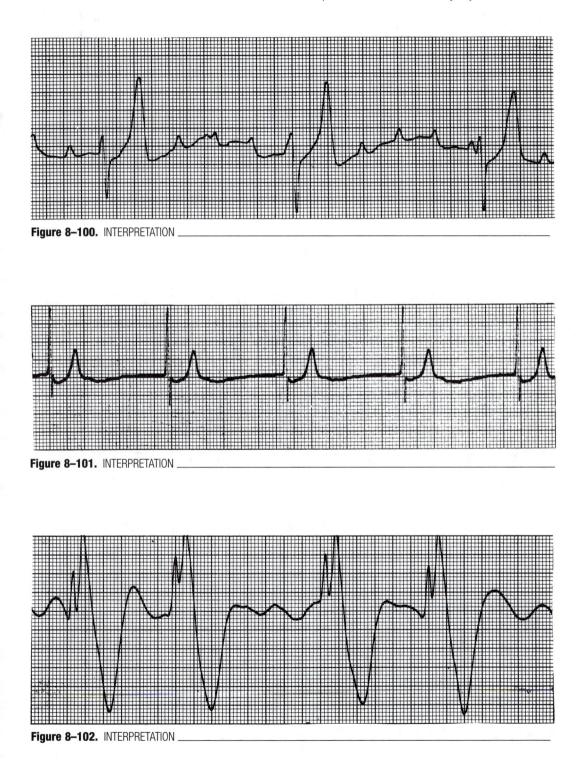

Figure 8–100. INTERPRETATION _____

Figure 8–101. INTERPRETATION _____

Figure 8–102. INTERPRETATION _____

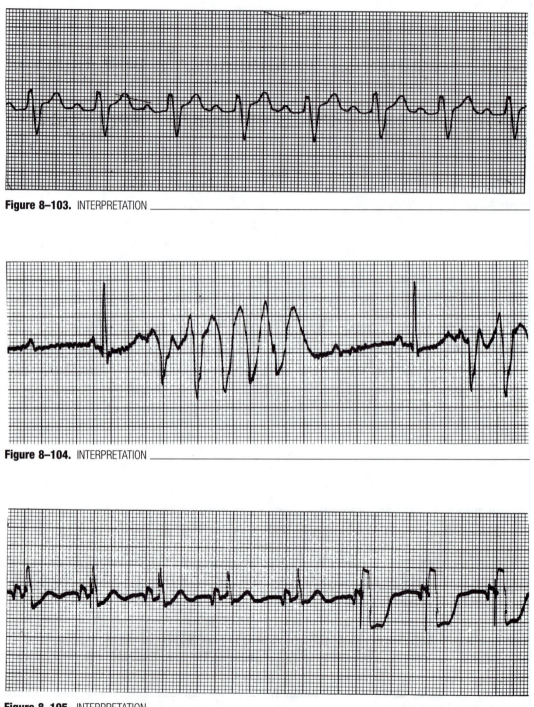

Figure 8–103. INTERPRETATION _____

Figure 8–104. INTERPRETATION _____

Figure 8–105. INTERPRETATION _____

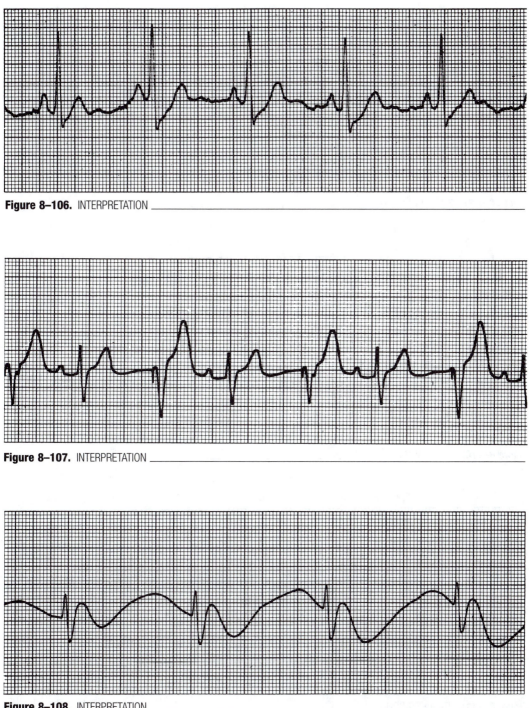

Figure 8–106. INTERPRETATION _____

Figure 8–107. INTERPRETATION _____

Figure 8–108. INTERPRETATION _____

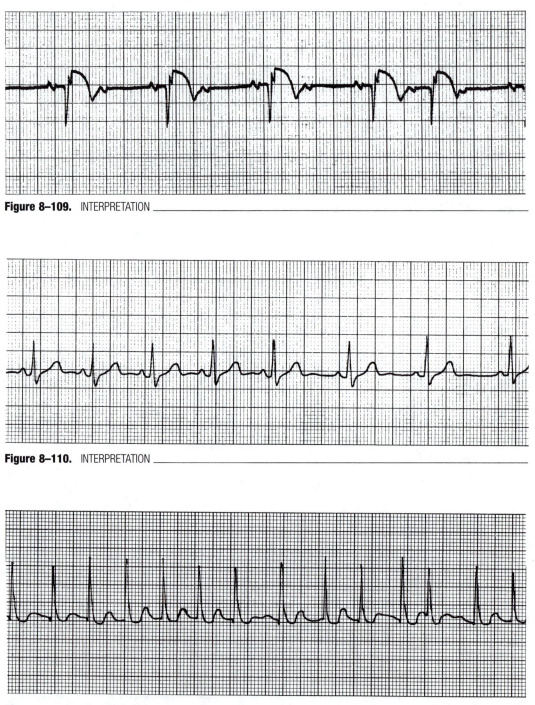

Figure 8–109. INTERPRETATION _____

Figure 8–110. INTERPRETATION _____

Figure 8–111. INTERPRETATION _____

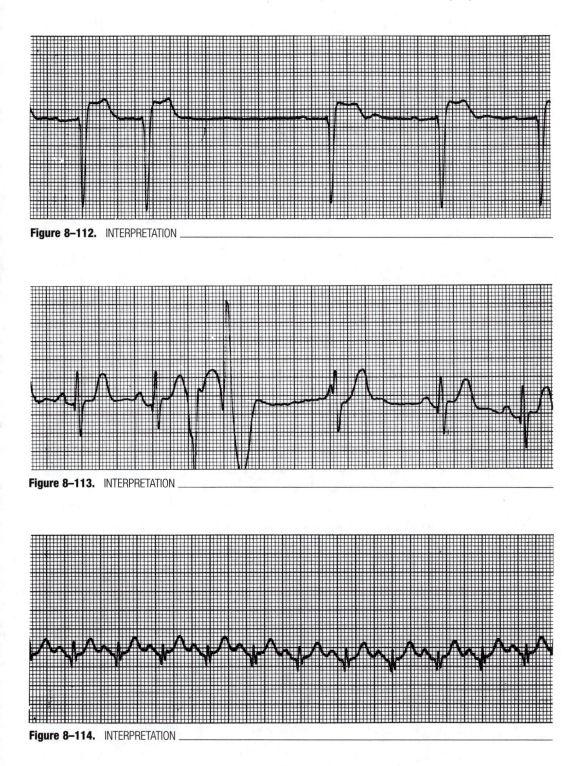

Figure 8–112. INTERPRETATION _____

Figure 8–113. INTERPRETATION _____

Figure 8–114. INTERPRETATION _____

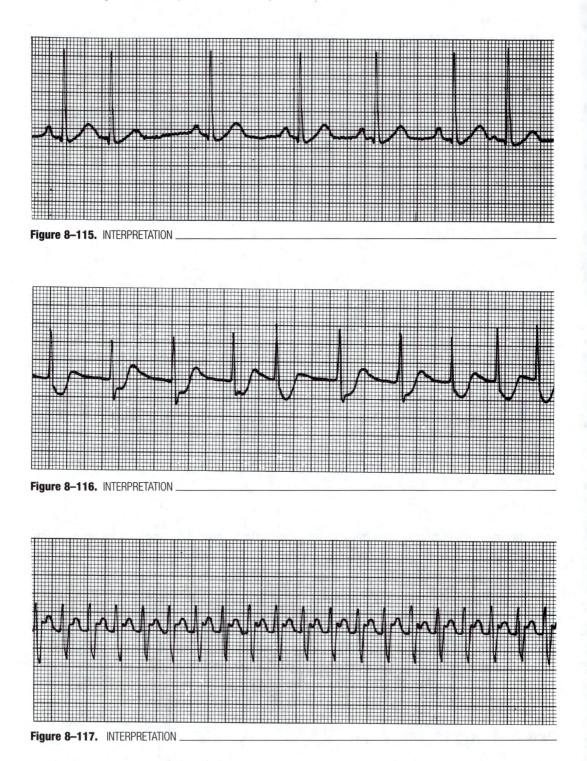

Figure 8–115. INTERPRETATION _____

Figure 8–116. INTERPRETATION _____

Figure 8–117. INTERPRETATION _____

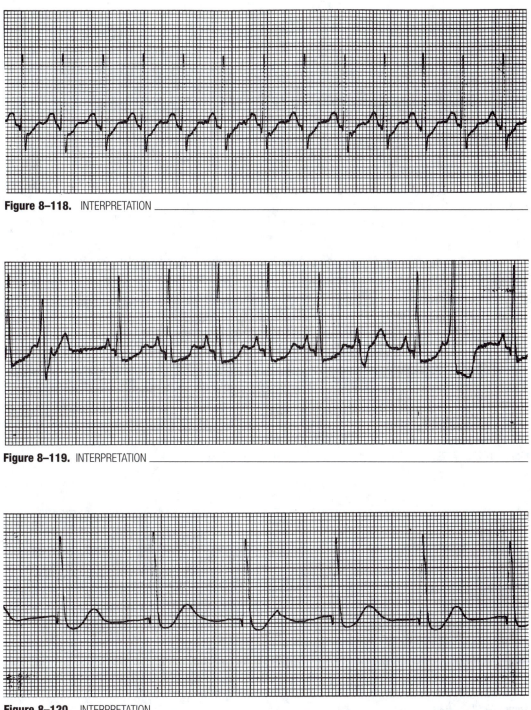

Figure 8–118. INTERPRETATION _____

Figure 8–119. INTERPRETATION _____

Figure 8–120. INTERPRETATION _____

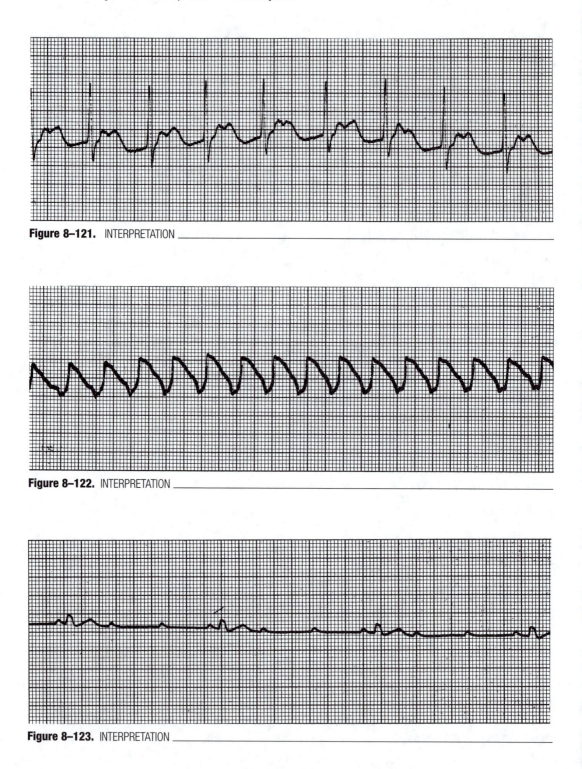

Figure 8–121. INTERPRETATION _____

Figure 8–122. INTERPRETATION _____

Figure 8–123. INTERPRETATION _____

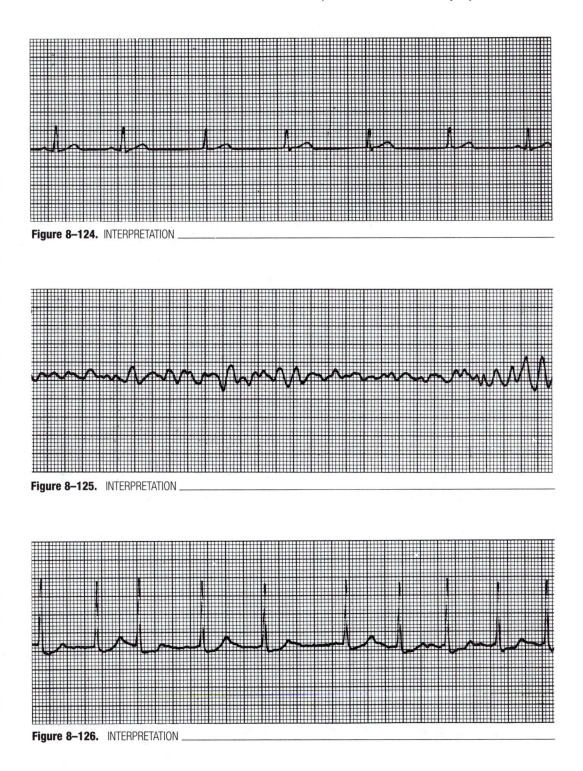

Figure 8–124. INTERPRETATION _____

Figure 8–125. INTERPRETATION _____

Figure 8–126. INTERPRETATION _____

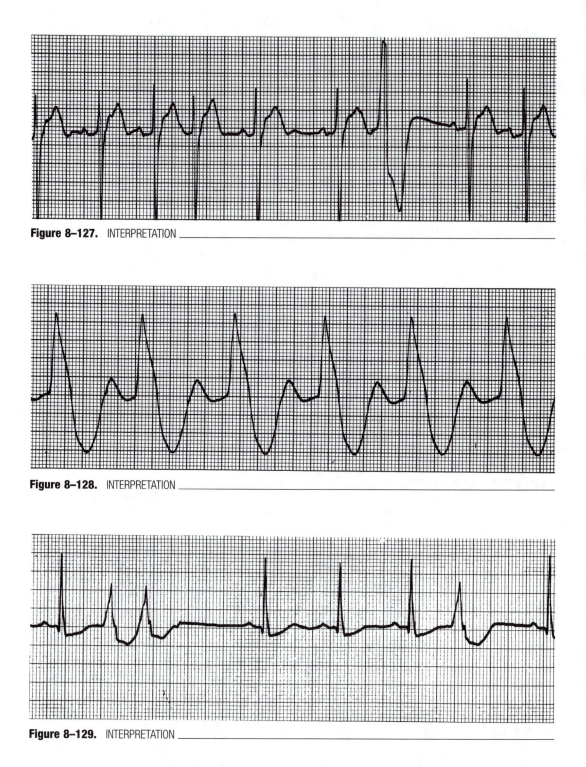

Figure 8–127. INTERPRETATION _____

Figure 8–128. INTERPRETATION _____

Figure 8–129. INTERPRETATION _____

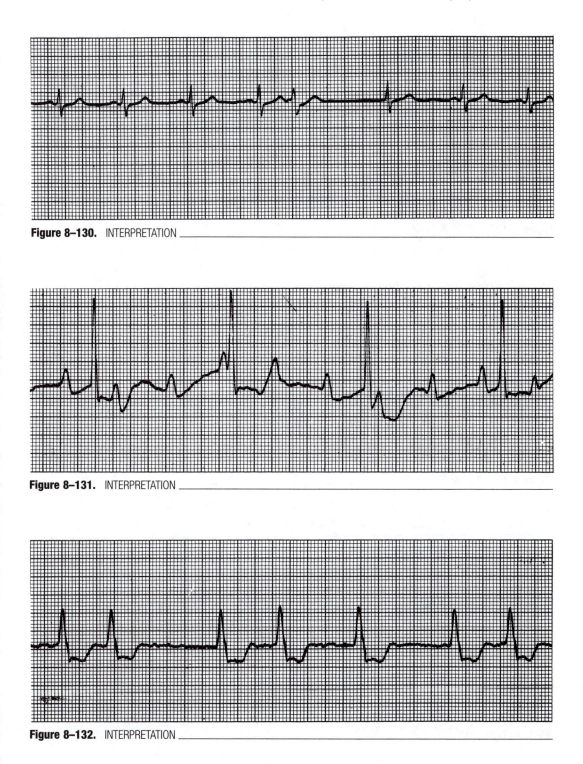

Figure 8–130. INTERPRETATION _____

Figure 8–131. INTERPRETATION _____

Figure 8–132. INTERPRETATION _____

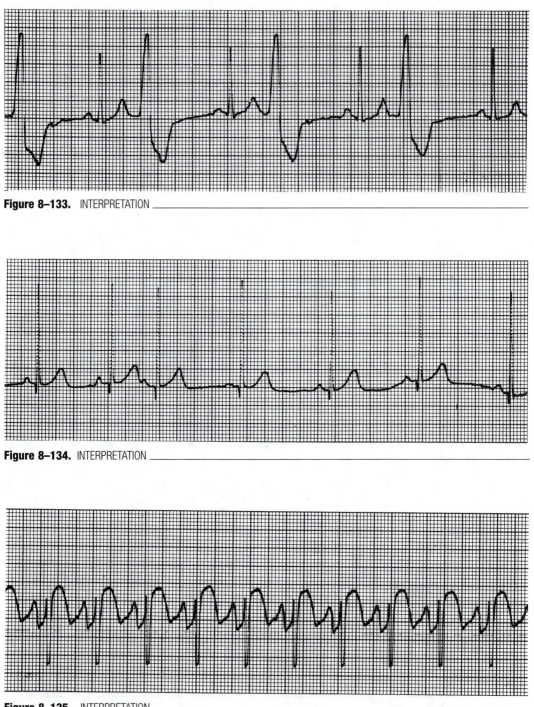

Figure 8–133. INTERPRETATION _____

Figure 8–134. INTERPRETATION _____

Figure 8–135. INTERPRETATION _____

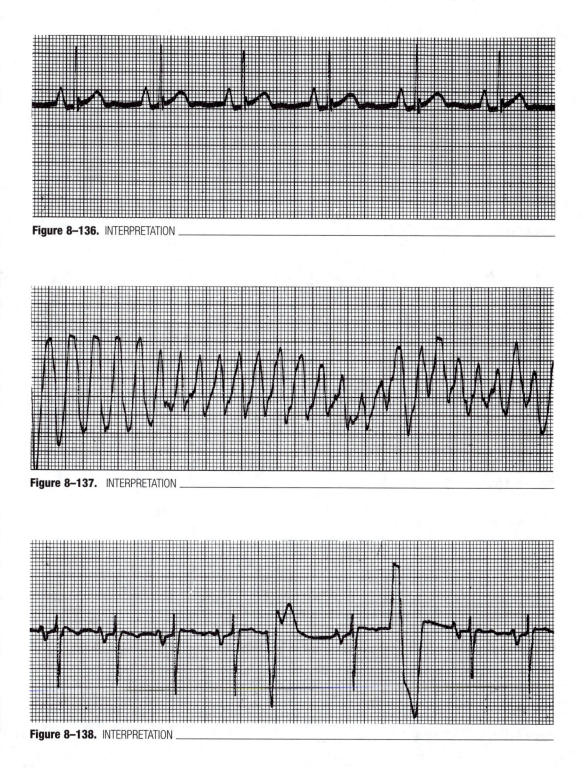

Figure 8–136. INTERPRETATION _____

Figure 8–137. INTERPRETATION _____

Figure 8–138. INTERPRETATION _____

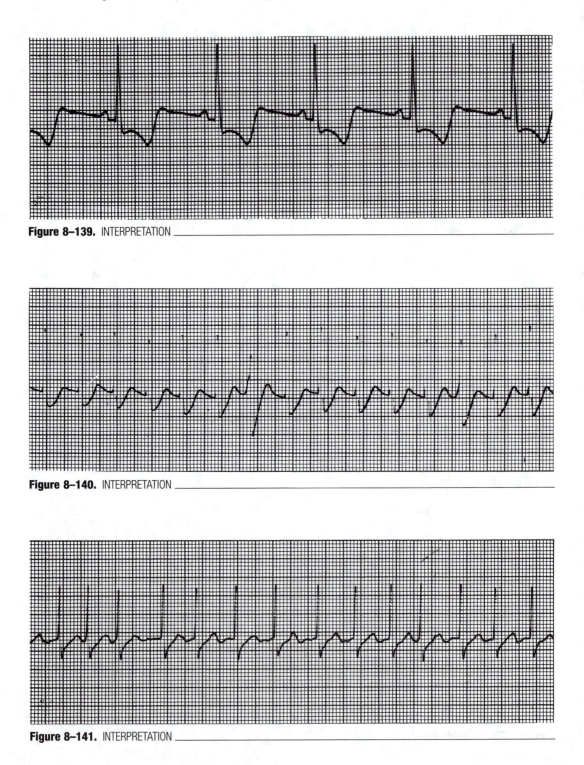

Figure 8–139. INTERPRETATION _____

Figure 8–140. INTERPRETATION _____

Figure 8–141. INTERPRETATION _____

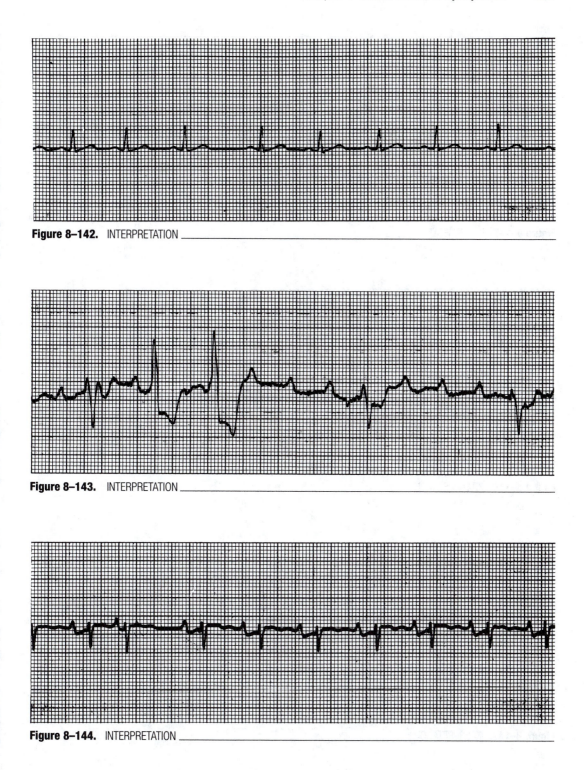

Figure 8–142. INTERPRETATION _____

Figure 8–143. INTERPRETATION _____

Figure 8–144. INTERPRETATION _____

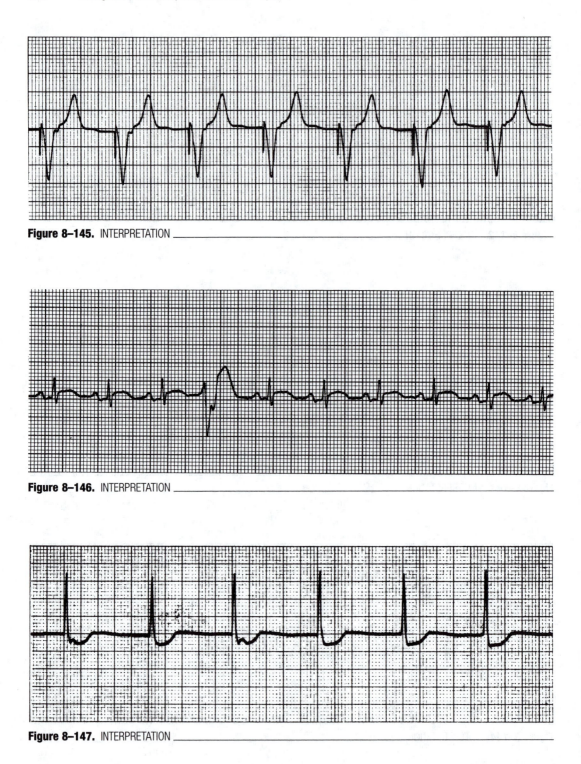

Figure 8–145. INTERPRETATION _____

Figure 8–146. INTERPRETATION _____

Figure 8–147. INTERPRETATION _____

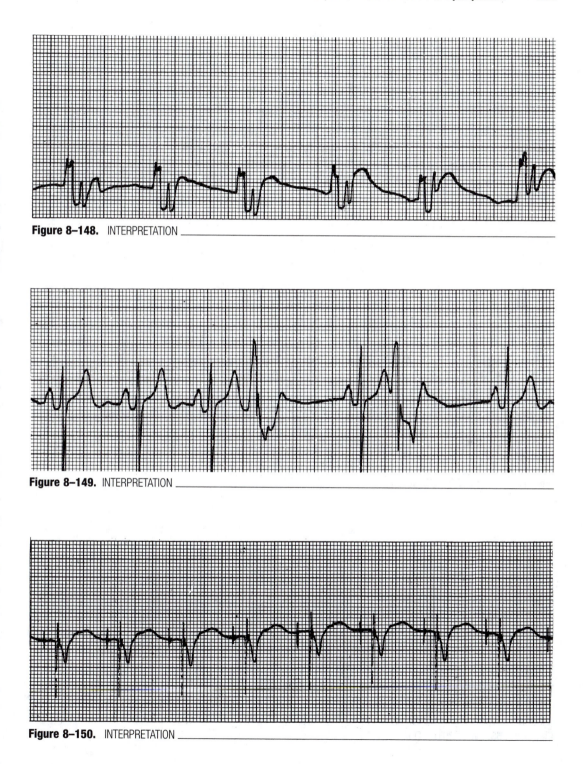

Figure 8–148. INTERPRETATION _____

Figure 8–149. INTERPRETATION _____

Figure 8–150. INTERPRETATION _____

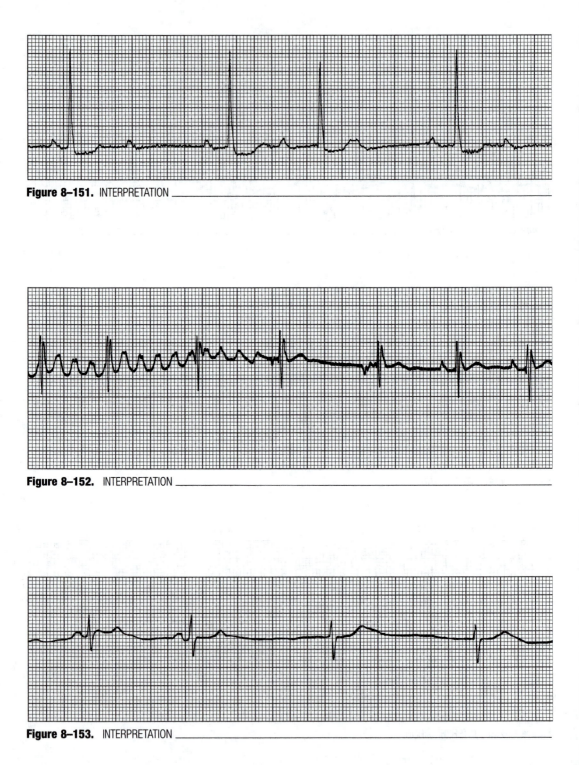

Figure 8–151. INTERPRETATION _____

Figure 8–152. INTERPRETATION _____

Figure 8–153. INTERPRETATION _____

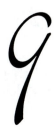

Treatment of Dysrhythmias

The treatment in this chapter is based upon current ACLS treatment algorithms. These algorithms were used because they are a national standard. However, it is important that you follow your local treatment guidelines/protocols if they differ from the ACLS standards.

To determine if treatment is necessary, *look at your patient*. Then ask yourself the following questions:

1. Is he or she experiencing signs and symptoms of decreased cardiac output?
   a. Chest pain
   b. Dyspnea
   c. Decreased level of consciousness
   d. Hypotension
   e. Congestive heart failure
2. Is the dysrhythmia potentially life threatening?
   a. Second degree A-V block, Type II
   b. Complete A-V block
   c. Ventricular tachycardia
   d. Ventricular fibrillation

If the answer to either of these questions is yes, you will need to treat the dysrhythmia.

Arrhythmias can be divided into four broad categories for determining treatment.

1. Bradycardias
2. Tachycardias

3. Ectopics
4. Cardiac arrest

As a general rule, if a dysrhythmia is causing a drop in cardiac output and it is too fast, you slow it down; if it is too slow, you speed it up. If ectopics are present, you suppress them by decreasing the irritability. If cardiac arrest is present, you generate a more viable rhythm.

BRADYCARDIA

The treatment of bradycardias depends upon the patient's ability to tolerate the dysrhythmia. If a patient is experiencing chest pain, dyspnea, lightheadedness, hypotension, or ventricular ectopy, treatment should be instituted.

Heart rates less than 60/min are considered bradycardic. Dysrhythmias that may have ventricular rates below 60/min include sinus bradycardia, junctional rhythm, A-V blocks, and idioventricular rhythm with a pulse. When treating these dysrhythmias, atropine is the medication of choice. However, if patients do not respond to atropine, a transcutaneous pacemaker (TCP) is preferred to multiple doses of atropine. If a transcutaneous pacemaker is unavailable, then atropine, dopamine, epinephrine, and isuprel may be used. With the exception of second degree A-V block Type II, complete A-V block and idioventricular rhythm, bradycardias usually respond to atropine without further interventions. Patients with second degree A-V block Type II, complete A-V block, or idioventricular dysrhythmias generally require transvenous pacing even if they temporarily respond to medications.

TACHYCARDIA

As with bradycardias, the treatment of tachycardias depends upon the patient's ability to tolerate the dysrhythmia. If a patient is experiencing an exacerbation of chest pain, hypotension, dyspnea, or congestive heart failure or has an altered level of consciousness, emergency treatment is warranted.

Tachycardic rhythms are divided into supraventricular (above the ventricles) and ventricular (originating in the ventricles). Heart rates greater than 100/min are considered tachycardic. However, a drop in cardiac output usually does not occur until the rate is greater than 140.

Supraventricular Tachycardias

Supraventricular tachycardias that may have heart rates greater than 100/min include junctional tachycardia, atrial fibrillation, atrial flutter, supraventricular tachycardia, and sinus tachycardia.

Sinus tachycardia is frequently a compensatory mechanism for underlying etiology. Therefore, the only treatment needed is to treat the underlying cause or abnormality (ie, fluid for shock, sedative for pain, etc.).

In supraventricular tachycardias that are more stable, treatment is less urgent. Therapy for these patients may include vagal maneuvers such as Valsalva's maneuver or carotid sinus massage. Adenosine is usually the medication of choice to treat these patients, but if the dysrhythmia is unresponsive, verapamil, cardioversion, digitalis, or beta blockers may be necessary.

Supraventricular tachycardias with a rate >150/min, with serious signs/symptoms are treated with immediate, synchronized cardioversion. The recommended watt-setting sequence is 100 joules, 200 joules, 300 joules, 360 joules, except in the case of PSVT and atrial flutter where 50 joules is the recommended initial setting. If the patient is awake and time permits, a short-acting sedative may be administered to relieve discomfort associated with the procedure.

Ventricular Tachycardia

Ventricular dysrhythmias that are tachycardic include accelerated idioventricular rhythm and ventricular tachycardia. Ventricular dysrhythmias that are tachycardic are divided into three categories to determine treatment priorities.

1. *Stable* patients with a pulse and no or borderline symptoms are treated with lidocaine as the medication of choice. Once the maximum dosage (3 mg/kg) of lidocaine is achieved, procainamide to a maximum of 17 mg/kg can be given. This may be followed by bretylium to a maximum dose of 30 mg/kg. If unsuccessful, cardioversion is recommended as outlined in the tachycardia algorithm. Sedation with a short-acting sedative may be needed.

2. *Unstable* patients with a pulse are treated with sedation, if appropriate, and synchronized cardioversion at 100 joules. The joules are doubled if repeat shocks are needed. If the patient has recurrent ventricular tachycardia, lidocaine, procainamide, or bretylium may be used to control the dysrhythmia. If necessary, repeat the synchronized cardioversion at the joules that were previously successful.

3. *Pulseless* ventricular tachycardia is treated as if the dysrhythmia were ventricular fibrillation (see ventricular fibrillation and treatment). Once ventricular tachycardia is corrected, an intravenous (IV)

infusion of the medication that corrected the problem should be started (eg, lidocaine drip).

ECTOPICS

Treatment of ectopics depends upon the focus of origin and the overall presentation of the patient. *Atrial* or *junctional ectopics* usually do not cause a drop in cardiac output and are considered benign. Premature atrial and junctional complexes usually respond to oxygen therapy as well as removal of stimulants such as caffeine and nicotine. Ventricular escape complexes are considered life saving and should not be suppressed. Ventricular ectopics can be considered benign and left untreated in some circumstances. However, they are treated when the following conditions exist: (1) frequent (more than six per minute), (2) bigeminy or trigeminy, (3) paired (couplets) or runs (three or more), (4) multiformed, (5) R on T, (6) in the presence of acute myocardial infarction (MI). Treatment for ventricular ectopics includes lidocaine as the medication of choice followed by procainamide, bretylium, and overdrive pacing if ectopics are not suppressed. Premature ventricular complexes in the presence of bradycardia are treated with atropine rather than lidocaine to override the irritable focus, thus suppressing the irritability.

CARDIAC ARREST

The patient who presents in cardiopulmonary arrest may have one of the following dysrhythmias: (1) ventricular fibrillation, (2) ventricular tachycardia, (3) asystole, (4) or pulseless electrical activity.

Ventricular fibrillation and *ventricular tachycardia* in the pulseless and apneic patient are treated the same. If the monitored patient is in ventricular tachycardia or ventricular fibrillation, a precordial thump can be administered if the defibrillator is not immediately available. Defibrillation and epinephrine are priorities for the initial treatment of the patient.

Once the IV has been established, epinephrine, lidocaine, and bretylium should be administered as indicated.

Asystole should be confirmed in at least two lead configurations. If the dysrhythmia is unclear and possibly ventricular fibrillation, treat as such. If asystole is confirmed, apply a transcutaneous pacemaker and follow with epinephrine and atropine.

Pulseless electrical activity (PEA) is not a dysrhythmia; instead it is a description of what is happening within the heart—electrical activity without mechanical response. Common dysrhythmias that may present with PEA include bradycardias with a heart rate less than 40/min, idioventricular rhythms, and tachycardias. The survival of patients in PEA is invariably poor unless an underlying etiology can be identified and corrected. The most common treatable causes of PEA include hypovolemia, cardiac tamponade, tension pneumothorax, hypoxia, and acidosis. While searching for a correctable etiology, the patient should be supported with CPR, intubation, initiation of an IV, and epinephrine.

See Figs. 9–1 through 9–7 for ACLS algorithms.

SELF-EVALUATION

Directions

Answer keys for the Self-Evaluation section begin on page 400.

1. *Fill-in.* In this section, fill in the blanks with the appropriate word(s) or statements. The length of

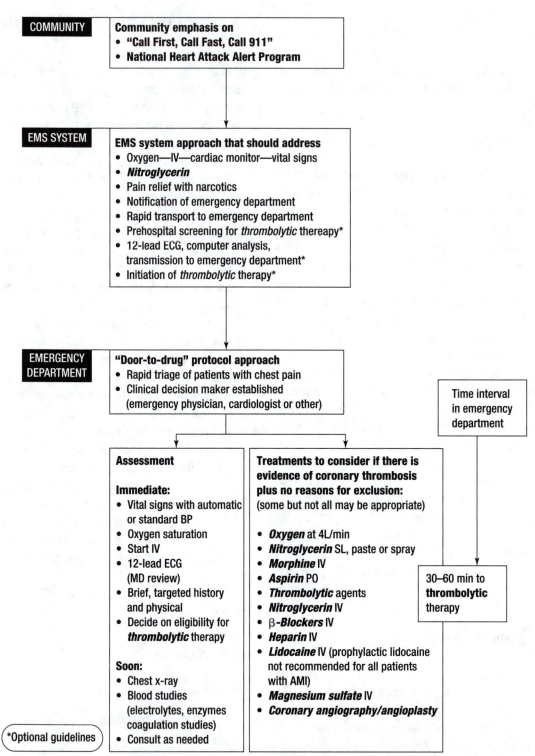

Figure 9–1. Acute myocardial infarction algorithm. Recommendations for early management of patients with chest pain and early AMI. (Reproduced with permission. *Journal of the American Medical Association*, 1992; 268: 2119–2240.)

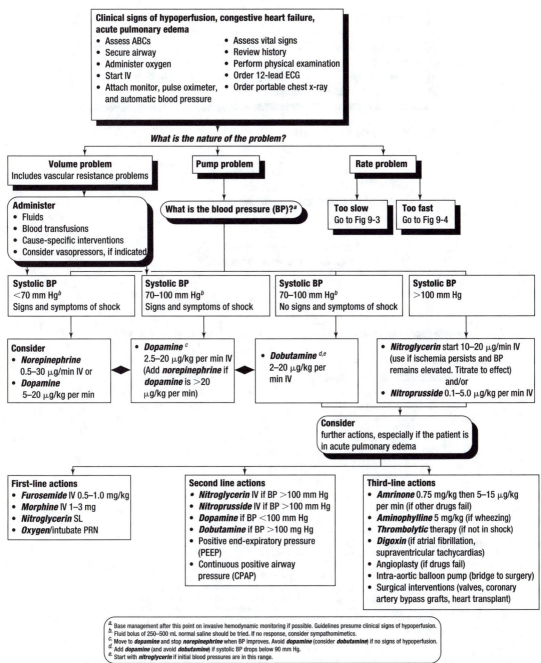

Figure 9–2. Acute pulmonary edema/hypotension/shock algorithm. (Reproduced with permission. *Journal of the American Medical Association,* 1992; 268: 2119–2240.)

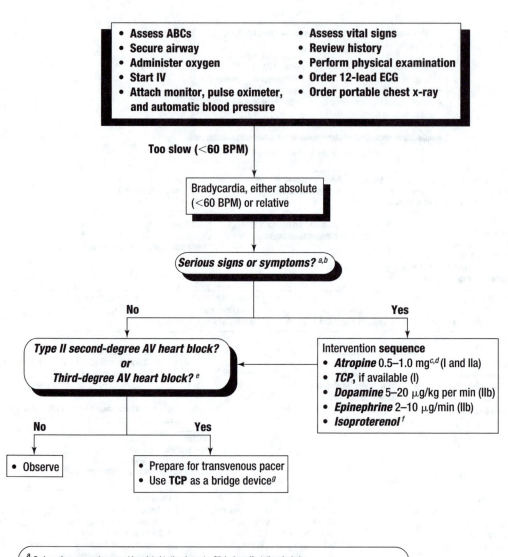

- Assess ABCs
- Secure airway
- Administer oxygen
- Start IV
- Attach monitor, pulse oximeter, and automatic blood pressure

- Assess vital signs
- Review history
- Perform physical examination
- Order 12-lead ECG
- Order portable chest x-ray

Too slow (<60 BPM)

Bradycardia, either absolute (<60 BPM) or relative

Serious signs or symptoms? [a,b]

No   **Yes**

Type II second-degree AV heart block?
or
Third-degree AV heart block? [e]

Intervention sequence
- *Atropine* 0.5–1.0 mg[c,d] (I and IIa)
- *TCP,* if available (I)
- *Dopamine* 5–20 μg/kg per min (IIb)
- *Epinephrine* 2–10 μg/min (IIb)
- *Isoproterenol* [f]

No   **Yes**

- Observe

- Prepare for transvenous pacer
- Use **TCP** as a bridge device[g]

[a.] Serious signs or symptoms must be related to the slow rate. Clinical manifestations include
  - Symptoms (chest pain, shortness of breath, decreased level of consciousness)
  - Signs (low BP, shock, pulmonary congestion, CHF, acute MI)

[b.] Do not delay TCP while awaiting IV access or for *atropine* to take effect if patient is symptomatic.

[c.] Denervated transplanted hearts will not respond to *atropine*. Go at once to pacing, *catecholamine* infusion, or both.

[d.] *Atropine* should be given in repeat doses every 3–5 min up to a total of 0.03–0.04 mg/kg. Use the shorter dosing interval (3 min) in severe clinical conditions. It has been suggested that *atropine* should be used with caution in atrioventricular (A-V) block at the His–Purkinje level (type II A-V block and new third-degree block with wide QRS complexes) (Class IIb).

[e.] Never treat third-degree heart block plus ventricular escape beats with *lidocaine*.

[f.] *Isoproterenol* should be used, if at all, with extreme caution. At low doses it is Class IIb (possibly helpful); at higher doses it is Class III (harmful).

[g.] Verify patient tolerance and mechanical capture. Use analgesia and sedation as needed.

Figure 9–3. Bradycardia algorithm. (Patient is not in cardiac arrest.) (Reproduced with permission. *Journal of the American Medical Association,* 1992; 268: 2119–2240.)

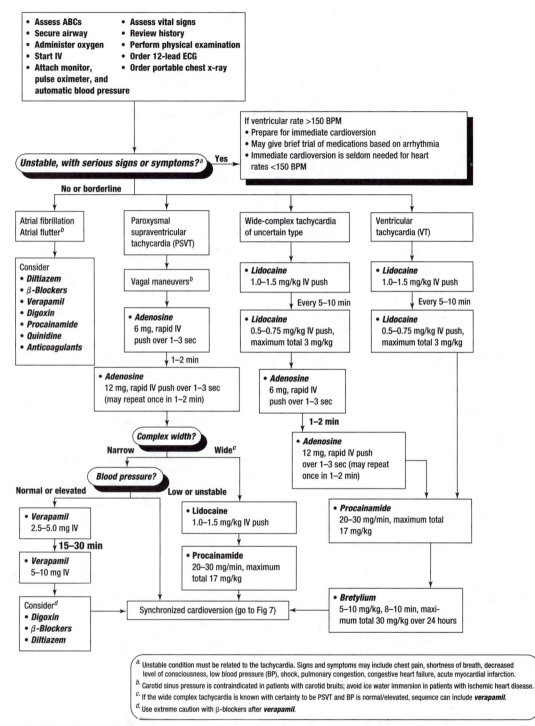

• Assess ABCs
• Secure airway
• Administer oxygen
• Start IV
• Attach monitor, pulse oximeter, and automatic blood pressure

• Assess vital signs
• Review history
• Perform physical examination
• Order 12-lead ECG
• Order portable chest x-ray

Unstable, with serious signs or symptoms?[a] —Yes→

If ventricular rate >150 BPM
• Prepare for immediate cardioversion
• May give brief trial of medications based on arrhythmia
• Immediate cardioversion is seldom needed for heart rates <150 BPM

No or borderline

Atrial fibrillation Atrial flutter[b]

Consider
• *Diltiazem*
• *β-Blockers*
• *Verapamil*
• *Digoxin*
• *Procainamide*
• *Quinidine*
• *Anticoagulants*

Paroxysmal supraventricular tachycardia (PSVT)

Vagal maneuvers[b]

• *Adenosine*
6 mg, rapid IV push over 1–3 sec

↓ 1–2 min

• *Adenosine*
12 mg, rapid IV push over 1–3 sec (may repeat once in 1–2 min)

Complex width?

Narrow — Wide[c]

Blood pressure?

Normal or elevated — Low or unstable

• *Verapamil*
2.5–5.0 mg IV

↓ 15–30 min

• *Verapamil*
5–10 mg IV

Consider[d]
• *Digoxin*
• *β-Blockers*
• *Diltiazem*

• Lidocaine
1.0–1.5 mg/kg IV push

• Procainamide
20–30 mg/min, maximum total 17 mg/kg

Synchronized cardioversion (go to Fig 7) ←

Wide-complex tachycardia of uncertain type

• *Lidocaine*
1.0–1.5 mg/kg IV push

↓ Every 5–10 min

• *Lidocaine*
0.5–0.75 mg/kg IV push, maximum total 3 mg/kg

• *Adenosine*
6 mg, rapid IV push over 1–3 sec

↓ 1–2 min

• *Adenosine*
12 mg, rapid IV push over 1–3 sec (may repeat once in 1–2 min)

Ventricular tachycardia (VT)

• *Lidocaine*
1.0–1.5 mg/kg IV push

↓ Every 5–10 min

• *Lidocaine*
0.5–0.75 mg/kg IV push, maximum total 3 mg/kg

• *Procainamide*
20–30 mg/min, maximum total 17 mg/kg

• *Bretylium*
5–10 mg/kg, 8–10 min, maximum total 30 mg/kg over 24 hours

[a.] Unstable condition must be related to the tachycardia. Signs and symptoms may include chest pain, shortness of breath, decreased level of consciousness, low blood pressure (BP), shock, pulmonary congestion, congestive heart failure, acute myocardial infarction.
[b.] Carotid sinus pressure is contraindicated in patients with carotid bruits; avoid ice water immersion in patients with ischemic heart disease.
[c.] If the wide complex tachycardia is known with certainty to be PSVT and BP is normal/elevated, sequence can include *verapamil*.
[d.] Use extreme caution with β-blockers after *verapamil*.

Figure 9–4. Tachycardia algorithm. (Reproduced with permission. *Journal of the American Medical Association,* 1992; 268: 2119–2240.)

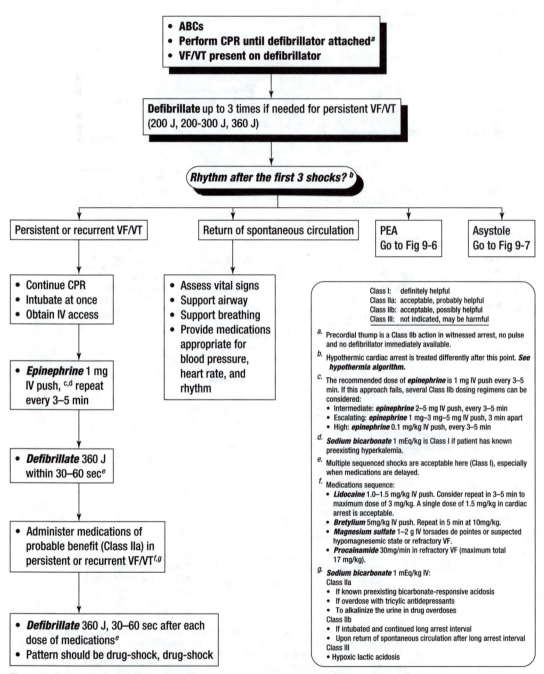

Figure 9–5. Ventricular fibrillation/pulseless ventricular tachycardia (VF/VT) algorithm. (Reproduced with permission. *Journal of the American Medical Association,* 1992; 268: 2119–2240.)

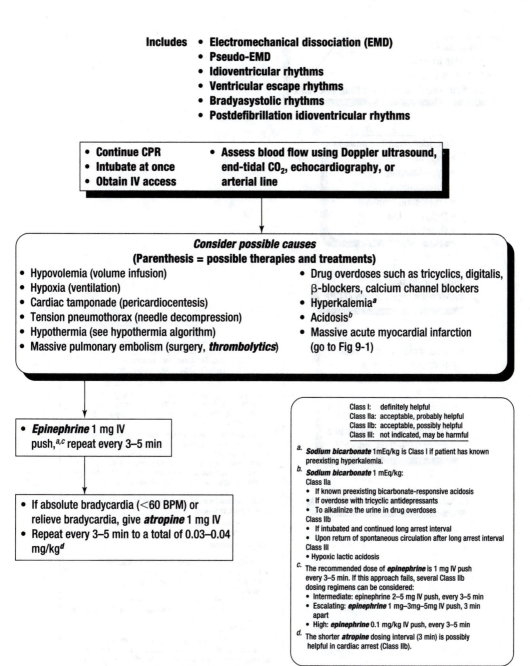

Includes
- **Electromechanical dissociation (EMD)**
- **Pseudo-EMD**
- **Idioventricular rhythms**
- **Ventricular escape rhythms**
- **Bradyasystolic rhythms**
- **Postdefibrillation idioventricular rhythms**

- **Continue CPR**
- **Intubate at once**
- **Obtain IV access**

- **Assess blood flow using Doppler ultrasound, end-tidal CO_2, echocardiography, or arterial line**

Consider possible causes
(Parenthesis = possible therapies and treatments)

- Hypovolemia (volume infusion)
- Hypoxia (ventilation)
- Cardiac tamponade (pericardiocentesis)
- Tension pneumothorax (needle decompression)
- Hypothermia (see hypothermia algorithm)
- Massive pulmonary embolism (surgery, ***thrombolytics***)

- Drug overdoses such as tricyclics, digitalis, β-blockers, calcium channel blockers
- Hyperkalemia[a]
- Acidosis[b]
- Massive acute myocardial infarction (go to Fig 9-1)

- ***Epinephrine*** 1 mg IV push,[a,c] repeat every 3–5 min

- If absolute bradycardia (<60 BPM) or relieve bradycardia, give ***atropine*** 1 mg IV
- Repeat every 3–5 min to a total of 0.03–0.04 mg/kg[d]

Class I: definitely helpful
Class IIa: acceptable, probably helpful
Class IIb: acceptable, possibly helpful
Class III: not indicated, may be harmful

a. ***Sodium bicarbonate*** 1mEq/kg is Class I if patient has known preexisting hyperkalemia.

b. ***Sodium bicarbonate*** 1 mEq/kg:
Class IIa
- If known preexisting bicarbonate-responsive acidosis
- If overdose with tricyclic antidepressants
- To alkalinize the urine in drug overdoses
Class IIb
- If intubated and continued long arrest interval
- Upon return of spontaneous circulation after long arrest interval
Class III
- Hypoxic lactic acidosis

c. The recommended dose of ***epinephrine*** is 1 mg IV push every 3–5 min. If this approach fails, several Class IIb dosing regimens can be considered:
- Intermediate: epinephrine 2–5 mg IV push, every 3–5 min
- Escalating: ***epinephrine*** 1 mg–3mg–5mg IV push, 3 min apart
- High: ***epinephrine*** 0.1 mg/kg IV push, every 3–5 min

d. The shorter ***atropine*** dosing interval (3 min) is possibly helpful in cardiac arrest (Class IIb).

Figure 9–6. Pulseless electrical activity (PEA) algorithm (electromechanical dissociation [EMD]). (Reproduced with permission. *Journal of the American Medical Association,* 1992; 268: 2119–2240.)

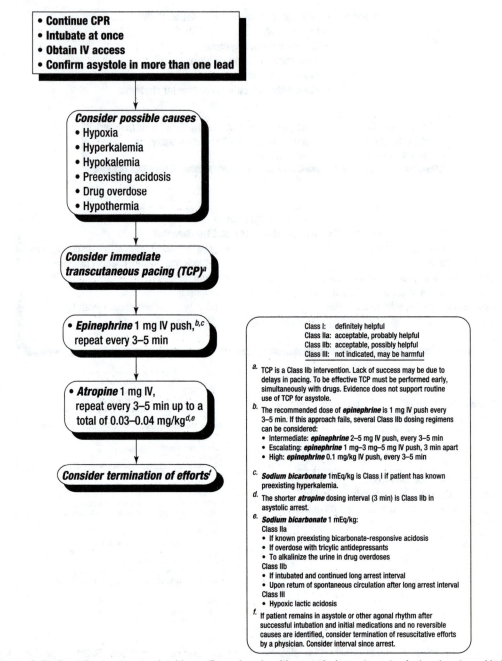

Figure 9–7. Asystole treatment algorithm. (Reproduced with permission. *Journal of the American Medical Association,* 1992; 268: 2119–2240.)

the line does not necessarily determine the length of the answer, and more than one word may be written on an unbroken line.

2. *ECG practice strips.* The practice strips in this section are accompanied by patient situations. When considering how to treat the dysrhythmia, look at the patient situation. Treatment is based upon the cause of the dysrhythmia and how the patient is tolerating it. Then identify which ACLS algorithm would be used to treat the patient in the treatment space.

FILL-IN

1. Dysrhythmias are treated if they
   a. _____ or
   b. _____

2. Signs and symptoms of decreased cardiac output include
   a. _____
   b. _____
   c. _____
   d. _____
   e. _____

3. List four potentially life-threatening dysrhythmias.
   a. _____
   b. _____
   c. _____
   d. _____

4. What are the four broad categories into which dysrhythmias can be divided?
   a. _____
   b. _____
   c. _____
   d. _____

5. As a general rule, if a dysrhythmia is causing a drop in cardiac output and it is too fast, you
   a. _____; too slow, you
   b. _____ .

6. To treat ectopics, you must _____ the irritability.

7. In cardiac arrest, treatment is aimed at generating a more _____ rhythm.

8. Dysrhythmias that may have heart rates less than 60/min include
   a. _____
   b. _____
   c. _____
   d. _____

9. The medication of choice to treat symptomatic bradycardias

10. If a patient has a symptomatic bradycardia that does not respond to atropine, what other treatments may be used?
    a. _____
    b. _____
    c. _____
    d. _____

11. What three bradycardic rhythms generally require pacing?
    a. _____
    b. _____
    c. _____

12. Supraventricular tachycardias that may have heart rates greater than 100/min include
    a. _____
    b. _____
    c. _____
    d. _____
    e. _____

13. What are the two treatment categories for supraventricular tachycardias?
    a. _____
    b. _____

14. Treatment of a stable supraventricular tachycardia consists of
    a. _____
    b. _____
    c. _____
    d. _____

15. Treatment of an unstable supraventricular tachycardia consists of _____ .

16. Identify the watts/second setting for cardioversion of the following dysrhythmias:
    a. atrial flutter _____
    b. paroxysmal supraventricular tachycardia
       _____
    c. atrial fibrillation _____

17. _____ is frequently a compensatory mechanism for an underlying etiology.

18. To treat a sinus tachycardia you treat the underlying _____ .

19. Some causes of sinus tachycardia include
    a. _____
    b. _____
    c. _____
    d. _____

20. List two ventricular dysrhythmias that are tachycardic.
    a. _____
    b. _____

21. What are the three treatment categories for ventricular tachycardias?
    a. _____
    b. _____
    c. _____

22. A patient who is conscious with a fluttering feeling in his or her chest and in ventricular tachycardia is treated with _____ and _____ .

23. A patient who is unconscious and in ventricular tachycardia is treated with _____ .

24. Unconscious, pulseless ventricular tachycardia is treated as if the dysrhythmia were _____ .

25. The main treatment of premature atrial complexes is _____ .

26. Premature ventricular complexes should be treated when
    a. _____
    b. _____
    c. _____
    d. _____

    e. _____
    f. _____

27. Treatment for runs of premature ventricular complexes includes
    a. _____
    b. _____
    c. _____

28. Premature ventricular complexes in a bradycardia are treated with _____ .

29. Patients who present in cardiac arrest have one of the following dysrhythmias:
    a. _____
    b. _____
    c. _____
    d. _____

30. If the defibrillator is not immediately available, the first treatment for witnessed ventricular fibrillation is _____ .

31. Initial treatment priorities for unwitnessed ventricular fibrillation includes
    a. _____
    b. _____

32. The treatment of asystole is
    a. _____
    b. _____
    c. _____

33. Dysrhythmias that may present in PEA include
    a. _____
    b. _____
    c. _____

34. Survival of patients in PEA is _____ .

35. What are five treatable causes of PEA?
    a. _____
    b. _____
    c. _____
    d. _____
    e. _____

36. While looking for a treatable cause of PEA, the initial medication used to treat PEA is _____ .

ECG PRACTICE STRIPS

This is the ECG of a 49-year-old female complaining of skipped beats.

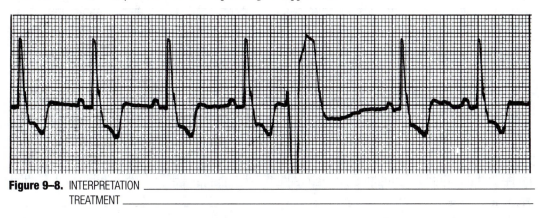

Figure 9–8. INTERPRETATION _____

TREATMENT _____

This is the ECG of a 55-year-old male with a blood pressure of 70/palpable.

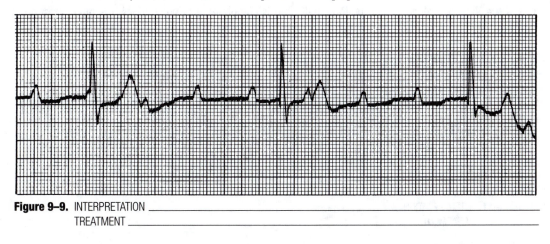

Figure 9–9. INTERPRETATION _____

TREATMENT _____

This is the ECG of a 60-year-old conscious female with a past history of heart disease and symptoms of a cerebrovascular accident. Her blood pressure is 160/90.

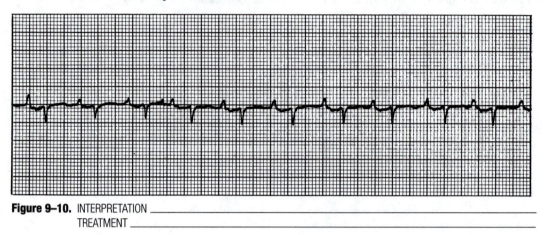

Figure 9–10. INTERPRETATION _____
              TREATMENT _____

This is the ECG of a 45-year-old conscious male who is complaining of palpitations. His blood pressure is 110/70.

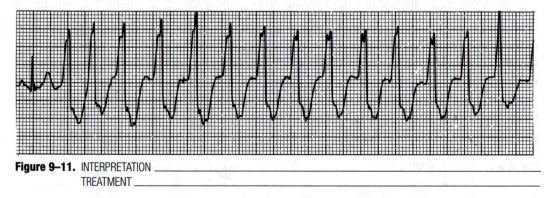

Figure 9–11. INTERPRETATION _____
              TREATMENT _____

This is the ECG of a 78-year-old conscious female who is feeling light-headed. Her blood pressure is 130/80.

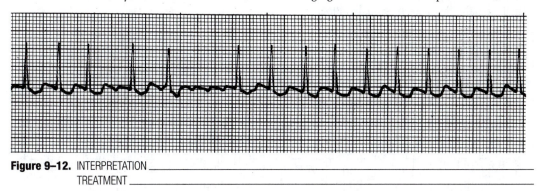

Figure 9–12. INTERPRETATION _____
TREATMENT _____

This is the ECG of an unconscious 78-year-old female with a blood pressure of 40/palpable.

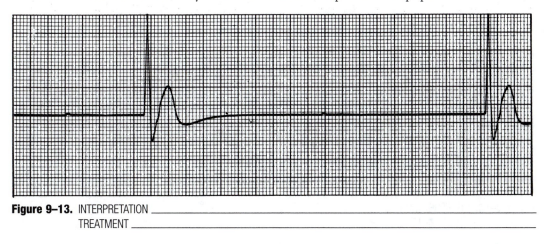

Figure 9–13. INTERPRETATION _____
TREATMENT _____

This is the ECG of a 47-year-old conscious female who was involved in a car accident. Her chief complaint is right thigh pain. Her blood pressure is 140/80.

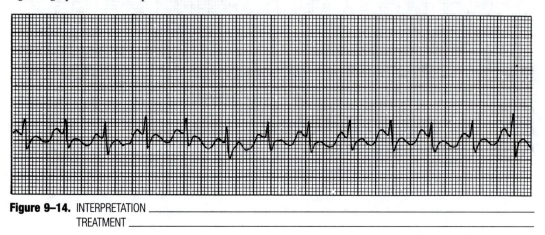

Figure 9–14. INTERPRETATION _____
               TREATMENT _____

This is the ECG of a 50-year-old unconscious, pulseless, and apneic male.

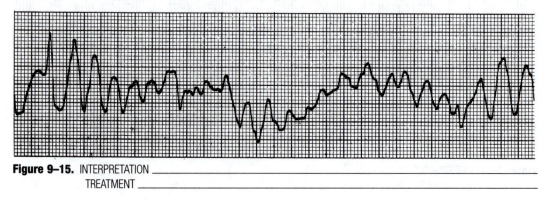

Figure 9–15. INTERPRETATION _____
               TREATMENT _____

This is the ECG of an unconscious, pulseless, and apneic 19-year-old male involved in an auto accident. His chest struck the steering wheel.

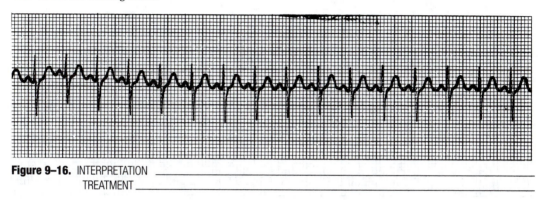

Figure 9–16. INTERPRETATION _____
                    TREATMENT _____

This is the ECG of a 30-year-old female who has a blood pressure of 40/palpable. She is unconscious and unresponsive.

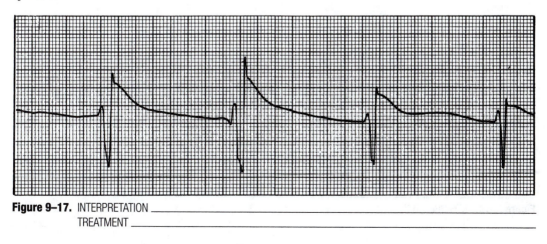

Figure 9–17. INTERPRETATION _____
                    TREATMENT _____

This is the ECG of a conscious 24-year-old male complaining of dyspnea. His blood pressure is 120/80; respirations are 28.

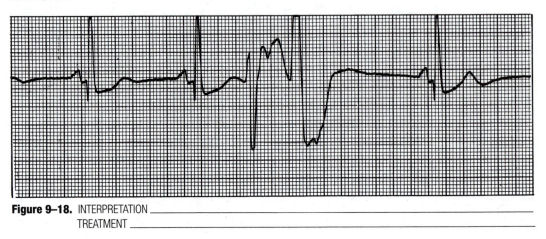

Figure 9–18. INTERPRETATION _____
                  TREATMENT _____

This is the ECG of a 92-year-old unconscious female with a blood pressure of 70/40.

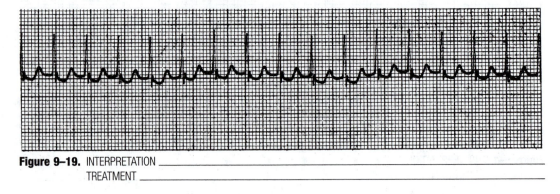

Figure 9–19. INTERPRETATION _____
                  TREATMENT _____

This is the ECG of a 45-year-old unconscious male who is pulseless and apneic.

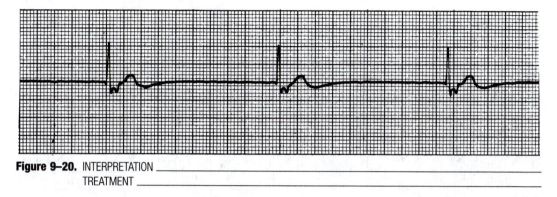

Figure 9–20. INTERPRETATION _____

TREATMENT _____

This is the ECG of a 54-year-old male complaining of a heavy feeling substernally with radiation into his left arm. His blood pressure is 80/50.

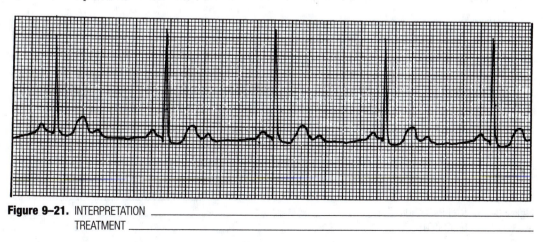

Figure 9–21. INTERPRETATION _____

TREATMENT _____

This is the ECG of a conscious 58-year-old female who slipped and fell and is complaining of right hip pain. Her blood pressure is 140/80.

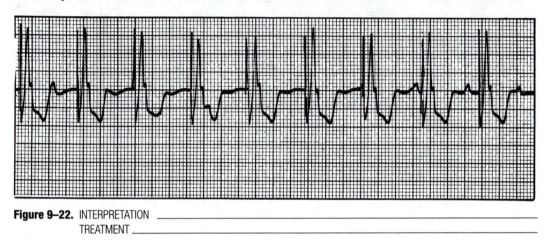

Figure 9–22. INTERPRETATION _____
                        TREATMENT _____

This is the ECG of a 54-year-old male complaining of severe chest pain. His blood pressure is 160/100.

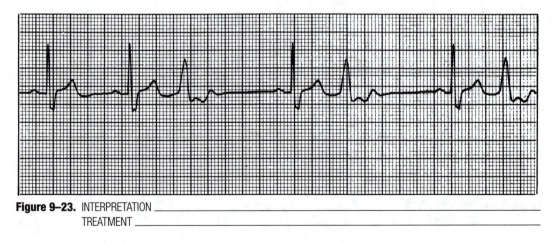

Figure 9–23. INTERPRETATION _____
                        TREATMENT _____

This is the ECG of an unconscious 24-year-old male. His blood pressure is 88/60.

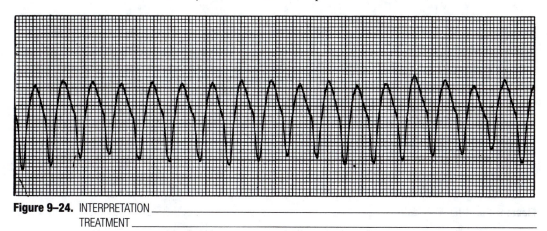

Figure 9–24. INTERPRETATION _____
TREATMENT _____

This is the ECG of a 54-year-old female who is pulseless and apneic. She has no known medical history.

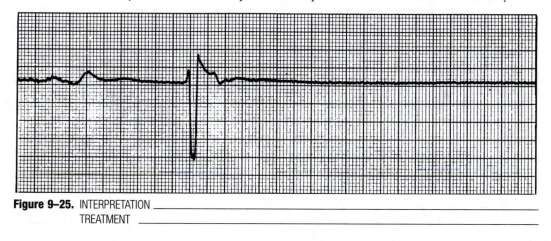

Figure 9–25. INTERPRETATION _____
TREATMENT _____

This is the ECG of an unconscious 60-year-old female. Her blood pressure is 80/50.

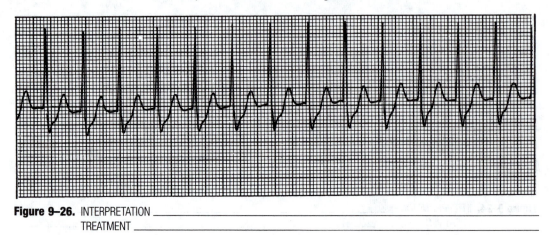

Figure 9–26. INTERPRETATION _____

                   TREATMENT _____

This is the ECG of a conscious 27-year-old male who overdosed. His blood pressure is 120/80.

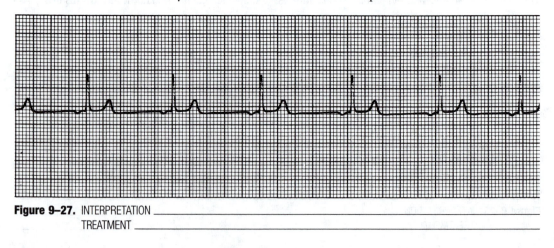

Figure 9–27. INTERPRETATION _____

                   TREATMENT _____

This is the ECG of a 69-year-old male with an acute MI. His blood pressure is 100/60.

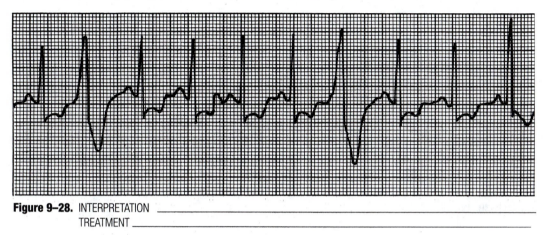

Figure 9–28. INTERPRETATION _____

TREATMENT _____

This is the ECG of a 54-year-old male. His blood pressure is 80/50.

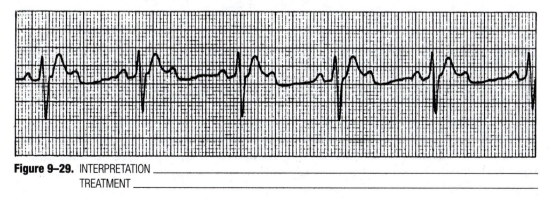

Figure 9–29. INTERPRETATION _____

TREATMENT _____

This is the ECG of a 75-year-old male who is pulseless and apneic.

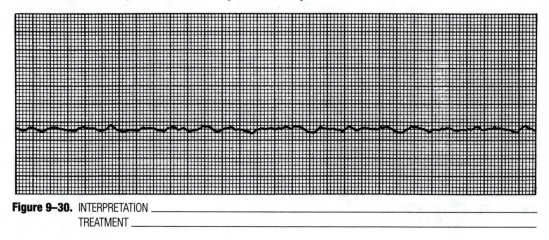

Figure 9–30. INTERPRETATION _____
                       TREATMENT _____

This is the ECG of a 72-year-old conscious female who has a known history of heart disease and is complaining of weakness. Vital signs are stable.

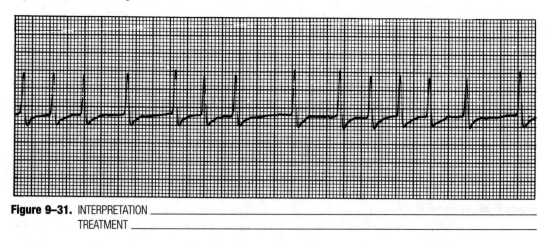

Figure 9–31. INTERPRETATION _____
                       TREATMENT _____

This is the ECG of a 60-year-old unconscious male who complained of chest pain and then collapsed. He is pulseless and apneic.

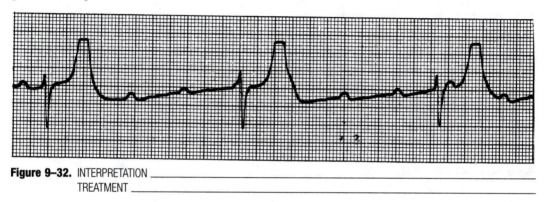

Figure 9–32. INTERPRETATION _____
TREATMENT _____

This is the ECG of a 52-year-old conscious male with an acute MI. His blood pressure is 110/70.

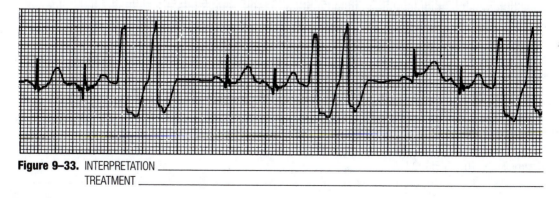

Figure 9–33. INTERPRETATION _____
TREATMENT _____

This is the ECG of a 70-year-old conscious male who has a "fluttering" feeling in his chest. His blood pressure is 138/80.

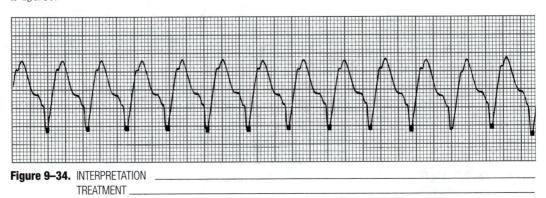

Figure 9–34. INTERPRETATION _____
                 TREATMENT _____

This is the ECG of a conscious 44-year-old male complaining of palpitations. His blood pressure is 140/60.

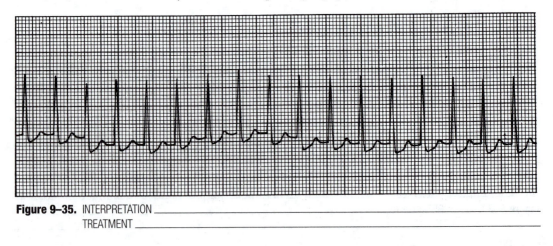

Figure 9–35. INTERPRETATION _____
                 TREATMENT _____

This is the ECG of a 65-year-old female who is complaining of feeling light-headed. Her blood pressure is 100/60.

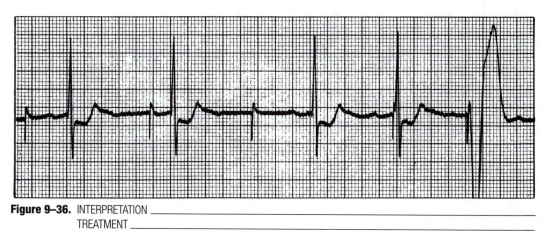

Figure 9–36. INTERPRETATION _____

   TREATMENT _____

This is the ECG of a 22-year-old female who was electrocuted. She is unresponsive, pulseless, and apneic.

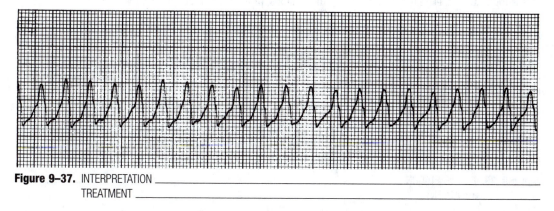

Figure 9–37. INTERPRETATION _____

   TREATMENT _____

This is the ECG of a conscious 62-year-old female complaining of shortness of breath and chest pain. Her blood pressure is 100/60.

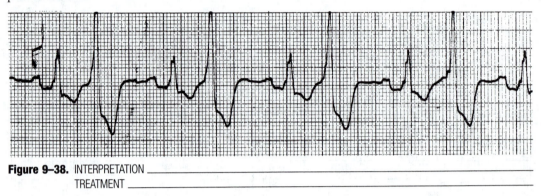

Figure 9–38. INTERPRETATION _____
                              TREATMENT _____

This is the ECG of a 44-year-old male found unconscious, pulseless, and apneic.

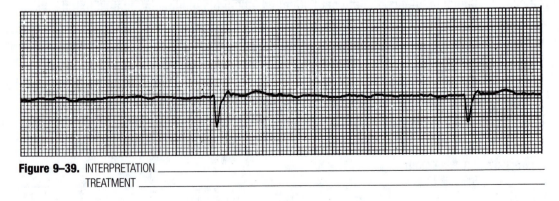

Figure 9–39. INTERPRETATION _____
                              TREATMENT _____

This is the ECG of a 33-year-old female complaining of severe substernal chest pain radiating into her left shoulder. Her blood pressure is 100/60.

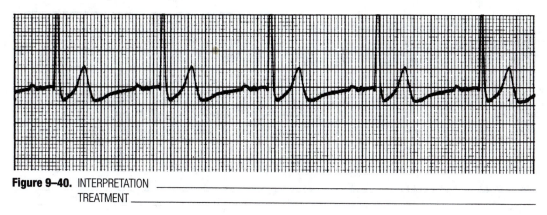

Figure 9–40. INTERPRETATION _____
                      TREATMENT _____

This is the ECG of an unconscious 80-year-old female with a blood pressure of 70/50.

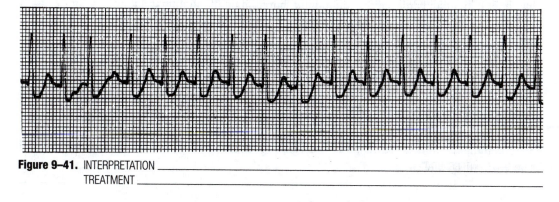

Figure 9–41. INTERPRETATION _____
                      TREATMENT _____

This is the ECG of a 22-year-old male who has had a history of diarrhea for three days. His blood pressure is 80/60.

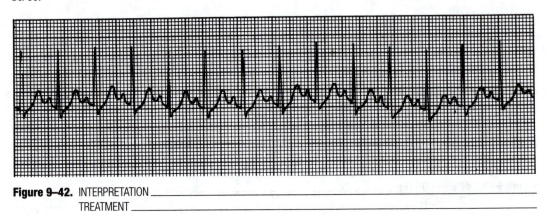

Figure 9–42. INTERPRETATION _____
                      TREATMENT _____

This is the ECG of an 18-year-old male involved in an automobile accident. He is pulseless, apneic, and cyanotic. He has no obvious signs of trauma.

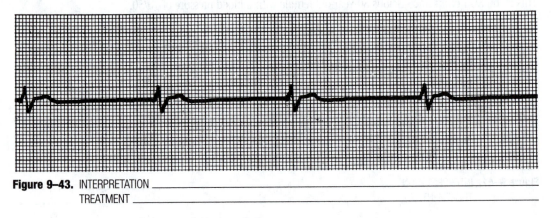

Figure 9–43. INTERPRETATION _____
                      TREATMENT _____

Chapter 9 Treatment of Dysrhythmias

This is the ECG of an unconscious 72-year-old female with a blood pressure of 60/40.

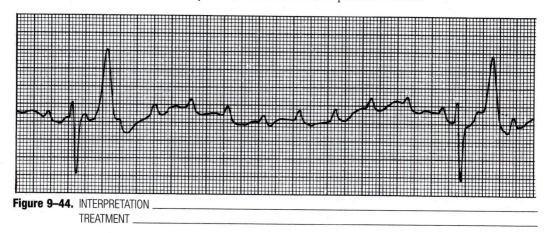

Figure 9–44. INTERPRETATION _____
TREATMENT _____

This is the ECG of an unconscious 35-year-old male who is pulseless and apneic.

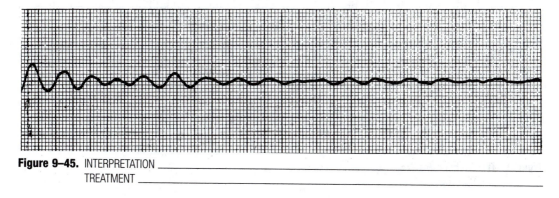

Figure 9–45. INTERPRETATION _____
TREATMENT _____

This is the ECG of a conscious 62-year-old female with a blood pressure of 80/50.

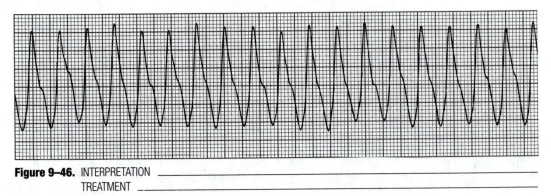

Figure 9–46. INTERPRETATION _____
                   TREATMENT _____

This is the ECG of an 88-year-old male who is pulseless and apneic.

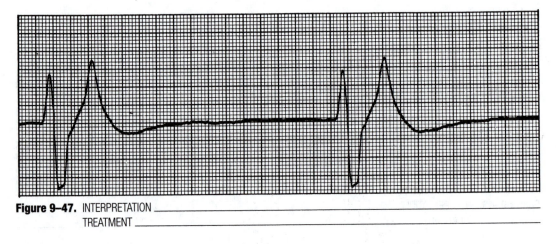

Figure 9–47. INTERPRETATION _____
                   TREATMENT _____

This is the ECG of a 45-year-old male complaining of severe substernal chest pain. His blood pressure is 70/50.

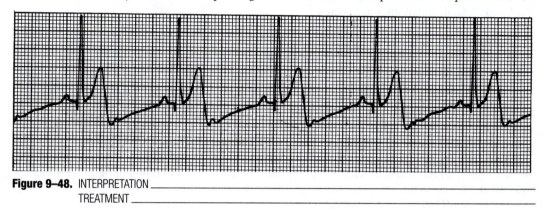

Figure 9–48. INTERPRETATION _____
                       TREATMENT _____

This is the ECG of a 74-year-old male with an acute MI. His blood pressure is 180/60.

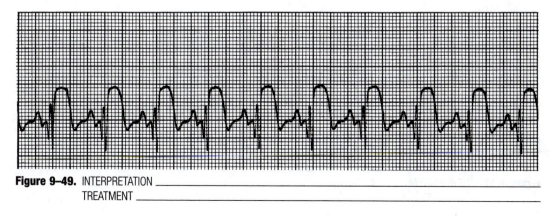

Figure 9–49. INTERPRETATION _____
                       TREATMENT _____

This is the ECG of a 20-year-old conscious male with a history of "rapid heart rate." His blood pressure is 110/70, and his only complaint is palpitations.

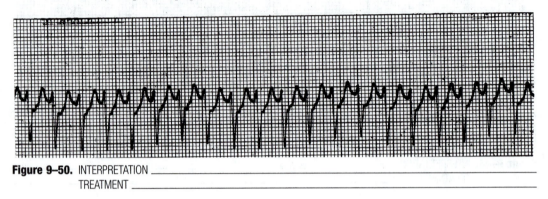

Figure 9–50. INTERPRETATION _____
                 TREATMENT _____

This is the ECG of a 42-year-old male who is complaining of chest pain and "skipped" beats. His blood pressure is 120/70.

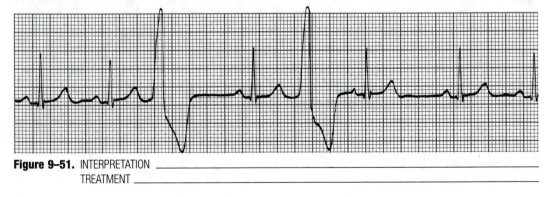

Figure 9–51. INTERPRETATION _____
                 TREATMENT _____

This is the ECG of a 62-year-old male complaining of dyspnea. His blood pressure is 88/60.

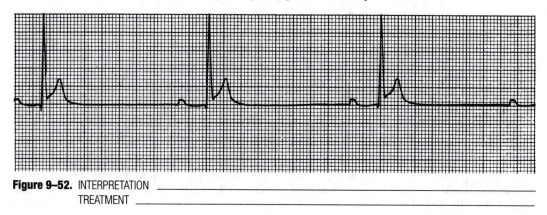

Figure 9–52. INTERPRETATION _____

TREATMENT _____

This is the ECG of a 52-year-old male who is unconscious, pulseless, and apneic.

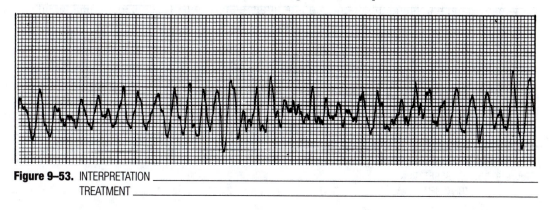

Figure 9–53. INTERPRETATION _____

TREATMENT _____

This is the ECG of a 90-year-old male who is pulseless and apneic.

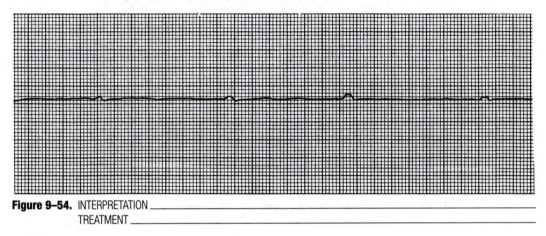

Figure 9–54. INTERPRETATION _____
                TREATMENT _____

This is the ECG of an 82-year-old male who has a blood pressure of 70/50.

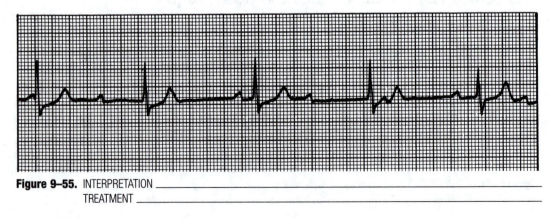

Figure 9–55. INTERPRETATION _____
                TREATMENT _____

This is the ECG of an unconscious 44-year-old male with a blood pressure of 80/52.

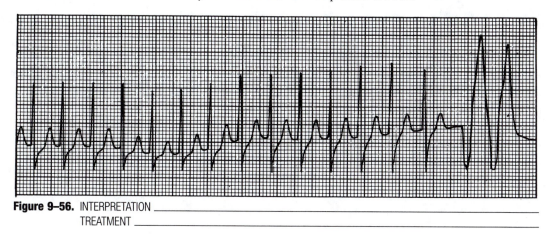

Figure 9–56. INTERPRETATION _____
TREATMENT _____

This is the ECG of an 18-year-old female who tried to commit suicide by turning on the gas heater. She is conscious with stable vital signs.

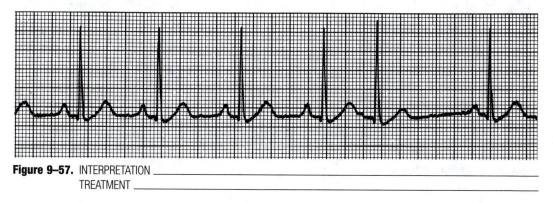

Figure 9–57. INTERPRETATION _____
TREATMENT _____

This is the ECG of an unconscious 63-year-old female with a blood pressure of 60/40.

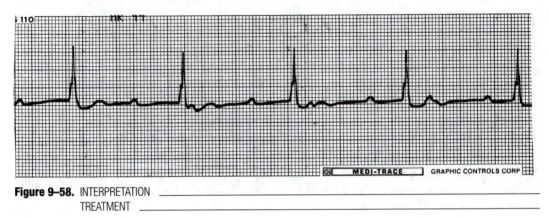

Figure 9–58. INTERPRETATION _____
TREATMENT _____

This is the ECG of a conscious 75-year-old female with shortness of breath and chest pain. Her blood pressure is 80/50.

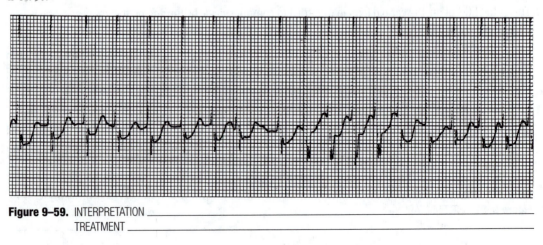

Figure 9–59. INTERPRETATION _____
TREATMENT _____

This is the ECG of a 65-year-old female; her blood pressure is 210/120; respirations are 20; and skin is pale, warm, and dry.

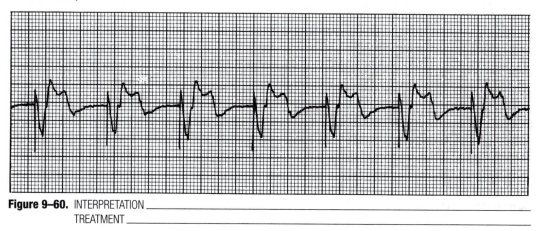

Figure 9–60. INTERPRETATION _____
TREATMENT _____

This is the ECG of a 65-year-old conscious female with a blood pressure of 130/80.

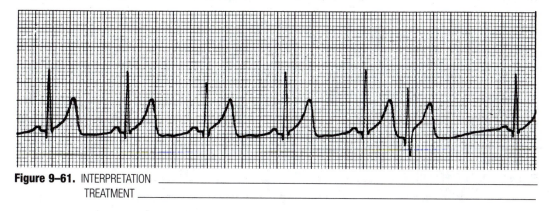

Figure 9–61. INTERPRETATION _____
TREATMENT _____

This is the ECG of a 45-year-old female who is complaining of feeling weak. While taking a history you see the following on the monitor.

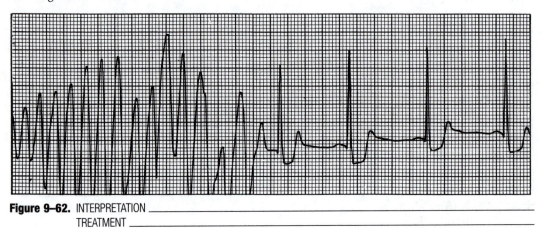

Figure 9–62. INTERPRETATION _____

TREATMENT _____

This is the ECG of a conscious 54-year-old female with a blood pressure of 130/80 and no chief complaint.

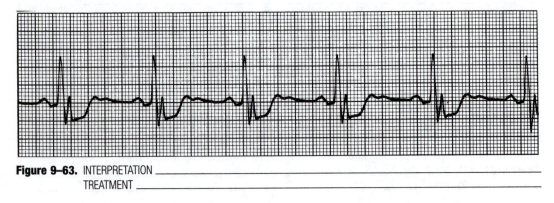

Figure 9–63. INTERPRETATION _____

TREATMENT _____

This is the ECG of a 45-year-old male with chest pain and a blood pressure of 88/60.

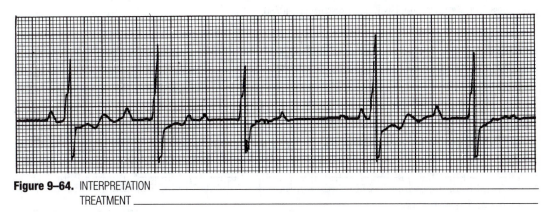

Figure 9–64. INTERPRETATION _____
TREATMENT _____

This is the ECG of an unconscious, pulseless, and apneic 84-year-old male.

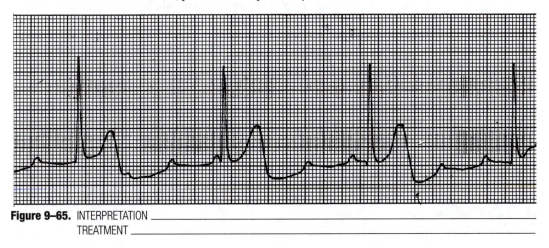

Figure 9–65. INTERPRETATION _____
TREATMENT _____

This is the ECG of a 45-year-old male who had valve surgery three weeks ago. He is complaining of pain and tenderness in his suture line. His blood pressure is 140/80.

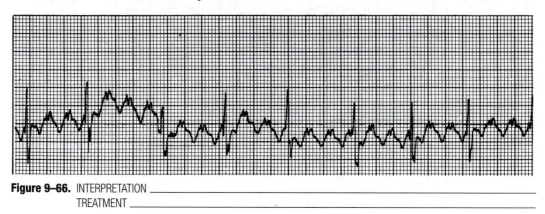

Figure 9–66. INTERPRETATION _____
TREATMENT _____

This is the ECG of a 55-year-old male complaining of feeling weak and light-headed. His blood pressure is 80/60.

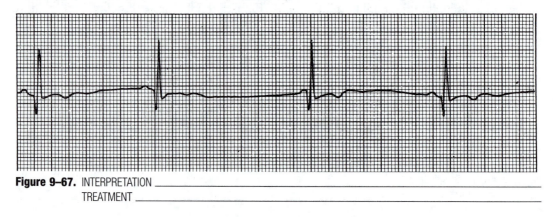

Figure 9–67. INTERPRETATION _____
TREATMENT _____

This is the ECG of a conscious 33-year-old male who has crushing substernal chest pain. His blood pressure is 120/80.

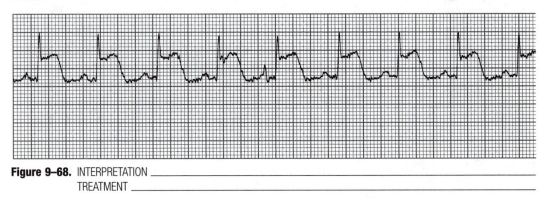

Figure 9–68. INTERPRETATION _____
             TREATMENT _____

This is the ECG of a conscious 51-year-old female who has "skipped" beats. Vital signs are stable.

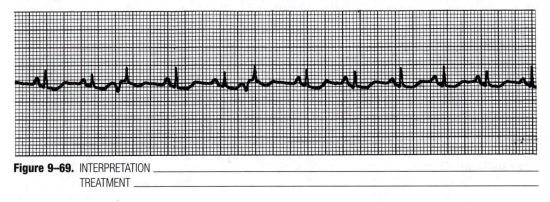

Figure 9–69. INTERPRETATION _____
             TREATMENT _____

This is the ECG of a conscious 72-year-old male who has bilateral rales and is complaining of shortness of breath. His blood pressure is 160/90.

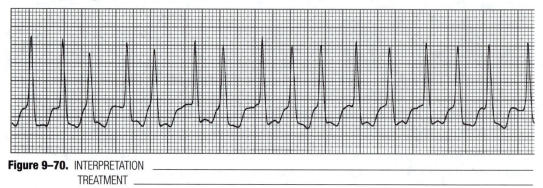

Figure 9–70. INTERPRETATION _____
                    TREATMENT _____

This is the ECG of a 62-year-old male who is on digitalis and complaining of skipped beats. Vital signs are stable.

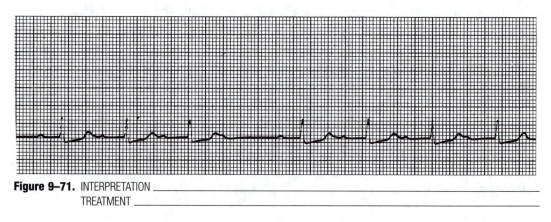

Figure 9–71. INTERPRETATION _____
                    TREATMENT _____

Answer Keys

CHAPTER 1

Answer Key—Matching

1.	b, i	9.	e	17.	l, p	25.	m	32.	e
2.	r	10.	m	18.	b	26.	o	33.	k
3.	a	11.	f	19.	i, n	27.	a	34.	g
4.	h	12.	o	20.	d	28.	j	35.	l
5.	n	13.	q	21.	f	29.	b	36.	h
6.	p	14.	l	22.	e	30.	j	37.	i
7.	k	15.	c	23.	k	31.	n	38.	m
8.	g	16.	g	24.	k				

Answer Key—ECG Practice Strips

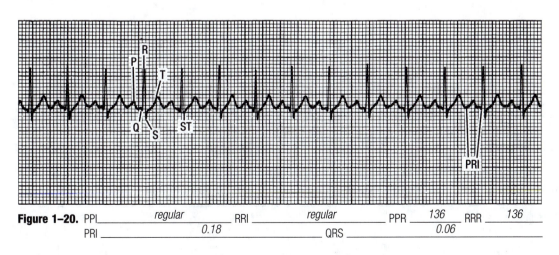

Figure 1–20. PPI _____ *regular* _____ RRI _____ *regular* _____ PPR _____ *136* _____ RRR _____ *136*
PRI _____ *0.18* _____ QRS _____ *0.06*

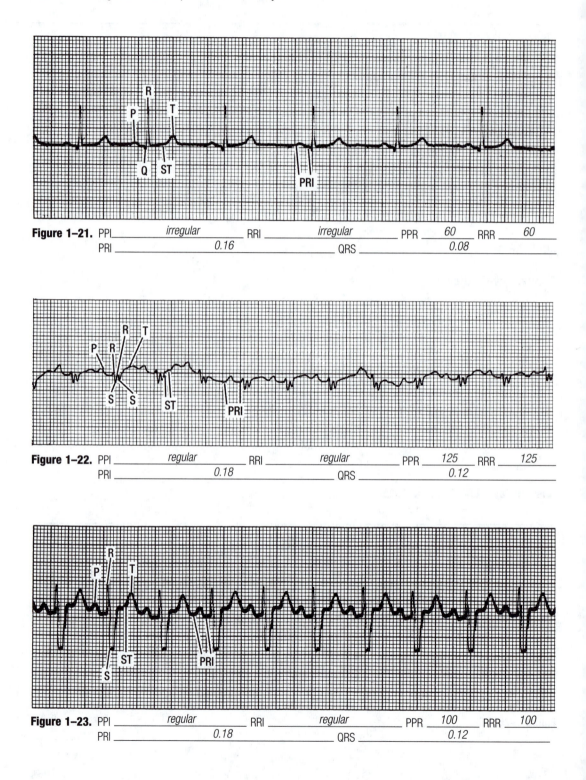

Figure 1–21. PPI _____ _irregular_ _____ RRI _____ _irregular_ _____ PPR __60__ RRR __60__
PRI _____ _0.16_ _____ QRS _____ _0.08_

Figure 1–22. PPI _____ _regular_ _____ RRI _____ _regular_ _____ PPR __125__ RRR __125__
PRI _____ _0.18_ _____ QRS _____ _0.12_

Figure 1–23. PPI _____ _regular_ _____ RRI _____ _regular_ _____ PPR __100__ RRR __100__
PRI _____ _0.18_ _____ QRS _____ _0.12_

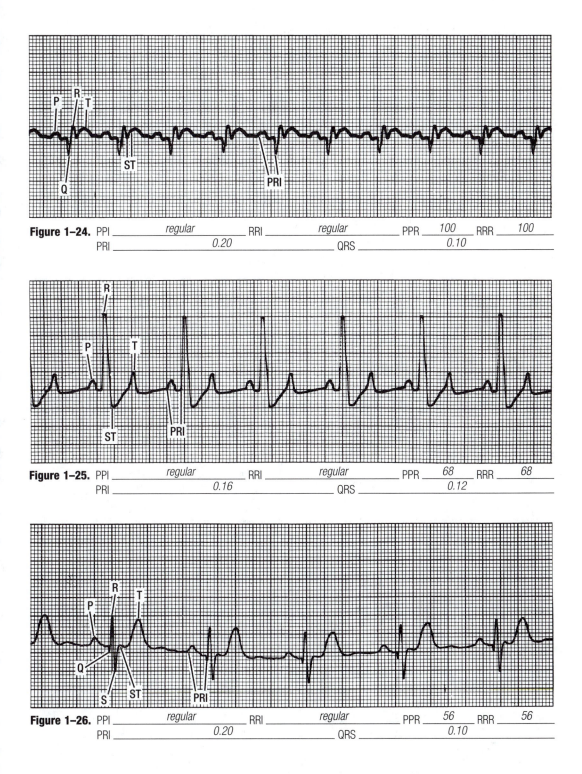

Figure 1–24. PPI _____ *regular* _____ RRI _____ *regular* _____ PPR _____ *100* _____ RRR _____ *100* _____
PRI _____ *0.20* _____ QRS _____ *0.10* _____

Figure 1–25. PPI _____ *regular* _____ RRI _____ *regular* _____ PPR _____ *68* _____ RRR _____ *68* _____
PRI _____ *0.16* _____ QRS _____ *0.12* _____

Figure 1–26. PPI _____ *regular* _____ RRI _____ *regular* _____ PPR _____ *56* _____ RRR _____ *56* _____
PRI _____ *0.20* _____ QRS _____ *0.10* _____

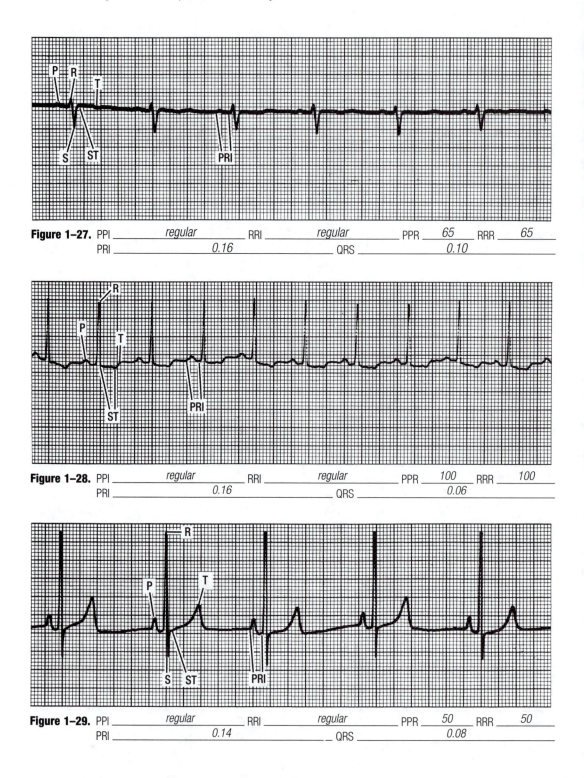

Figure 1–27. PPI _____ *regular* _____ RRI _____ *regular* _____ PPR __ *65* __ RRR __ *65* __
PRI _____ *0.16* _____ QRS _____ *0.10* _____

Figure 1–28. PPI _____ *regular* _____ RRI _____ *regular* _____ PPR __ *100* __ RRR __ *100* __
PRI _____ *0.16* _____ QRS _____ *0.06* _____

Figure 1–29. PPI _____ *regular* _____ RRI _____ *regular* _____ PPR __ *50* __ RRR __ *50* __
PRI _____ *0.14* _____ QRS _____ *0.08* _____

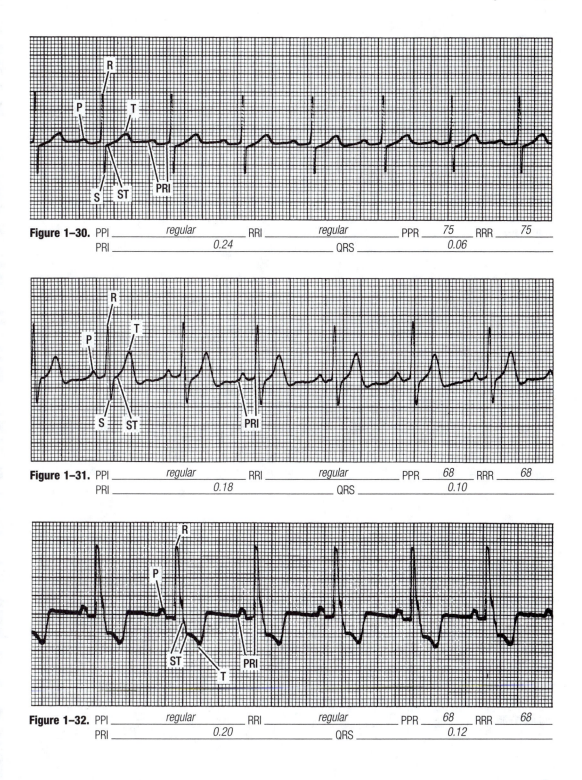

Figure 1–30. PPI _____ *regular* _____ RRI _____ *regular* _____ PPR ___ *75* ___ RRR ___ *75* ___
PRI _____ *0.24* _____ QRS _____ *0.06* _____

Figure 1–31. PPI _____ *regular* _____ RRI _____ *regular* _____ PPR ___ *68* ___ RRR ___ *68* ___
PRI _____ *0.18* _____ QRS _____ *0.10* _____

Figure 1–32. PPI _____ *regular* _____ RRI _____ *regular* _____ PPR ___ *68* ___ RRR ___ *68* ___
PRI _____ *0.20* _____ QRS _____ *0.12* _____

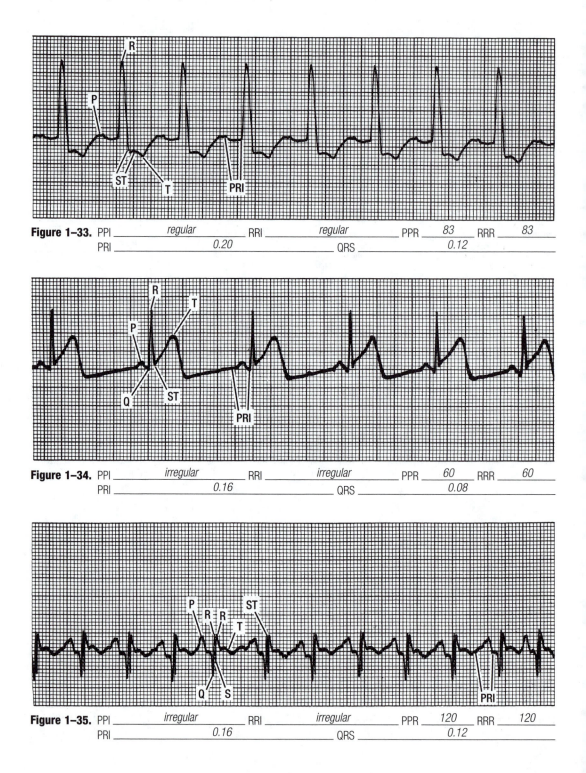

Figure 1–33. PPI _____ *regular* _____ RRI _____ *regular* _____ PPR ___ *83* ___ RRR ___ *83* ___
PRI _____ *0.20* _____ QRS _____ *0.12* _____

Figure 1–34. PPI _____ *irregular* _____ RRI _____ *irregular* _____ PPR ___ *60* ___ RRR ___ *60* ___
PRI _____ *0.16* _____ QRS _____ *0.08* _____

Figure 1–35. PPI _____ *irregular* _____ RRI _____ *irregular* _____ PPR ___ *120* ___ RRR ___ *120* ___
PRI _____ *0.16* _____ QRS _____ *0.12* _____

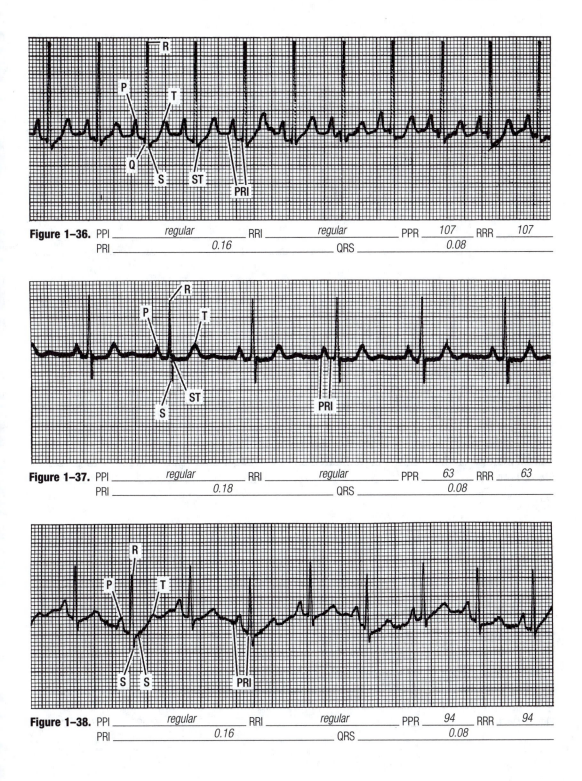

Figure 1–36. PPI _____ *regular* _____ RRI _____ *regular* _____ PPR ___ *107* ___ RRR ___ *107* ___
PRI _____ *0.16* _____ QRS _____ *0.08* _____

Figure 1–37. PPI _____ *regular* _____ RRI _____ *regular* _____ PPR ___ *63* ___ RRR ___ *63* ___
PRI _____ *0.18* _____ QRS _____ *0.08* _____

Figure 1–38. PPI _____ *regular* _____ RRI _____ *regular* _____ PPR ___ *94* ___ RRR ___ *94* ___
PRI _____ *0.16* _____ QRS _____ *0.08* _____

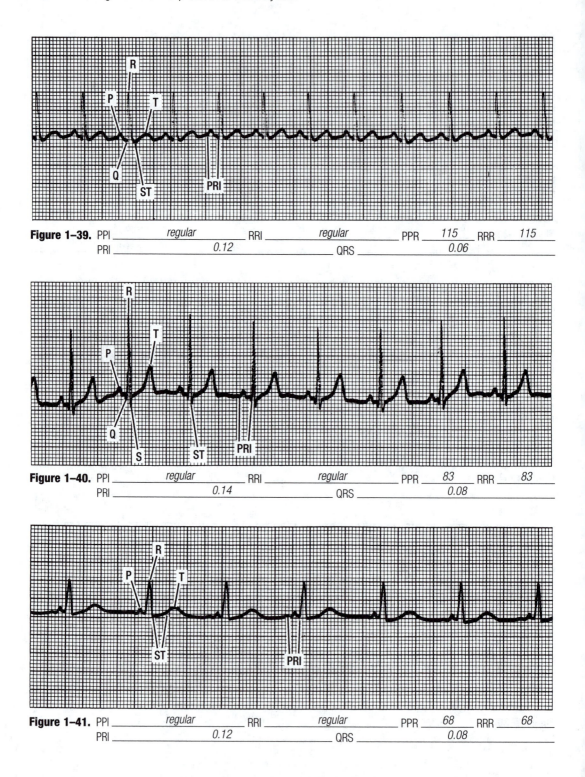

Figure 1–39. PPI _____ *regular* _____ RRI _____ *regular* _____ PPR __ *115* __ RRR __ *115*
PRI _____ *0.12* _____ QRS _____ *0.06*

Figure 1–40. PPI _____ *regular* _____ RRI _____ *regular* _____ PPR __ *83* __ RRR __ *83*
PRI _____ *0.14* _____ QRS _____ *0.08*

Figure 1–41. PPI _____ *regular* _____ RRI _____ *regular* _____ PPR __ *68* __ RRR __ *68*
PRI _____ *0.12* _____ QRS _____ *0.08*

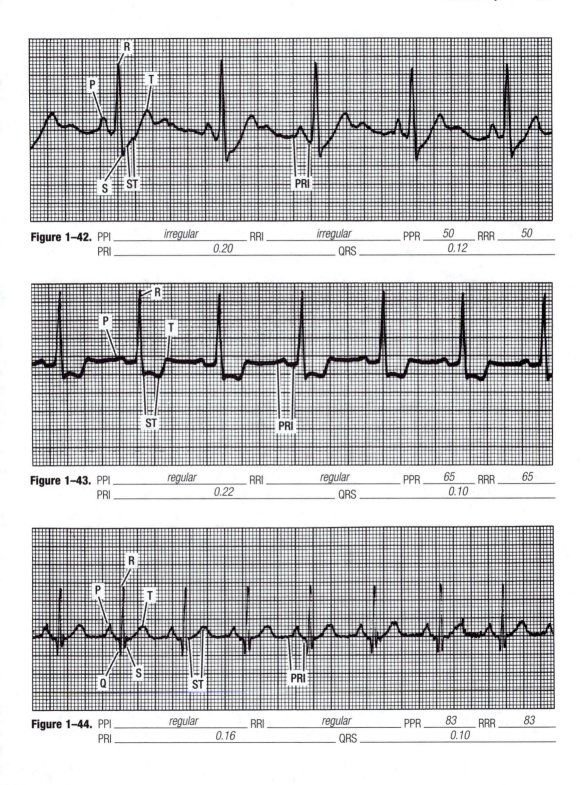

Figure 1–42. PPI _____ *irregular* _____ RRI _____ *irregular* _____ PPR __ *50* __ RRR __ *50*
PRI _____ *0.20* _____ QRS _____ *0.12*

Figure 1–43. PPI _____ *regular* _____ RRI _____ *regular* _____ PPR __ *65* __ RRR __ *65*
PRI _____ *0.22* _____ QRS _____ *0.10*

Figure 1–44. PPI _____ *regular* _____ RRI _____ *regular* _____ PPR __ *83* __ RRR __ *83*
PRI _____ *0.16* _____ QRS _____ *0.10*

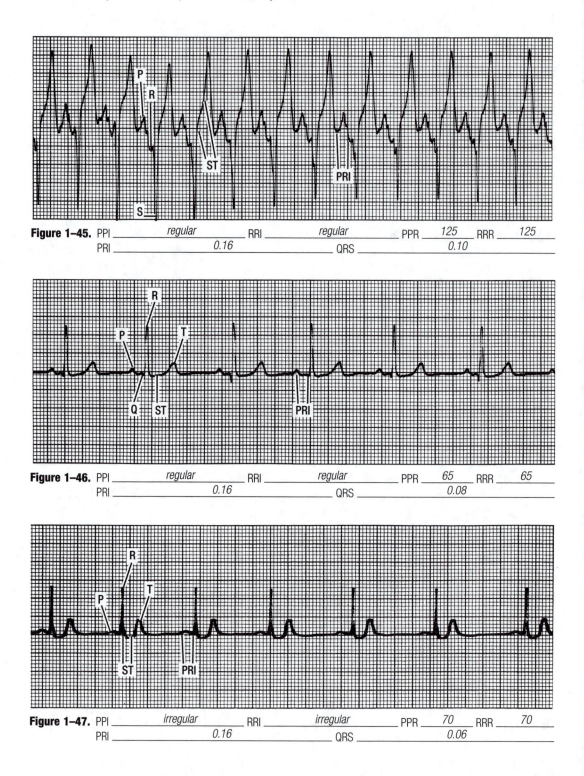

Figure 1–45. PPI _____ *regular* _____ RRI _____ *regular* _____ PPR __ *125* __ RRR __ *125*
PRI _____ *0.16* _____ QRS _____ *0.10*

Figure 1–46. PPI _____ *regular* _____ RRI _____ *regular* _____ PPR __ *65* __ RRR __ *65*
PRI _____ *0.16* _____ QRS _____ *0.08*

Figure 1–47. PPI _____ *irregular* _____ RRI _____ *irregular* _____ PPR __ *70* __ RRR __ *70*
PRI _____ *0.16* _____ QRS _____ *0.06*

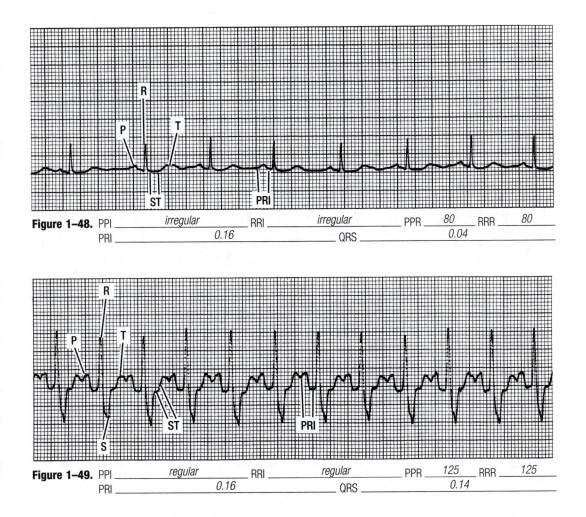

Figure 1–48. PPI _____ *irregular* _____ RRI _____ *irregular* _____ PPR ___80___ RRR ___80___
PRI _____ *0.16* _____ QRS _____ *0.04*

Figure 1–49. PPI _____ *regular* _____ RRI _____ *regular* _____ PPR ___125___ RRR ___125___
PRI _____ *0.16* _____ QRS _____ *0.14*

CHAPTER 2

Answer Key—Matching

1. h	10. a	18. i, c	26. k	34. (a) n
2. c	11. e	19. b	27. d	(b) o
3. a	12. d	20. c	28. h	(c) m
4. i	13. f	21. e	29. g	(d) j
5. j	14. g	22. k	30. d	35. k
6. k	15. s	23. l	31. i	36. f
7. b	16. f	24. o	32. g	37. c
8. b	17. a, h, j, n	25. g	33. b	38. e
9. c				

Answer Key—ECG Practice Strips

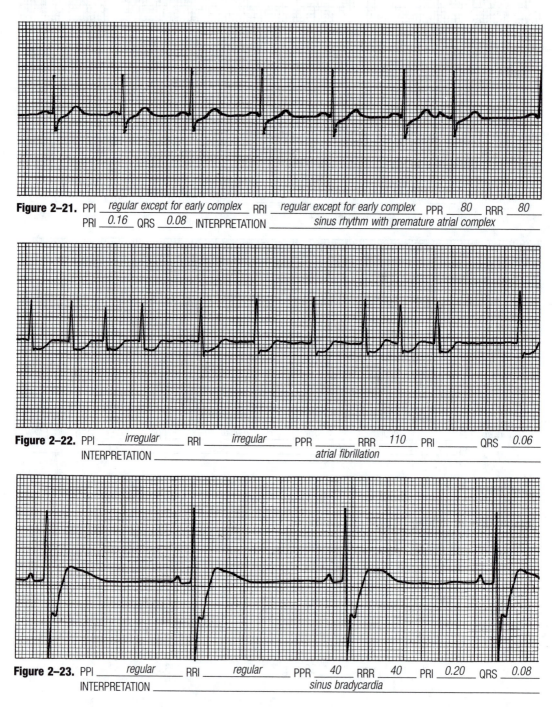

Figure 2–21. PPI _regular except for early complex_ RRI _regular except for early complex_ PPR _80_ RRR _80_
PRI _0.16_ QRS _0.08_ INTERPRETATION _____ sinus rhythm with premature atrial complex _____

Figure 2–22. PPI _____ irregular _____ RRI _____ irregular _____ PPR _____ RRR _110_ PRI _____ QRS _0.06_
INTERPRETATION _____ atrial fibrillation _____

Figure 2–23. PPI _____ regular _____ RRI _____ regular _____ PPR _40_ RRR _40_ PRI _0.20_ QRS _0.08_
INTERPRETATION _____ sinus bradycardia _____

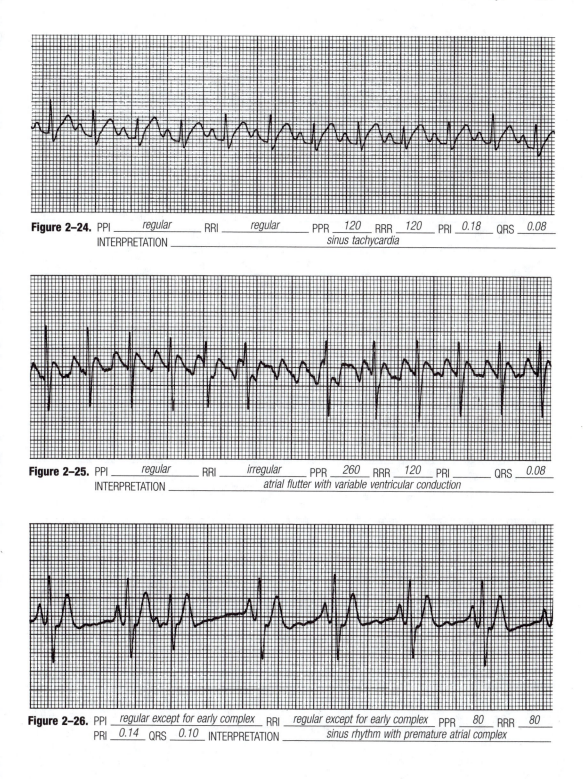

Figure 2–24. PPI _____*regular*_____ RRI _____*regular*_____ PPR __*120*__ RRR __*120*__ PRI _*0.18*_ QRS _*0.08*_
INTERPRETATION _____ *sinus tachycardia*

Figure 2–25. PPI _____*regular*_____ RRI _____*irregular*_____ PPR __*260*__ RRR __*120*__ PRI _____ QRS _*0.08*_
INTERPRETATION _____ *atrial flutter with variable ventricular conduction*

Figure 2–26. PPI _*regular except for early complex*_ RRI _*regular except for early complex*_ PPR __*80*__ RRR __*80*__
PRI _*0.14*_ QRS _*0.10*_ INTERPRETATION _____ *sinus rhythm with premature atrial complex*

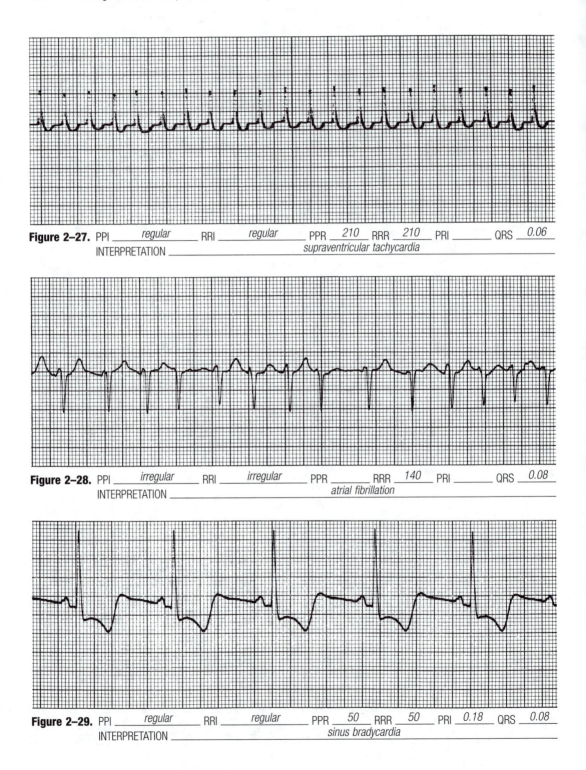

Figure 2–27. PPI _____regular_____ RRI _____regular_____ PPR __210__ RRR __210__ PRI _____ QRS __0.06__
INTERPRETATION _____supraventricular tachycardia_____

Figure 2–28. PPI _____irregular_____ RRI _____irregular_____ PPR _____ RRR __140__ PRI _____ QRS __0.08__
INTERPRETATION _____atrial fibrillation_____

Figure 2–29. PPI _____regular_____ RRI _____regular_____ PPR __50__ RRR __50__ PRI __0.18__ QRS __0.08__
INTERPRETATION _____sinus bradycardia_____

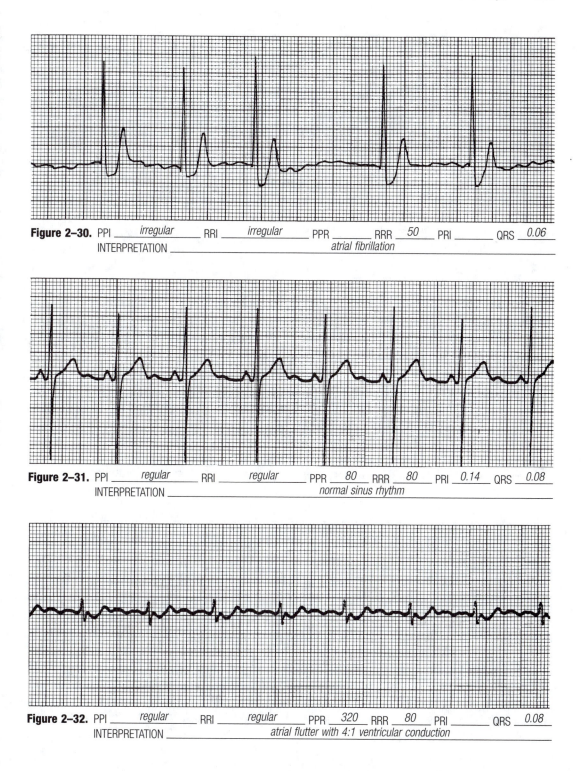

Figure 2–30. PPI ___*irregular*___ RRI ___*irregular*___ PPR _____ RRR ___*50*___ PRI _____ QRS ___*0.06*___
INTERPRETATION _____*atrial fibrillation*_____

Figure 2–31. PPI ___*regular*___ RRI ___*regular*___ PPR ___*80*___ RRR ___*80*___ PRI ___*0.14*___ QRS ___*0.08*___
INTERPRETATION _____*normal sinus rhythm*_____

Figure 2–32. PPI ___*regular*___ RRI ___*regular*___ PPR ___*320*___ RRR ___*80*___ PRI _____ QRS ___*0.08*___
INTERPRETATION _____*atrial flutter with 4:1 ventricular conduction*_____

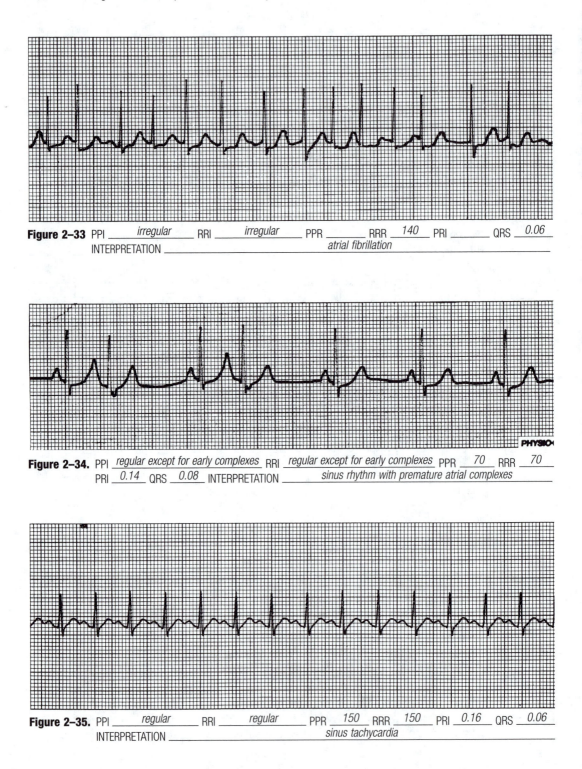

Figure 2–33 PPI _____*irregular*_____ RRI _____*irregular*_____ PPR _____ RRR __*140*__ PRI _____ QRS __*0.06*__
INTERPRETATION _____*atrial fibrillation*_____

Figure 2–34. PPI _*regular except for early complexes*_ RRI _*regular except for early complexes*_ PPR __*70*__ RRR __*70*__
PRI _*0.14*_ QRS _*0.08*_ INTERPRETATION _____*sinus rhythm with premature atrial complexes*_____

Figure 2–35. PPI _____*regular*_____ RRI _____*regular*_____ PPR _*150*_ RRR _*150*_ PRI _*0.16*_ QRS _*0.06*_
INTERPRETATION _____*sinus tachycardia*_____

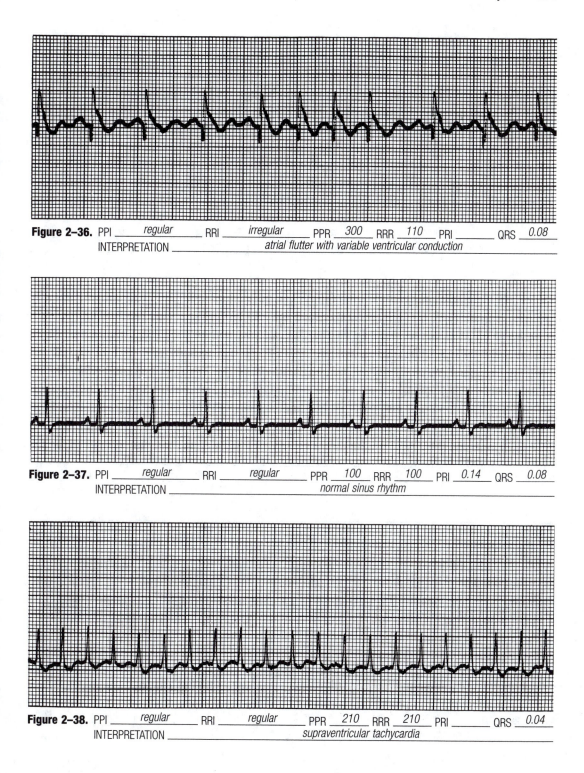

Figure 2–36. PPI _____*regular*_____ RRI _____*irregular*_____ PPR __*300*__ RRR __*110*__ PRI _____ QRS __*0.08*__
INTERPRETATION _____*atrial flutter with variable ventricular conduction*_____

Figure 2–37. PPI _____*regular*_____ RRI _____*regular*_____ PPR __*100*__ RRR __*100*__ PRI __*0.14*__ QRS __*0.08*__
INTERPRETATION _____*normal sinus rhythm*_____

Figure 2–38. PPI _____*regular*_____ RRI _____*regular*_____ PPR __*210*__ RRR __*210*__ PRI _____ QRS __*0.04*__
INTERPRETATION _____*supraventricular tachycardia*_____

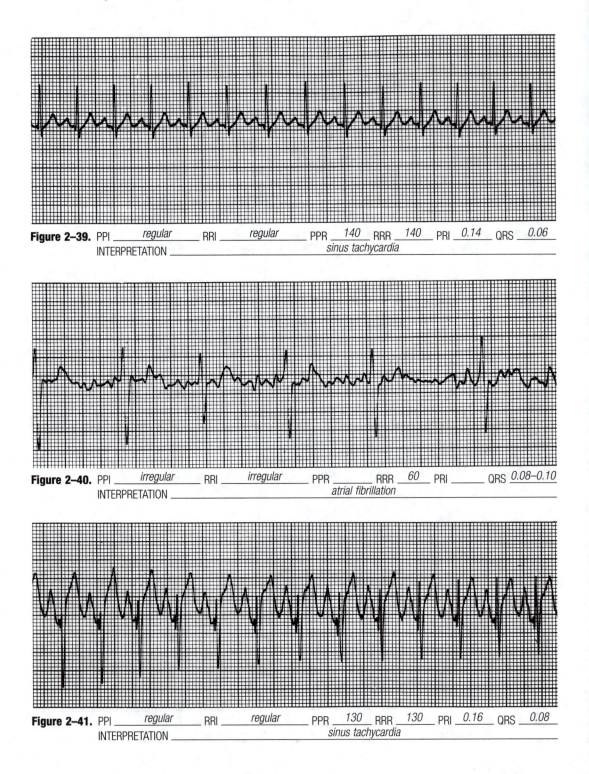

Figure 2–39. PPI _____*regular*_____ RRI _____*regular*_____ PPR __*140*__ RRR __*140*__ PRI __*0.14*__ QRS __*0.06*__
INTERPRETATION _____*sinus tachycardia*_____

Figure 2–40. PPI _____*irregular*_____ RRI _____*irregular*_____ PPR _____ RRR __*60*__ PRI _____ QRS *0.08–0.10*
INTERPRETATION _____*atrial fibrillation*_____

Figure 2–41. PPI _____*regular*_____ RRI _____*regular*_____ PPR __*130*__ RRR __*130*__ PRI __*0.16*__ QRS __*0.08*__
INTERPRETATION _____*sinus tachycardia*_____

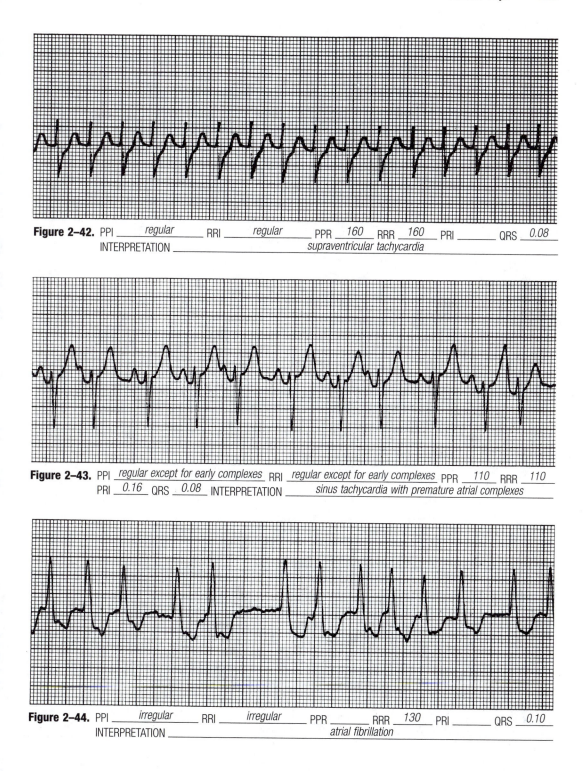

Figure 2–42. PPI _____regular_____ RRI _____regular_____ PPR __160__ RRR __160__ PRI _____ QRS __0.08__
INTERPRETATION _____ supraventricular tachycardia _____

Figure 2–43. PPI _regular except for early complexes_ RRI _regular except for early complexes_ PPR __110__ RRR __110__
PRI _0.16_ QRS _0.08_ INTERPRETATION ____ sinus tachycardia with premature atrial complexes ____

Figure 2–44. PPI _____irregular_____ RRI _____irregular_____ PPR _____ RRR __130__ PRI _____ QRS __0.10__
INTERPRETATION _____ atrial fibrillation _____

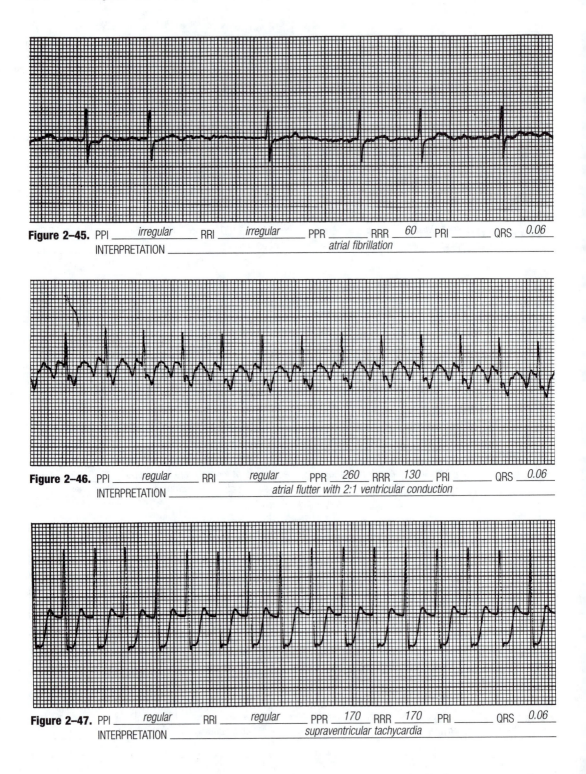

Figure 2–45. PPI _____*irregular*_____ RRI _____*irregular*_____ PPR _____ RRR __*60*__ PRI _____ QRS __*0.06*__
INTERPRETATION _____*atrial fibrillation*_____

Figure 2–46. PPI _____*regular*_____ RRI _____*regular*_____ PPR __*260*__ RRR __*130*__ PRI _____ QRS __*0.06*__
INTERPRETATION _____*atrial flutter with 2:1 ventricular conduction*_____

Figure 2–47. PPI _____*regular*_____ RRI _____*regular*_____ PPR __*170*__ RRR __*170*__ PRI _____ QRS __*0.06*__
INTERPRETATION _____*supraventricular tachycardia*_____

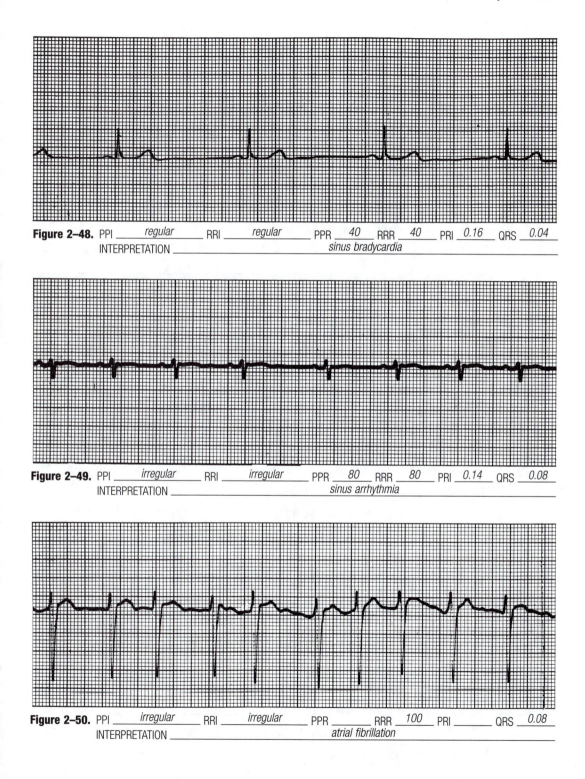

Figure 2–48. PPI _____regular_____ RRI _____regular_____ PPR __40__ RRR __40__ PRI _0.16_ QRS _0.04_
INTERPRETATION _____ _sinus bradycardia_ _____

Figure 2–49. PPI _____irregular_____ RRI _____irregular_____ PPR __80__ RRR __80__ PRI _0.14_ QRS _0.08_
INTERPRETATION _____ _sinus arrhythmia_ _____

Figure 2–50. PPI _____irregular_____ RRI _____irregular_____ PPR _____ RRR _100_ PRI _____ QRS _0.08_
INTERPRETATION _____ _atrial fibrillation_ _____

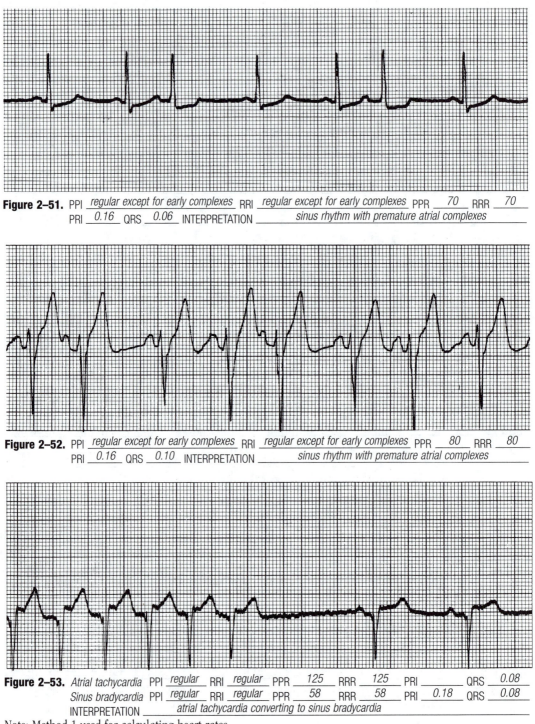

Figure 2–51. PPI _regular except for early complexes_ RRI _regular except for early complexes_ PPR _70_ RRR _70_
PRI _0.16_ QRS _0.06_ INTERPRETATION _sinus rhythm with premature atrial complexes_

Figure 2–52. PPI _regular except for early complexes_ RRI _regular except for early complexes_ PPR _80_ RRR _80_
PRI _0.16_ QRS _0.10_ INTERPRETATION _sinus rhythm with premature atrial complexes_

Figure 2–53. _Atrial tachycardia_ PPI _regular_ RRI _regular_ PPR _125_ RRR _125_ PRI _____ QRS _0.08_
Sinus bradycardia PPI _regular_ RRI _regular_ PPR _58_ RRR _58_ PRI _0.18_ QRS _0.08_
INTERPRETATION _atrial tachycardia converting to sinus bradycardia_

Note: Method 1 used for calculating heart rates.

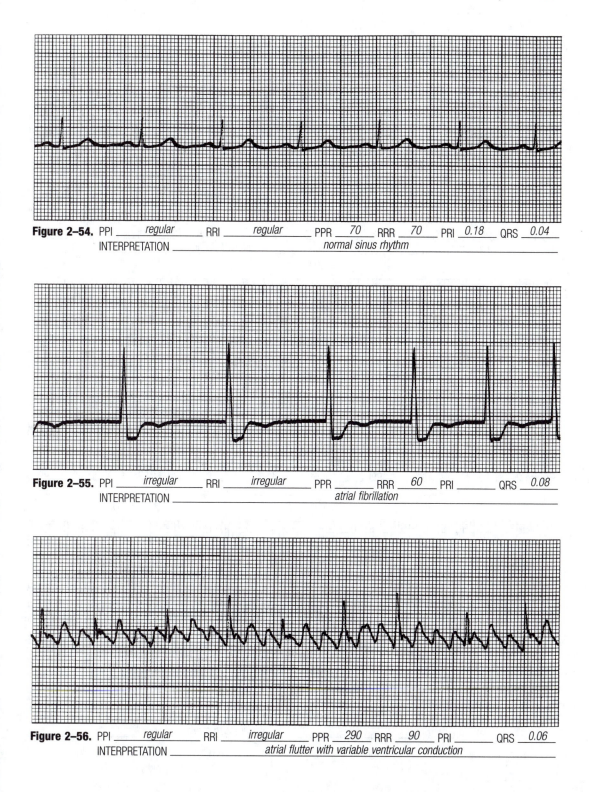

Figure 2–54. PPI _____*regular*_____ RRI _____*regular*_____ PPR __*70*__ RRR __*70*__ PRI _*0.18*_ QRS _*0.04*_
INTERPRETATION _____*normal sinus rhythm*_____

Figure 2–55. PPI _____*irregular*_____ RRI _____*irregular*_____ PPR _____ RRR __*60*__ PRI _____ QRS _*0.08*_
INTERPRETATION _____*atrial fibrillation*_____

Figure 2–56. PPI _____*regular*_____ RRI _____*irregular*_____ PPR __*290*__ RRR __*90*__ PRI _____ QRS _*0.06*_
INTERPRETATION _____*atrial flutter with variable ventricular conduction*_____

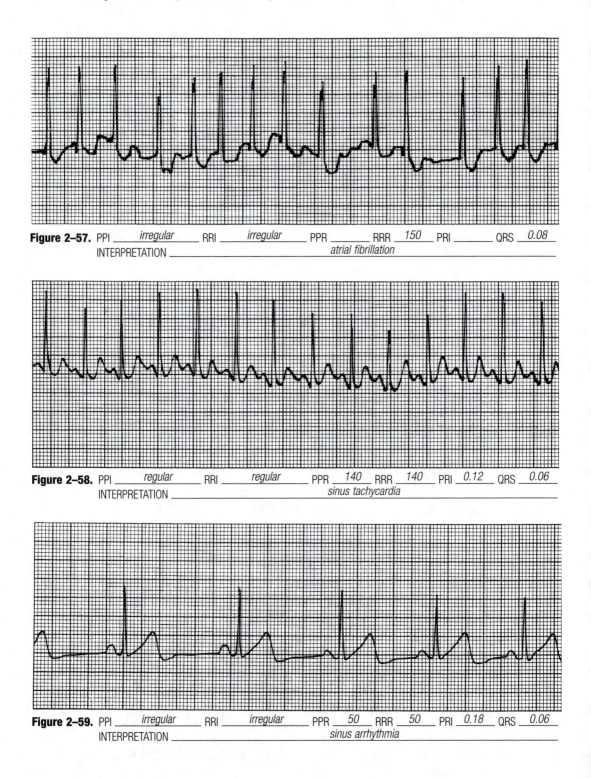

Figure 2–57. PPI _____*irregular*_____ RRI _____*irregular*_____ PPR _____ RRR _*150*_ PRI _____ QRS _*0.08*_
INTERPRETATION _____*atrial fibrillation*_____

Figure 2–58. PPI _____*regular*_____ RRI _____*regular*_____ PPR _*140*_ RRR _*140*_ PRI _*0.12*_ QRS _*0.06*_
INTERPRETATION _____*sinus tachycardia*_____

Figure 2–59. PPI _____*irregular*_____ RRI _____*irregular*_____ PPR _*50*_ RRR _*50*_ PRI _*0.18*_ QRS _*0.06*_
INTERPRETATION _____*sinus arrhythmia*_____

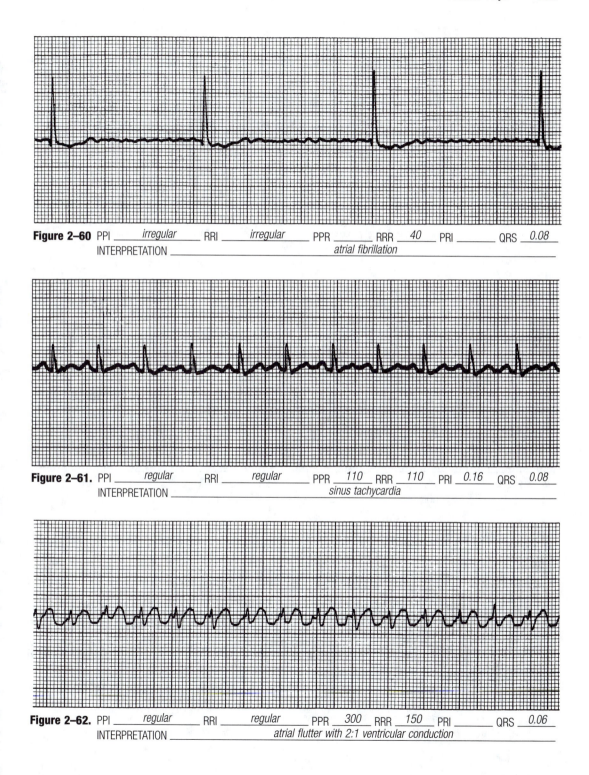

Figure 2–60 PPI ___*irregular*___ RRI ___*irregular*___ PPR _____ RRR __*40*__ PRI _____ QRS __*0.08*__
INTERPRETATION _____*atrial fibrillation*_____

Figure 2–61. PPI ___*regular*___ RRI ___*regular*___ PPR __*110*__ RRR __*110*__ PRI __*0.16*__ QRS __*0.08*__
INTERPRETATION _____*sinus tachycardia*_____

Figure 2–62. PPI ___*regular*___ RRI ___*regular*___ PPR __*300*__ RRR __*150*__ PRI _____ QRS __*0.06*__
INTERPRETATION _____*atrial flutter with 2:1 ventricular conduction*_____

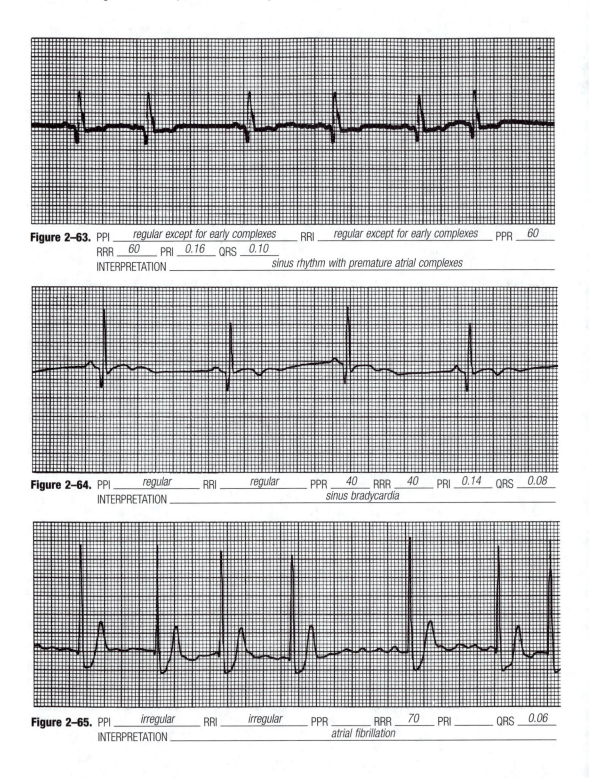

Figure 2–63. PPI _regular except for early complexes_ RRI _regular except for early complexes_ PPR _60_
RRR _60_ PRI _0.16_ QRS _0.10_
INTERPRETATION _sinus rhythm with premature atrial complexes_

Figure 2–64. PPI _regular_ RRI _regular_ PPR _40_ RRR _40_ PRI _0.14_ QRS _0.08_
INTERPRETATION _sinus bradycardia_

Figure 2–65. PPI _irregular_ RRI _irregular_ PPR _____ RRR _70_ PRI _____ QRS _0.06_
INTERPRETATION _atrial fibrillation_

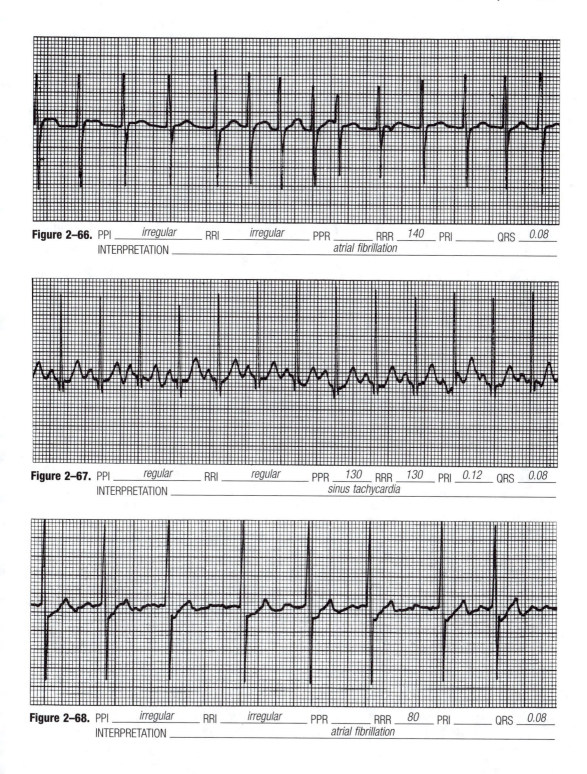

Figure 2–66. PPI _____*irregular*_____ RRI _____*irregular*_____ PPR _____ RRR __*140*__ PRI _____ QRS __*0.08*__
INTERPRETATION _____*atrial fibrillation*_____

Figure 2–67. PPI _____*regular*_____ RRI _____*regular*_____ PPR __*130*__ RRR __*130*__ PRI __*0.12*__ QRS __*0.08*__
INTERPRETATION _____*sinus tachycardia*_____

Figure 2–68. PPI _____*irregular*_____ RRI _____*irregular*_____ PPR _____ RRR __*80*__ PRI _____ QRS __*0.08*__
INTERPRETATION _____*atrial fibrillation*_____

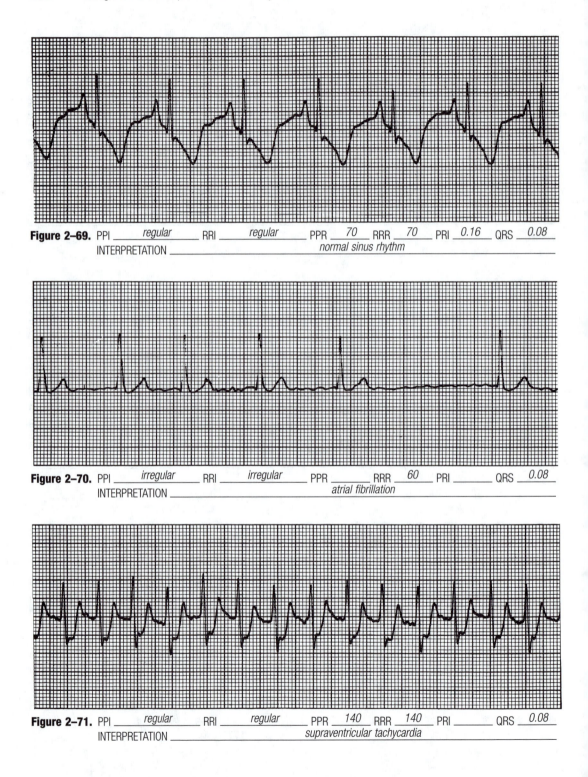

Figure 2–69. PPI _____*regular*_____ RRI _____*regular*_____ PPR __*70*__ RRR __*70*__ PRI _*0.16*_ QRS _*0.08*_
INTERPRETATION _____*normal sinus rhythm*_____

Figure 2–70. PPI _____*irregular*_____ RRI _____*irregular*_____ PPR _____ RRR __*60*__ PRI _____ QRS _*0.08*_
INTERPRETATION _____*atrial fibrillation*_____

Figure 2–71. PPI _____*regular*_____ RRI _____*regular*_____ PPR __*140*__ RRR __*140*__ PRI _____ QRS _*0.08*_
INTERPRETATION _____*supraventricular tachycardia*_____

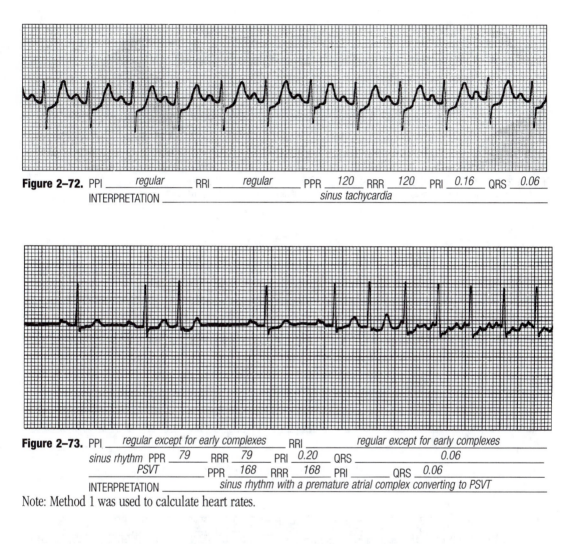

Figure 2–72. PPI _____*regular*_____ RRI _____*regular*_____ PPR __120__ RRR __120__ PRI __0.16__ QRS __0.06__
INTERPRETATION _____*sinus tachycardia*_____

Figure 2–73. PPI ___*regular except for early complexes*___ RRI _____*regular except for early complexes*_____
sinus rhythm PPR __79__ RRR __79__ PRI __0.20__ QRS _____*0.06*_____
_____*PSVT*_____ PPR __168__ RRR __168__ PRI _____ QRS __0.06__
INTERPRETATION _____*sinus rhythm with a premature atrial complex converting to PSVT*_____

Note: Method 1 was used to calculate heart rates.

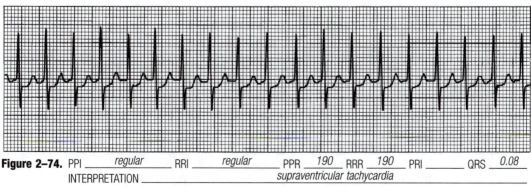

Figure 2–74. PPI _____*regular*_____ RRI _____*regular*_____ PPR __190__ RRR __190__ PRI _____ QRS __0.08__
INTERPRETATION _____*supraventricular tachycardia*_____

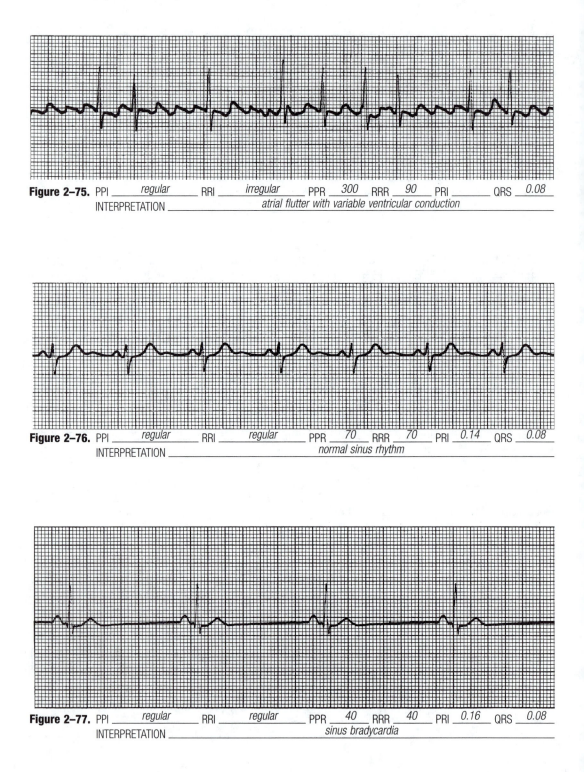

Figure 2–75. PPI _____*regular*_____ RRI _____*irregular*_____ PPR __*300*__ RRR __*90*__ PRI _____ QRS __*0.08*__
INTERPRETATION _____*atrial flutter with variable ventricular conduction*_____

Figure 2–76. PPI _____*regular*_____ RRI _____*regular*_____ PPR __*70*__ RRR __*70*__ PRI _*0.14*_ QRS __*0.08*__
INTERPRETATION _____*normal sinus rhythm*_____

Figure 2–77. PPI _____*regular*_____ RRI _____*regular*_____ PPR __*40*__ RRR __*40*__ PRI _*0.16*_ QRS __*0.08*__
INTERPRETATION _____*sinus bradycardia*_____

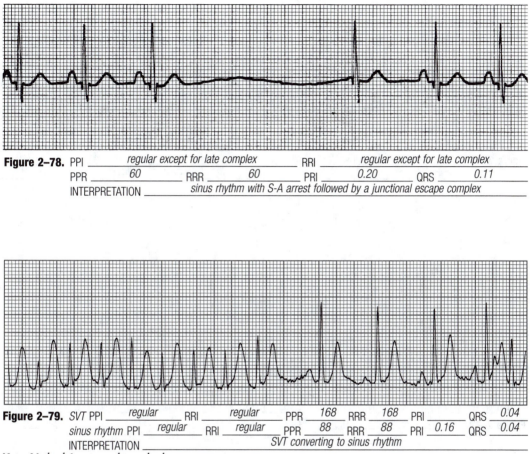

Figure 2–78. PPI _____ *regular except for late complex* _____ RRI _____ *regular except for late complex* _____
PPR _____ *60* _____ RRR _____ *60* _____ PRI _____ *0.20* _____ QRS _____ *0.11* _____
INTERPRETATION _____ *sinus rhythm with S-A arrest followed by a junctional escape complex* _____

Figure 2–79. *SVT* PPI _____ *regular* _____ RRI _____ *regular* _____ PPR _____ *168* _____ RRR _____ *168* _____ PRI _____ QRS _____ *0.04* _____
sinus rhythm PPI _____ *regular* _____ RRI _____ *regular* _____ PPR _____ *88* _____ RRR _____ *88* _____ PRI _____ *0.16* _____ QRS _____ *0.04* _____
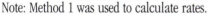
INTERPRETATION _____ *SVT converting to sinus rhythm* _____

Note: Method 1 was used to calculate rates.

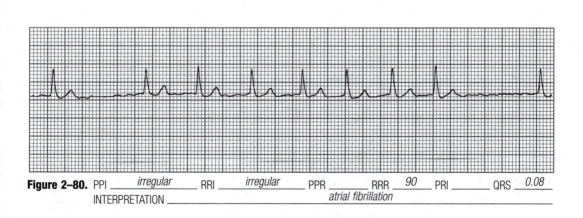

Figure 2–80. PPI _____ *irregular* _____ RRI _____ *irregular* _____ PPR _____ RRR _____ *90* _____ PRI _____ QRS _____ *0.08* _____
INTERPRETATION _____ *atrial fibrillation* _____

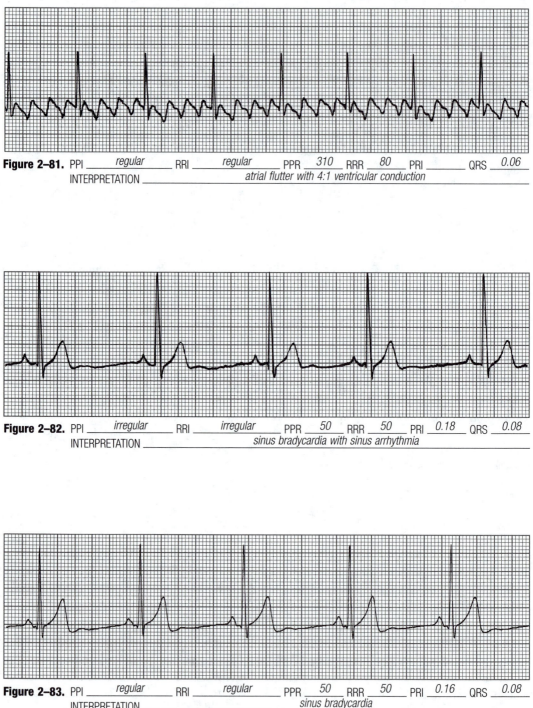

Figure 2–81. PPI _____*regular*_____ RRI _____*regular*_____ PPR __*310*__ RRR __*80*__ PRI _____ QRS __*0.06*__
INTERPRETATION _____*atrial flutter with 4:1 ventricular conduction*_____

Figure 2–82. PPI _____*irregular*_____ RRI _____*irregular*_____ PPR __*50*__ RRR __*50*__ PRI __*0.18*__ QRS __*0.08*__
INTERPRETATION _____*sinus bradycardia with sinus arrhythmia*_____

Figure 2–83. PPI _____*regular*_____ RRI _____*regular*_____ PPR __*50*__ RRR __*50*__ PRI __*0.16*__ QRS __*0.08*__
INTERPRETATION _____*sinus bradycardia*_____

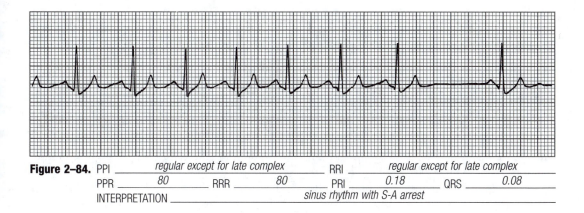

Figure 2–84. PPI _____ *regular except for late complex* _____ RRI _____ *regular except for late complex* _____
PPR _____ *80* _____ RRR _____ *80* _____ PRI _____ *0.18* _____ QRS _____ *0.08* _____
INTERPRETATION _____ *sinus rhythm with S-A arrest* _____

CHAPTER 3

Answer Key—Matching

1. f
2. d
3. g
4. a, i, p
5. b
6. j
7. c
8. l
9. r
10. n
11. h

Answer Key—ECG Practice Strips

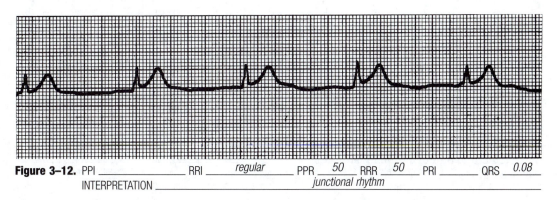

Figure 3–12. PPI _____ RRI _____ *regular* _____ PPR _____ *50* _____ RRR _____ *50* _____ PRI _____ QRS _____ *0.08* _____
INTERPRETATION _____ *junctional rhythm* _____

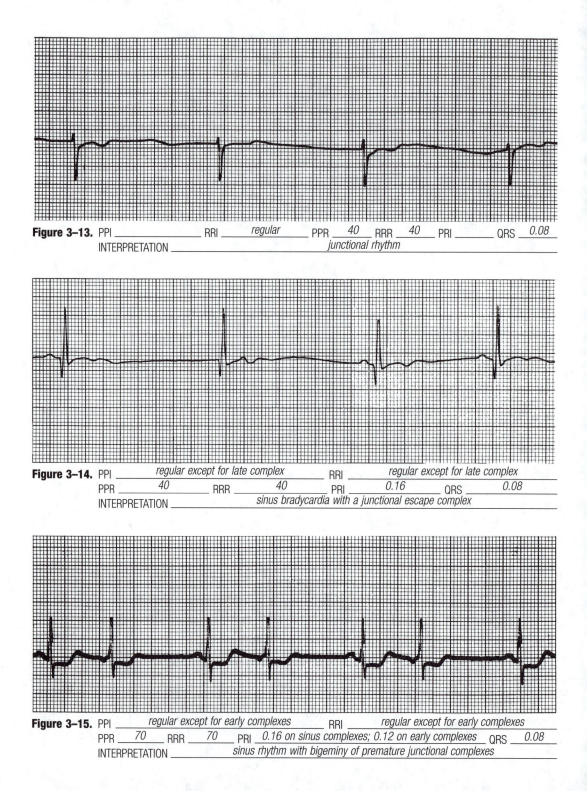

Figure 3–13. PPI _____ RRI ____*regular*____ PPR __*40*__ RRR __*40*__ PRI _____ QRS __*0.08*__
INTERPRETATION _____*junctional rhythm*_____

Figure 3–14. PPI ____*regular except for late complex*____ RRI ____*regular except for late complex*____
PPR ____*40*____ RRR ____*40*____ PRI ____*0.16*____ QRS ____*0.08*____
INTERPRETATION ____*sinus bradycardia with a junctional escape complex*____

Figure 3–15. PPI ____*regular except for early complexes*____ RRI ____*regular except for early complexes*____
PPR __*70*__ RRR __*70*__ PRI _*0.16 on sinus complexes; 0.12 on early complexes*_ QRS __*0.08*__
INTERPRETATION ____*sinus rhythm with bigeminy of premature junctional complexes*____

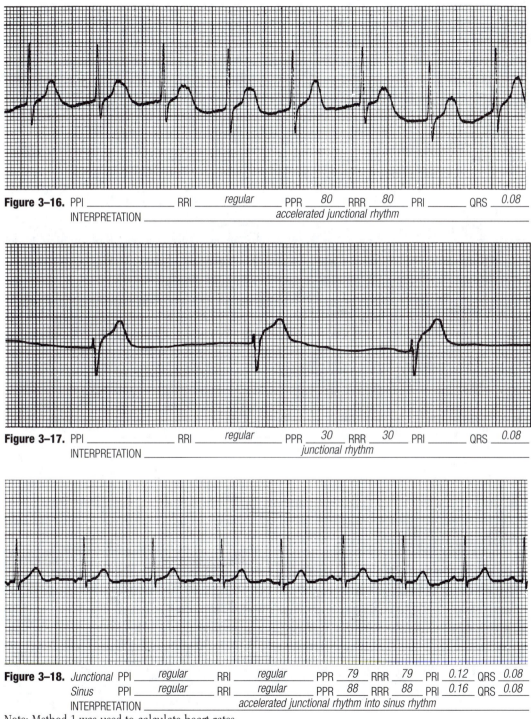

Figure 3–16. PPI _____ RRI ___*regular*___ PPR __*80*__ RRR __*80*__ PRI _____ QRS __*0.08*__
INTERPRETATION _____*accelerated junctional rhythm*_____

Figure 3–17. PPI _____ RRI ___*regular*___ PPR __*30*__ RRR __*30*__ PRI _____ QRS __*0.08*__
INTERPRETATION _____*junctional rhythm*_____

Figure 3–18. *Junctional* PPI ___*regular*___ RRI ___*regular*___ PPR __*79*__ RRR __*79*__ PRI _*0.12*_ QRS _*0.08*_
Sinus PPI ___*regular*___ RRI ___*regular*___ PPR __*88*__ RRR __*88*__ PRI _*0.16*_ QRS _*0.08*_
INTERPRETATION _____*accelerated junctional rhythm into sinus rhythm*_____
Note: Method 1 was used to calculate heart rates.

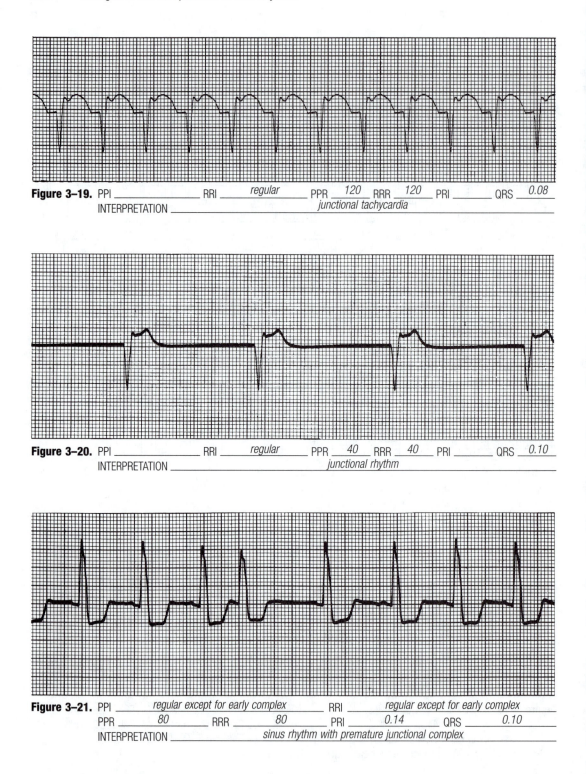

Figure 3–19. PPI _____ RRI _____*regular*_____ PPR __*120*__ RRR __*120*__ PRI _____ QRS __*0.08*__
INTERPRETATION _____*junctional tachycardia*_____

Figure 3–20. PPI _____ RRI _____*regular*_____ PPR __*40*__ RRR __*40*__ PRI _____ QRS __*0.10*__
INTERPRETATION _____*junctional rhythm*_____

Figure 3–21. PPI _____*regular except for early complex*_____ RRI _____*regular except for early complex*_____
PPR __*80*__ RRR __*80*__ PRI __*0.14*__ QRS __*0.10*__
INTERPRETATION _____*sinus rhythm with premature junctional complex*_____

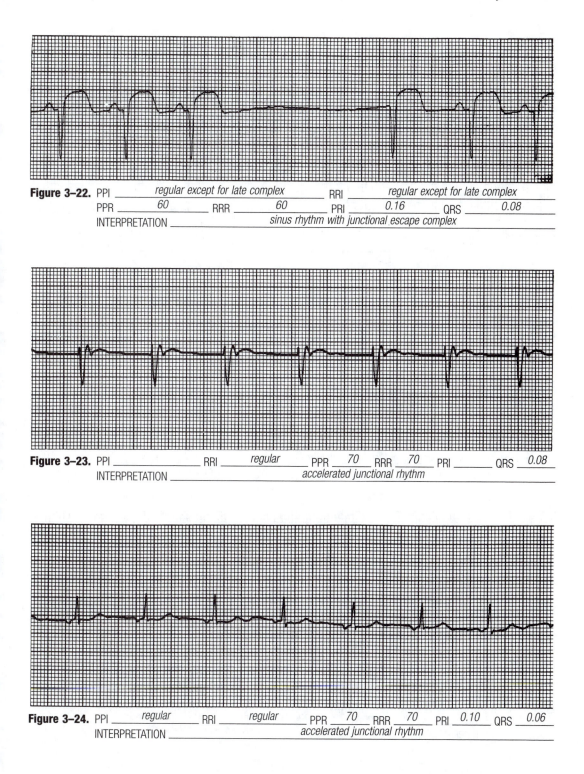

Figure 3–22. PPI _____ _regular except for late complex_ _____ RRI _____ _regular except for late complex_ _____
PPR _____ _60_ _____ RRR _____ _60_ _____ PRI _____ _0.16_ _____ QRS _____ _0.08_ _____
INTERPRETATION _____ _sinus rhythm with junctional escape complex_ _____

Figure 3–23. PPI _____ _____ RRI _____ _regular_ _____ PPR _____ _70_ _____ RRR _____ _70_ _____ PRI _____ _____ QRS _____ _0.08_ _____
INTERPRETATION _____ _accelerated junctional rhythm_ _____

Figure 3–24. PPI _____ _regular_ _____ RRI _____ _regular_ _____ PPR _____ _70_ _____ RRR _____ _70_ _____ PRI _____ _0.10_ _____ QRS _____ _0.06_ _____
INTERPRETATION _____ _accelerated junctional rhythm_ _____

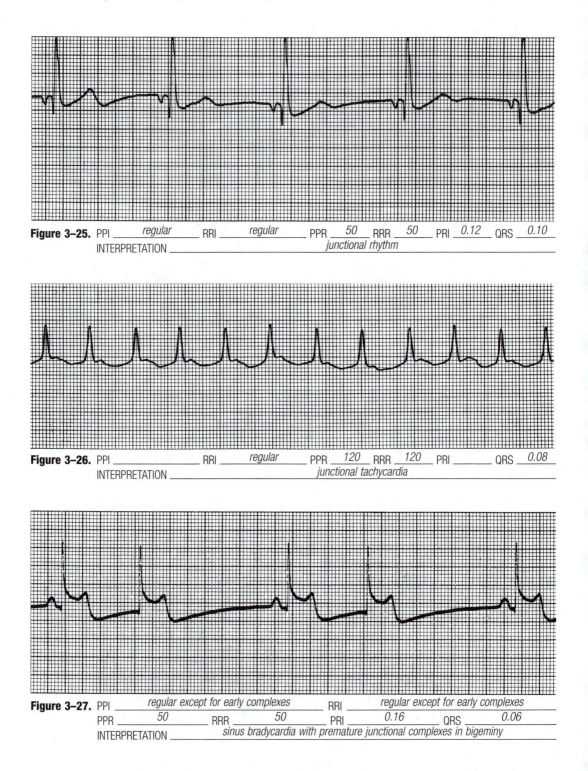

Figure 3–25. PPI _____*regular*_____ RRI _____*regular*_____ PPR __*50*__ RRR __*50*__ PRI _*0.12*_ QRS _*0.10*_
INTERPRETATION _____*junctional rhythm*_____

Figure 3–26. PPI _____ RRI _____*regular*_____ PPR __*120*__ RRR __*120*__ PRI _____ QRS _*0.08*_
INTERPRETATION _____*junctional tachycardia*_____

Figure 3–27. PPI _____*regular except for early complexes*_____ RRI _____*regular except for early complexes*_____
PPR __*50*__ RRR __*50*__ PRI __*0.16*__ QRS __*0.06*__
INTERPRETATION _____*sinus bradycardia with premature junctional complexes in bigeminy*_____

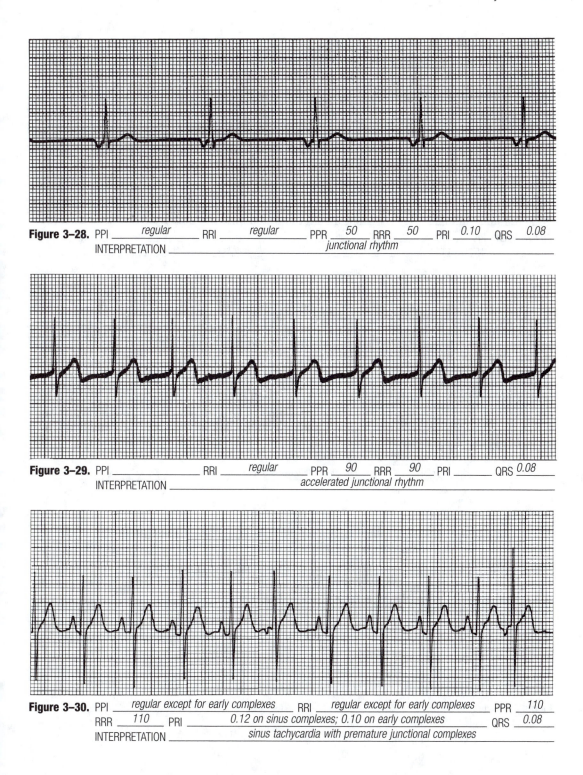

Figure 3–28. PPI _____regular_____ RRI _____regular_____ PPR __50__ RRR __50__ PRI _0.10_ QRS _0.08_
INTERPRETATION _____junctional rhythm_____

Figure 3–29. PPI _____ RRI _____regular_____ PPR __90__ RRR __90__ PRI _____ QRS _0.08_
INTERPRETATION _____accelerated junctional rhythm_____

Figure 3–30. PPI __regular except for early complexes__ RRI __regular except for early complexes__ PPR __110__
RRR __110__ PRI __0.12 on sinus complexes; 0.10 on early complexes__ QRS _0.08_
INTERPRETATION _____sinus tachycardia with premature junctional complexes_____

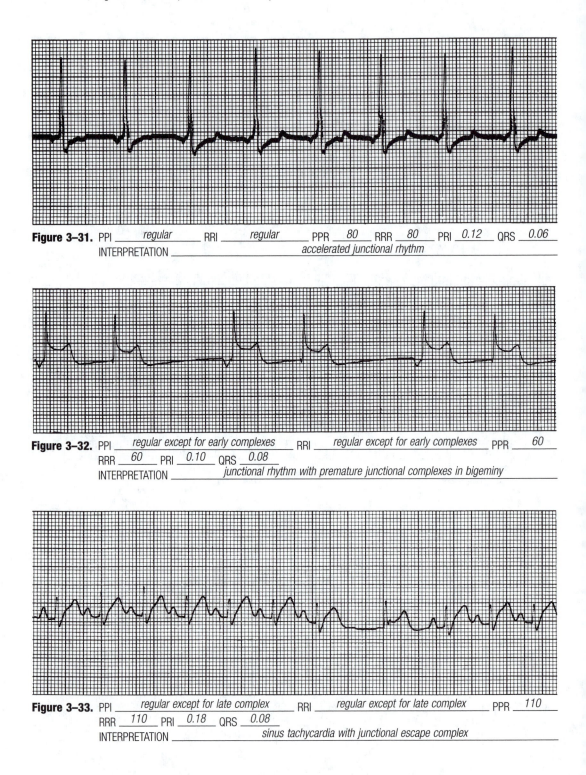

Figure 3–31. PPI _____ *regular* _____ RRI _____ *regular* _____ PPR __ *80* __ RRR __ *80* __ PRI __ *0.12* __ QRS __ *0.06* __
INTERPRETATION _____ *accelerated junctional rhythm* _____

Figure 3–32. PPI __ *regular except for early complexes* __ RRI __ *regular except for early complexes* __ PPR __ *60* __
RRR __ *60* __ PRI __ *0.10* __ QRS __ *0.08* __
INTERPRETATION _____ *junctional rhythm with premature junctional complexes in bigeminy* _____

Figure 3–33. PPI __ *regular except for late complex* __ RRI __ *regular except for late complex* __ PPR __ *110* __
RRR __ *110* __ PRI __ *0.18* __ QRS __ *0.08* __
INTERPRETATION _____ *sinus tachycardia with junctional escape complex* _____

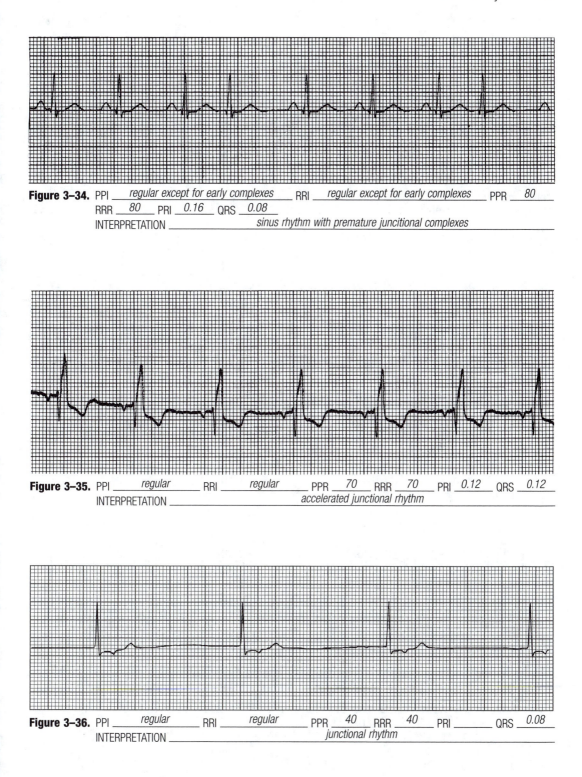

Figure 3–34. PPI ___*regular except for early complexes*___ RRI ___*regular except for early complexes*___ PPR __*80*__
RRR __*80*__ PRI __*0.16*__ QRS __*0.08*__
INTERPRETATION _____*sinus rhythm with premature juncitional complexes*_____

Figure 3–35. PPI _____*regular*_____ RRI _____*regular*_____ PPR __*70*__ RRR __*70*__ PRI __*0.12*__ QRS __*0.12*__
INTERPRETATION _____*accelerated junctional rhythm*_____

Figure 3–36. PPI _____*regular*_____ RRI _____*regular*_____ PPR __*40*__ RRR __*40*__ PRI _____ QRS __*0.08*__
INTERPRETATION _____*junctional rhythm*_____

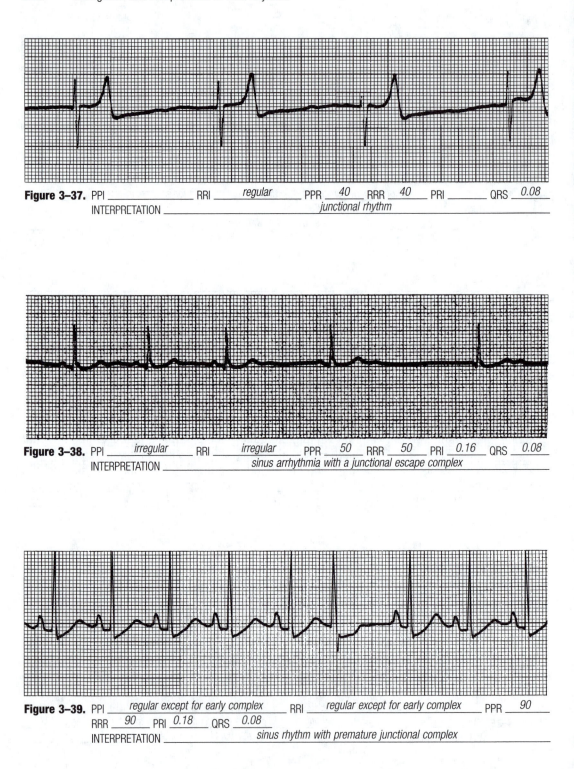

Figure 3–37. PPI _____ RRI _____*regular*_____ PPR __*40*__ RRR __*40*__ PRI _____ QRS __*0.08*__
INTERPRETATION _____*junctional rhythm*_____

Figure 3–38. PPI ___*irregular*___ RRI _____*irregular*_____ PPR __*50*__ RRR __*50*__ PRI _*0.16*_ QRS __*0.08*__
INTERPRETATION _____*sinus arrhythmia with a junctional escape complex*_____

Figure 3–39. PPI ____*regular except for early complex*____ RRI ____*regular except for early complex*____ PPR __*90*__
RRR __*90*__ PRI _*0.18*_ QRS __*0.08*__
INTERPRETATION _____*sinus rhythm with premature junctional complex*_____

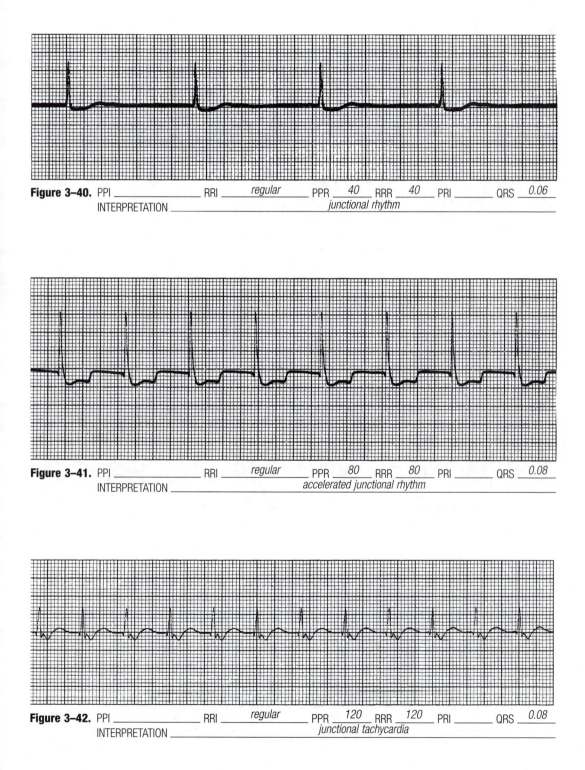

Figure 3–40. PPI _____ RRI _____ *regular* _____ PPR __*40*__ RRR __*40*__ PRI _____ QRS __*0.06*__
INTERPRETATION _____ *junctional rhythm* _____

Figure 3–41. PPI _____ RRI _____ *regular* _____ PPR __*80*__ RRR __*80*__ PRI _____ QRS __*0.08*__
INTERPRETATION _____ *accelerated junctional rhythm* _____

Figure 3–42. PPI _____ RRI _____ *regular* _____ PPR __*120*__ RRR __*120*__ PRI _____ QRS __*0.08*__
INTERPRETATION _____ *junctional tachycardia* _____

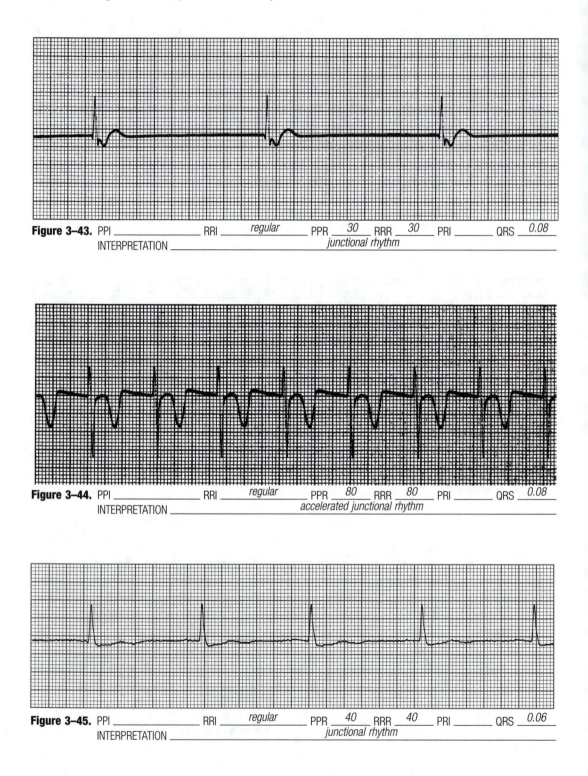

Figure 3–43. PPI _____ RRI ___*regular*___ PPR ___*30*___ RRR ___*30*___ PRI _____ QRS ___*0.08*___
INTERPRETATION _____*junctional rhythm*_____

Figure 3–44. PPI _____ RRI ___*regular*___ PPR ___*80*___ RRR ___*80*___ PRI _____ QRS ___*0.08*___
INTERPRETATION _____*accelerated junctional rhythm*_____

Figure 3–45. PPI _____ RRI ___*regular*___ PPR ___*40*___ RRR ___*40*___ PRI _____ QRS ___*0.06*___
INTERPRETATION _____*junctional rhythm*_____

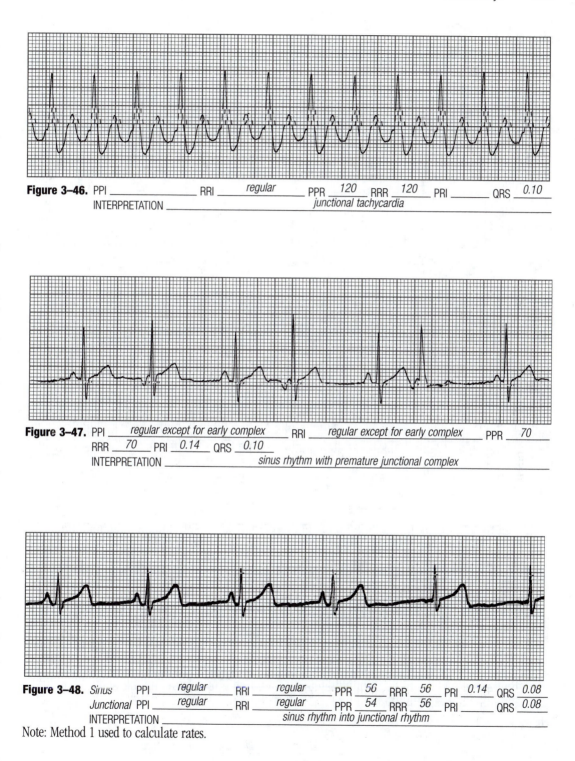

Figure 3–46. PPI _____ RRI ___*regular*___ PPR _*120*_ RRR _*120*_ PRI _____ QRS _*0.10*_
INTERPRETATION _____*junctional tachycardia*_____

Figure 3–47. PPI ___*regular except for early complex*___ RRI ___*regular except for early complex*___ PPR _*70*_
RRR _*70*_ PRI _*0.14*_ QRS _*0.10*_
INTERPRETATION _____*sinus rhythm with premature junctional complex*_____

Figure 3–48. *Sinus* PPI ___*regular*___ RRI ___*regular*___ PPR _*56*_ RRR _*56*_ PRI _*0.14*_ QRS _*0.08*_
Junctional PPI ___*regular*___ RRI ___*regular*___ PPR _*54*_ RRR _*56*_ PRI _____ QRS _*0.08*_
INTERPRETATION _____*sinus rhythm into junctional rhythm*_____

Note: Method 1 used to calculate rates.

CHAPTER 4

Answer Key—ECG Practice Strips

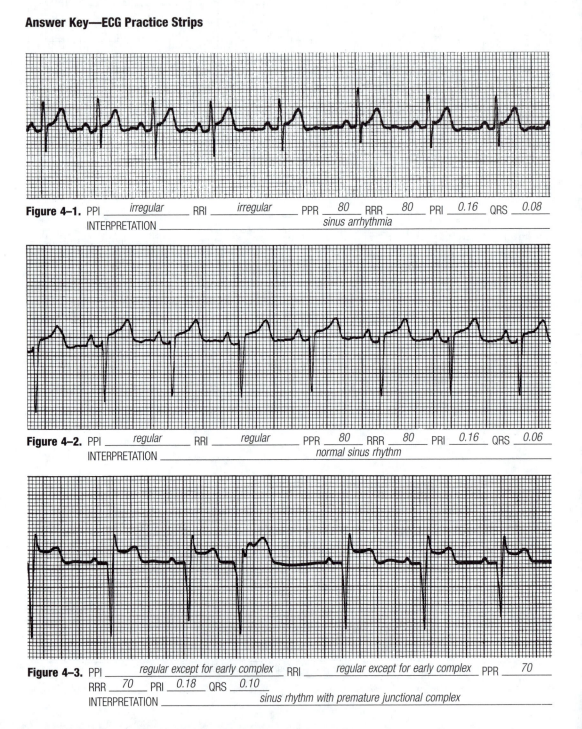

Figure 4–1. PPI _____ *irregular* _____ RRI _____ *irregular* _____ PPR __*80*__ RRR __*80*__ PRI __*0.16*__ QRS __*0.08*__
INTERPRETATION _____ *sinus arrhythmia* _____

Figure 4–2. PPI _____ *regular* _____ RRI _____ *regular* _____ PPR __*80*__ RRR __*80*__ PRI __*0.16*__ QRS __*0.06*__
INTERPRETATION _____ *normal sinus rhythm* _____

Figure 4–3. PPI _____ *regular except for early complex* _____ RRI _____ *regular except for early complex* _____ PPR __*70*__
RRR __*70*__ PRI __*0.18*__ QRS __*0.10*__
INTERPRETATION _____ *sinus rhythm with premature junctional complex*

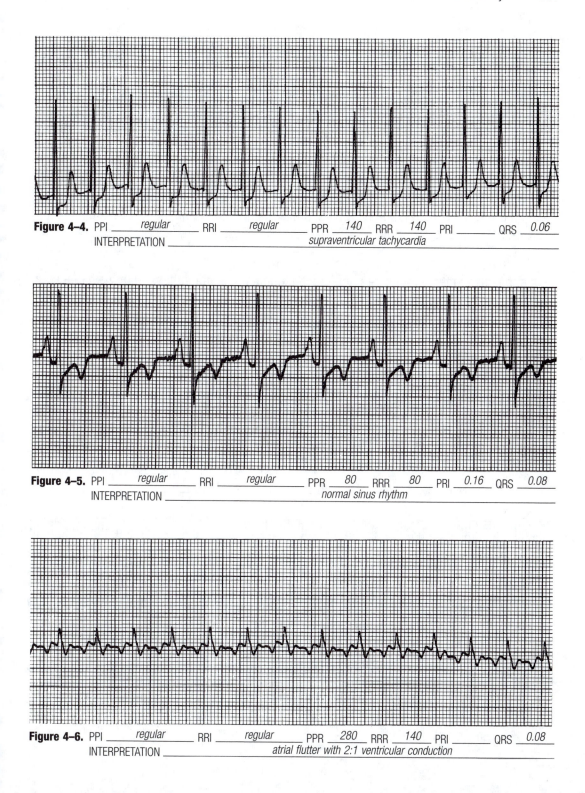

Figure 4–4. PPI _____ *regular* _____ RRI _____ *regular* _____ PPR __*140*__ RRR __*140*__ PRI _____ QRS __*0.06*__
INTERPRETATION _____ *supraventricular tachycardia* _____

Figure 4–5. PPI _____ *regular* _____ RRI _____ *regular* _____ PPR __*80*__ RRR __*80*__ PRI __*0.16*__ QRS __*0.08*__
INTERPRETATION _____ *normal sinus rhythm* _____

Figure 4–6. PPI _____ *regular* _____ RRI _____ *regular* _____ PPR __*280*__ RRR __*140*__ PRI _____ QRS __*0.08*__
INTERPRETATION _____ *atrial flutter with 2:1 ventricular conduction* _____

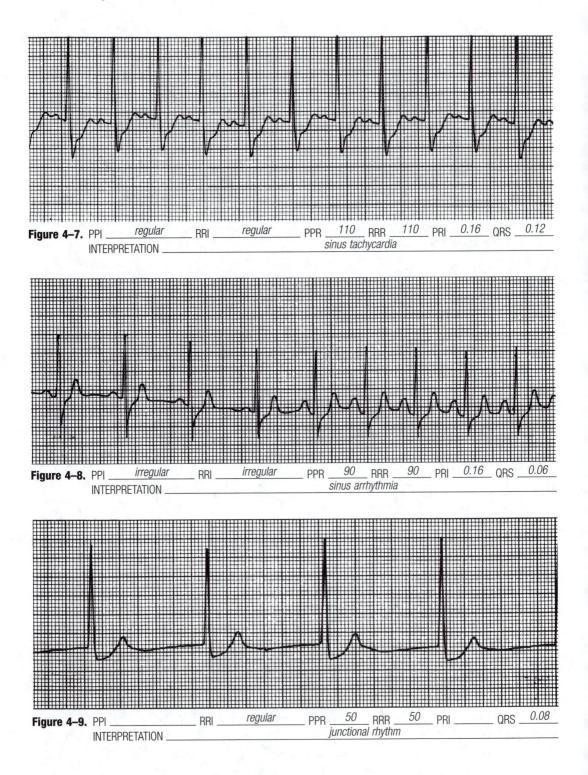

Figure 4–7. PPI _____*regular*_____ RRI _____*regular*_____ PPR __*110*__ RRR __*110*__ PRI __*0.16*__ QRS __*0.12*__
INTERPRETATION _____*sinus tachycardia*_____

Figure 4–8. PPI _____*irregular*_____ RRI _____*irregular*_____ PPR __*90*__ RRR __*90*__ PRI __*0.16*__ QRS __*0.06*__
INTERPRETATION _____*sinus arrhythmia*_____

Figure 4–9. PPI _____ RRI _____*regular*_____ PPR __*50*__ RRR __*50*__ PRI _____ QRS __*0.08*__
INTERPRETATION _____*junctional rhythm*_____

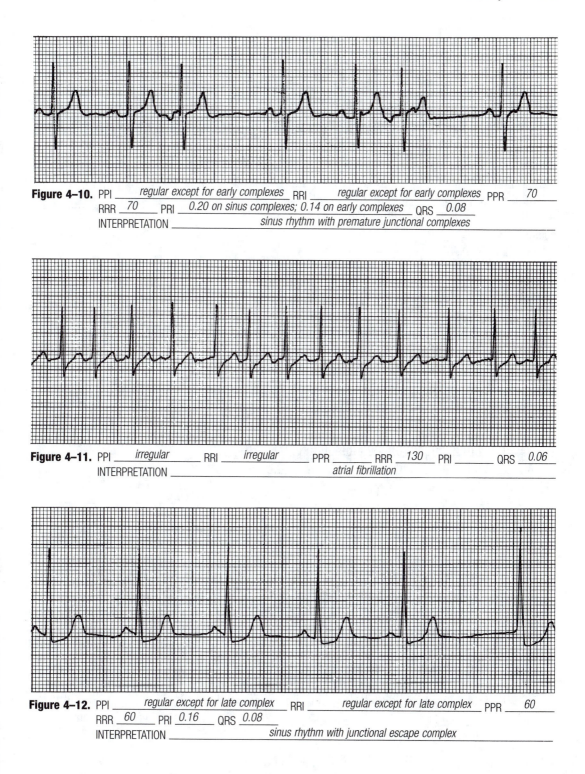

Figure 4–10. PPI ___*regular except for early complexes*___ RRI ___*regular except for early complexes*___ PPR ___*70*___
RRR ___*70*___ PRI ___*0.20 on sinus complexes; 0.14 on early complexes*___ QRS ___*0.08*___
INTERPRETATION ___*sinus rhythm with premature junctional complexes*___

Figure 4–11. PPI ___*irregular*___ RRI ___*irregular*___ PPR ___ RRR ___*130*___ PRI ___ QRS ___*0.06*___
INTERPRETATION ___*atrial fibrillation*___

Figure 4–12. PPI ___*regular except for late complex*___ RRI ___*regular except for late complex*___ PPR ___*60*___
RRR ___*60*___ PRI ___*0.16*___ QRS ___*0.08*___
INTERPRETATION ___*sinus rhythm with junctional escape complex*___

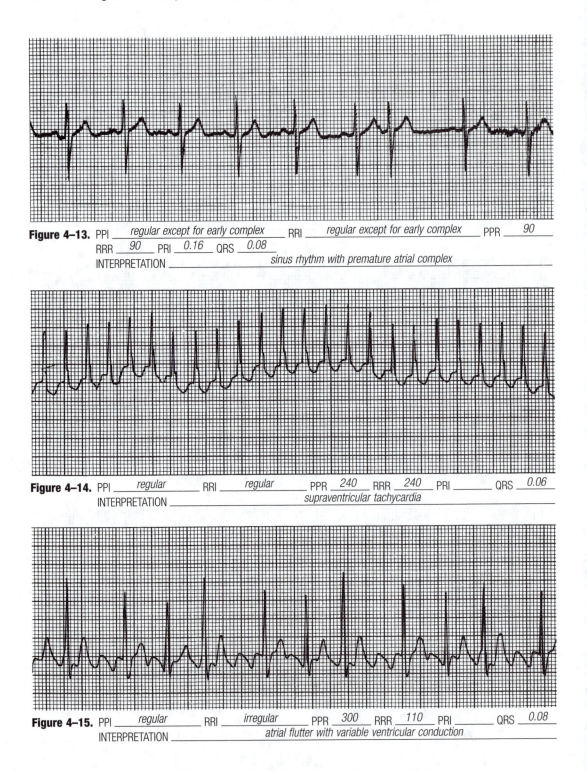

Figure 4–13. PPI ___*regular except for early complex*___ RRI ___*regular except for early complex*___ PPR ___*90*___
RRR ___*90*___ PRI ___*0.16*___ QRS ___*0.08*___
INTERPRETATION _____*sinus rhythm with premature atrial complex*_____

Figure 4–14. PPI ___*regular*___ RRI ___*regular*___ PPR ___*240*___ RRR ___*240*___ PRI _____ QRS ___*0.06*___
INTERPRETATION _____*supraventricular tachycardia*_____

Figure 4–15. PPI ___*regular*___ RRI ___*irregular*___ PPR ___*300*___ RRR ___*110*___ PRI _____ QRS ___*0.08*___
INTERPRETATION _____*atrial flutter with variable ventricular conduction*_____

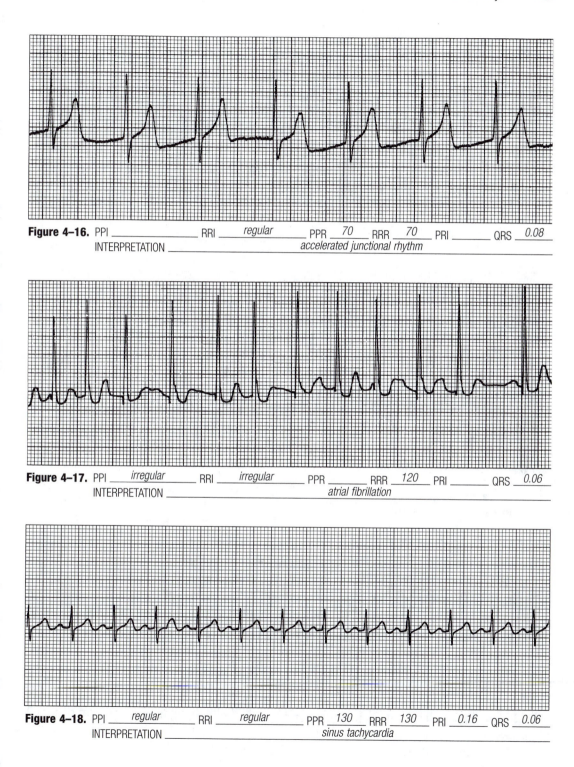

Figure 4–16. PPI _____ RRI _____*regular*_____ PPR __*70*__ RRR __*70*__ PRI _____ QRS __*0.08*__
INTERPRETATION _____*accelerated junctional rhythm*_____

Figure 4–17. PPI ___*irregular*___ RRI ___*irregular*___ PPR _____ RRR __*120*__ PRI _____ QRS __*0.06*__
INTERPRETATION _____*atrial fibrillation*_____

Figure 4–18. PPI ___*regular*___ RRI ___*regular*___ PPR __*130*__ RRR __*130*__ PRI __*0.16*__ QRS __*0.06*__
INTERPRETATION _____*sinus tachycardia*_____

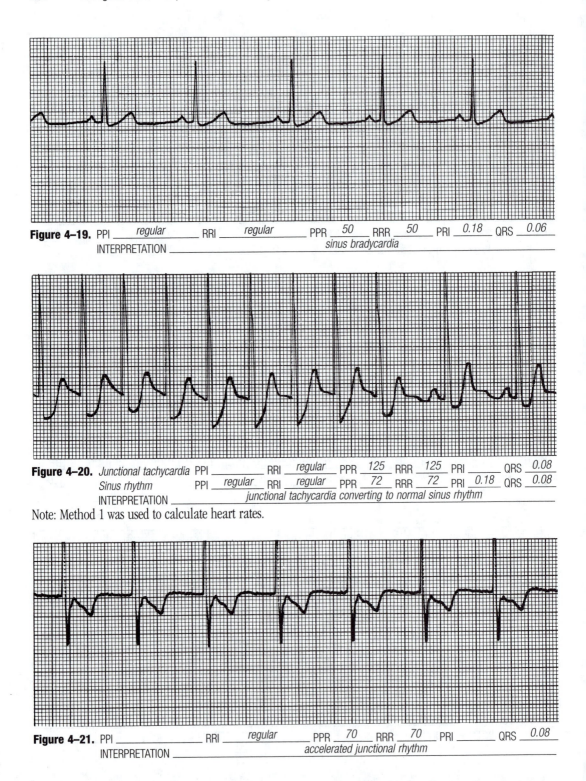

Figure 4–19. PPI _____regular_____ RRI _____regular_____ PPR __50__ RRR __50__ PRI __0.18__ QRS __0.06__
INTERPRETATION _____sinus bradycardia_____

Figure 4–20. Junctional tachycardia PPI _____ RRI __regular__ PPR __125__ RRR __125__ PRI ____ QRS __0.08__
Sinus rhythm PPI __regular__ RRI __regular__ PPR __72__ RRR __72__ PRI __0.18__ QRS __0.08__
INTERPRETATION _____junctional tachycardia converting to normal sinus rhythm_____

Note: Method 1 was used to calculate heart rates.

Figure 4–21. PPI _____ RRI __regular__ PPR __70__ RRR __70__ PRI _____ QRS __0.08__
INTERPRETATION _____accelerated junctional rhythm_____

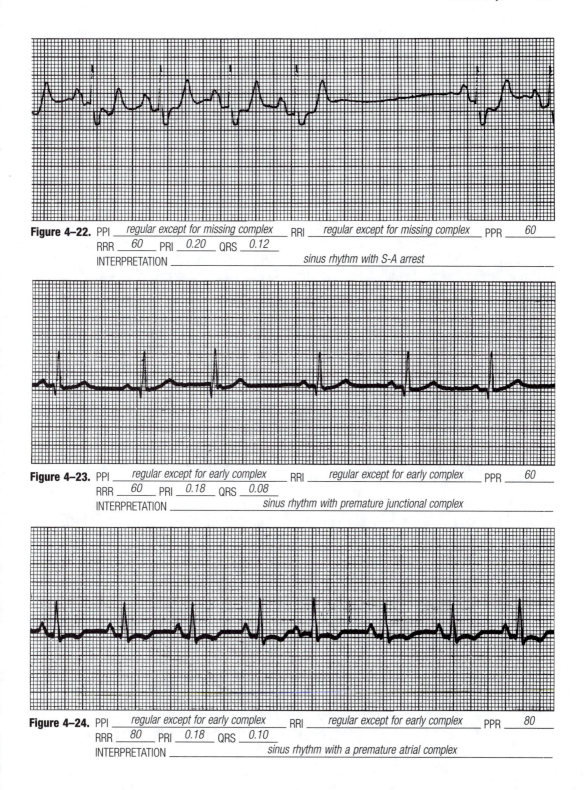

Figure 4–22. PPI _regular except for missing complex_ RRI _regular except for missing complex_ PPR _60_
RRR _60_ PRI _0.20_ QRS _0.12_
INTERPRETATION _sinus rhythm with S-A arrest_

Figure 4–23. PPI _regular except for early complex_ RRI _regular except for early complex_ PPR _60_
RRR _60_ PRI _0.18_ QRS _0.08_
INTERPRETATION _sinus rhythm with premature junctional complex_

Figure 4–24. PPI _regular except for early complex_ RRI _regular except for early complex_ PPR _80_
RRR _80_ PRI _0.18_ QRS _0.10_
INTERPRETATION _sinus rhythm with a premature atrial complex_

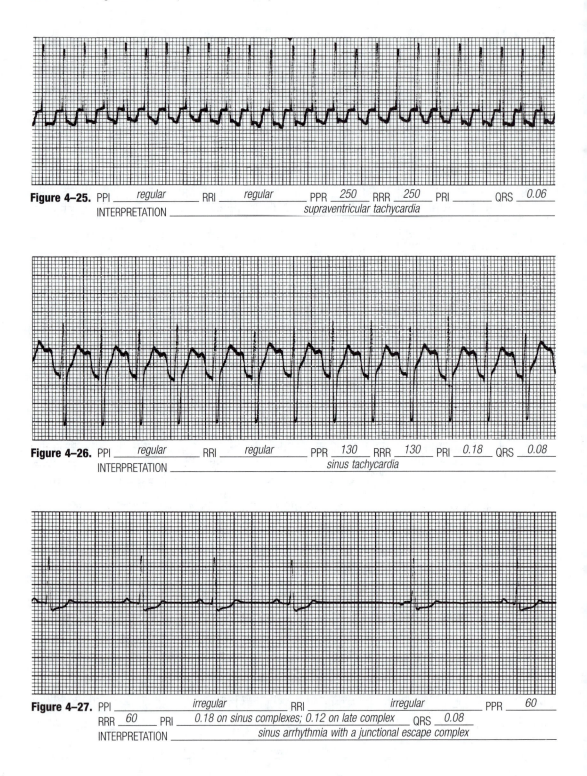

Figure 4–25. PPI _____*regular*_____ RRI _____*regular*_____ PPR __*250*__ RRR __*250*__ PRI _____ QRS __*0.06*__
INTERPRETATION _____*supraventricular tachycardia*_____

Figure 4–26. PPI _____*regular*_____ RRI _____*regular*_____ PPR __*130*__ RRR __*130*__ PRI __*0.18*__ QRS __*0.08*__
INTERPRETATION _____*sinus tachycardia*_____

Figure 4–27. PPI _____*irregular*_____ RRI _____*irregular*_____ PPR __*60*__
RRR __*60*__ PRI __*0.18 on sinus complexes; 0.12 on late complex*__ QRS __*0.08*__
INTERPRETATION _____*sinus arrhythmia with a junctional escape complex*_____

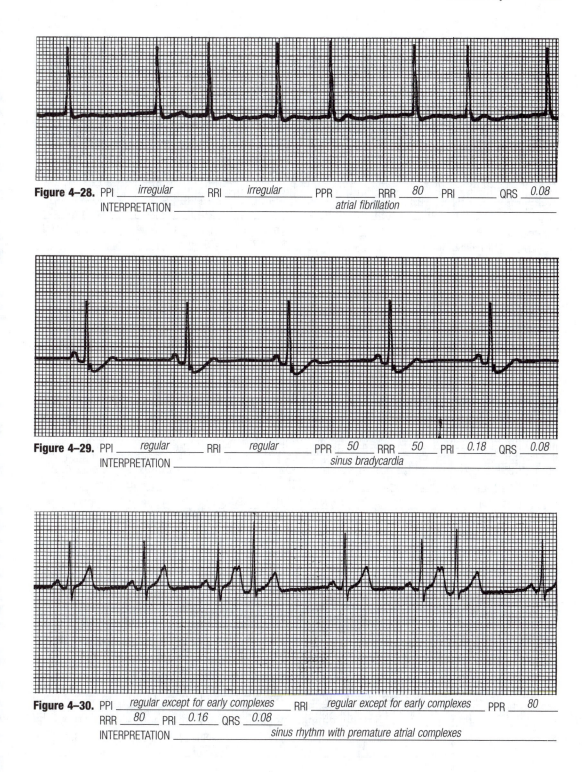

Figure 4–28. PPI _____irregular_____ RRI _____irregular_____ PPR _____ RRR __80__ PRI _____ QRS __0.08__
INTERPRETATION _____atrial fibrillation_____

Figure 4–29. PPI _____regular_____ RRI _____regular_____ PPR __50__ RRR __50__ PRI __0.18__ QRS __0.08__
INTERPRETATION _____sinus bradycardia_____

Figure 4–30. PPI __regular except for early complexes__ RRI __regular except for early complexes__ PPR __80__
RRR __80__ PRI __0.16__ QRS __0.08__
INTERPRETATION _____sinus rhythm with premature atrial complexes_____

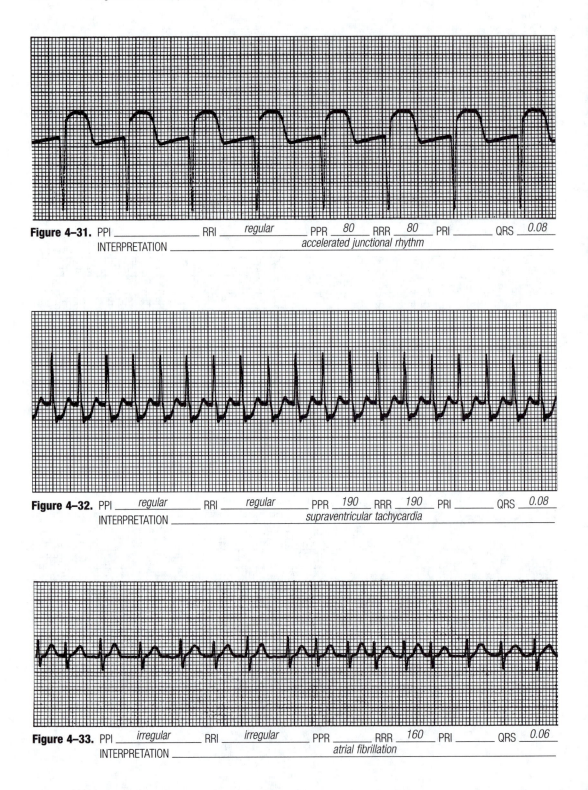

Figure 4–31. PPI _____ RRI ____*regular*____ PPR __*80*__ RRR __*80*__ PRI _____ QRS _*0.08*_
INTERPRETATION _____*accelerated junctional rhythm*_____

Figure 4–32. PPI ___*regular*___ RRI ___*regular*___ PPR _*190*_ RRR _*190*_ PRI _____ QRS _*0.08*_
INTERPRETATION _____*supraventricular tachycardia*_____

Figure 4–33. PPI ___*irregular*___ RRI ___*irregular*___ PPR _____ RRR _*160*_ PRI _____ QRS _*0.06*_
INTERPRETATION _____*atrial fibrillation*_____

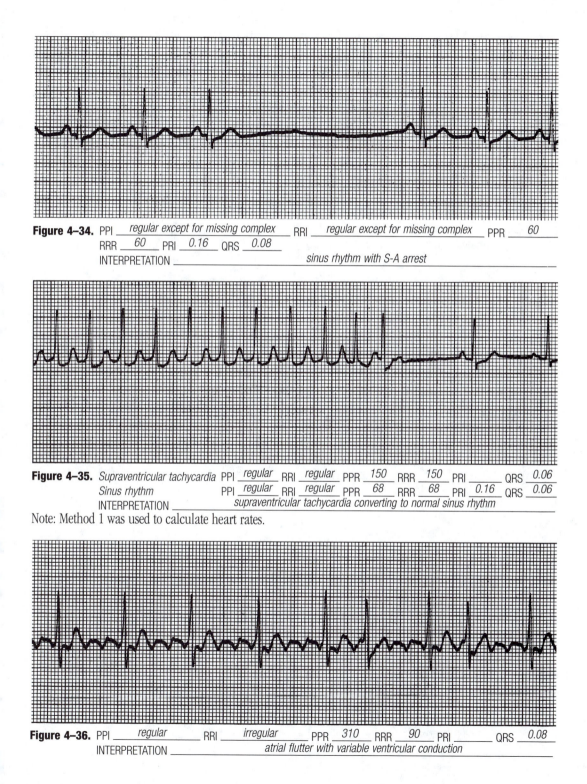

Figure 4–34. PPI _regular except for missing complex_ RRI _regular except for missing complex_ PPR _60_
RRR _60_ PRI _0.16_ QRS _0.08_
INTERPRETATION _sinus rhythm with S-A arrest_

Figure 4–35. _Supraventricular tachycardia_ PPI _regular_ RRI _regular_ PPR _150_ RRR _150_ PRI _____ QRS _0.06_
Sinus rhythm PPI _regular_ RRI _regular_ PPR _68_ RRR _68_ PRI _0.16_ QRS _0.06_
INTERPRETATION _supraventricular tachycardia converting to normal sinus rhythm_

Note: Method 1 was used to calculate heart rates.

Figure 4–36. PPI _regular_ RRI _irregular_ PPR _310_ RRR _90_ PRI _____ QRS _0.08_
INTERPRETATION _atrial flutter with variable ventricular conduction_

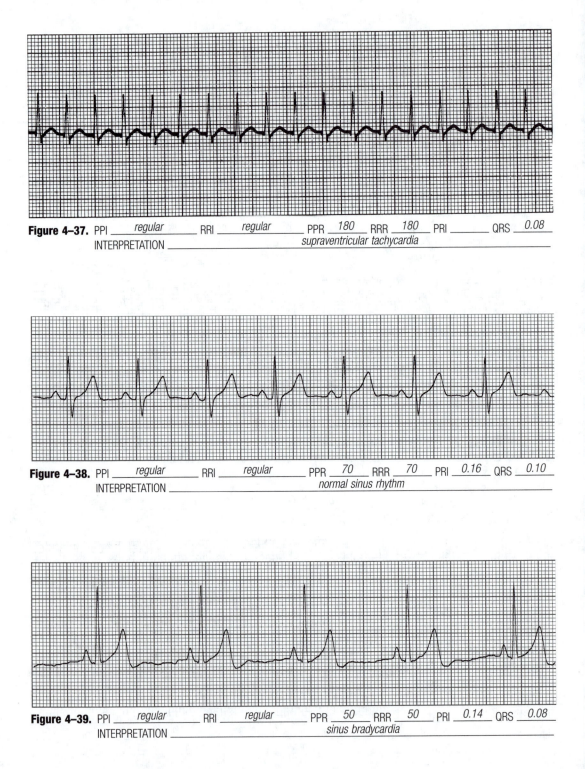

Figure 4–37. PPI _____ *regular* _____ RRI _____ *regular* _____ PPR __*180*__ RRR __*180*__ PRI _____ QRS __*0.08*__
INTERPRETATION _____ *supraventricular tachycardia* _____

Figure 4–38. PPI _____ *regular* _____ RRI _____ *regular* _____ PPR __*70*__ RRR __*70*__ PRI __*0.16*__ QRS __*0.10*__
INTERPRETATION _____ *normal sinus rhythm* _____

Figure 4–39. PPI _____ *regular* _____ RRI _____ *regular* _____ PPR __*50*__ RRR __*50*__ PRI __*0.14*__ QRS __*0.08*__
INTERPRETATION _____ *sinus bradycardia* _____

CHAPTER 5

Answer Key—Matching

1.	i	6.	j	11.	h	16.	c	21.	j, k
2.	b	7.	k	12.	d	17.	b, d	22.	j
3.	e	8.	g	13.	d, e	18.	d	23.	k
4.	k	9.	c	14.	b	19.	h	24.	d
5.	c	10.	c	15.	a, b, c, d	20.	g		

Answer Key—ECG Practice Strips

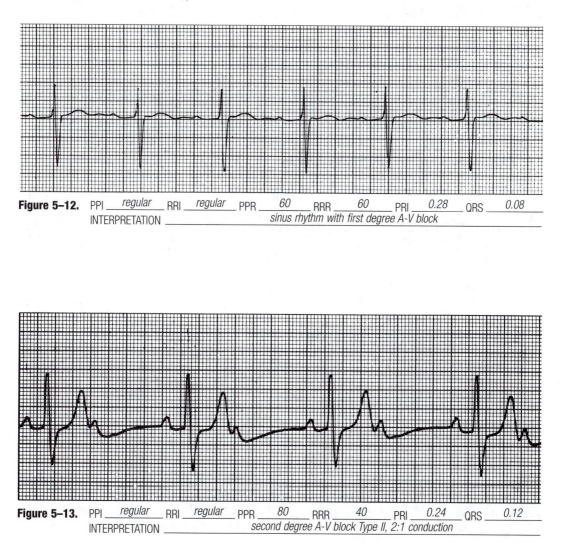

Figure 5–12. PPI _regular_ RRI _regular_ PPR _60_ RRR _60_ PRI _0.28_ QRS _0.08_
INTERPRETATION _sinus rhythm with first degree A-V block_

Figure 5–13. PPI _regular_ RRI _regular_ PPR _80_ RRR _40_ PRI _0.24_ QRS _0.12_
INTERPRETATION _second degree A-V block Type II, 2:1 conduction_

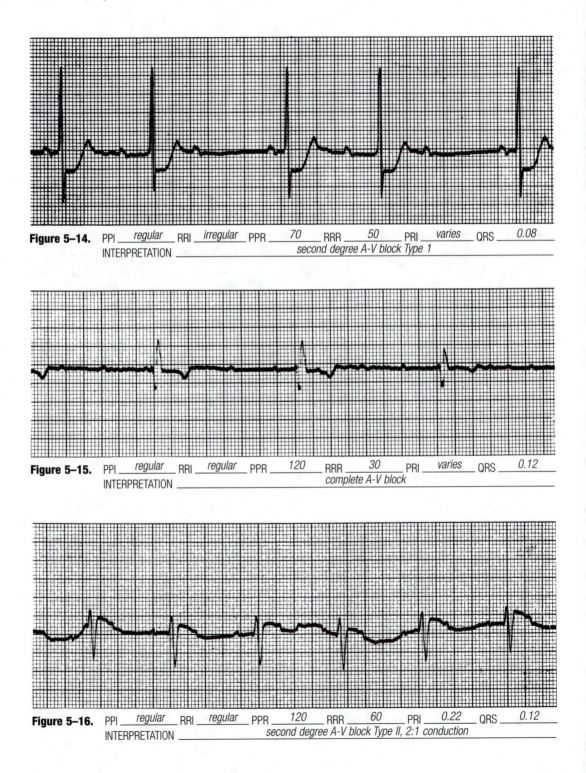

Figure 5–14.   PPI _____*regular*_____ RRI _____*irregular*_____ PPR _____*70*_____ RRR _____*50*_____ PRI _____*varies*_____ QRS _____*0.08*_____
INTERPRETATION _____*second degree A-V block Type 1*_____

Figure 5–15.   PPI _____*regular*_____ RRI _____*regular*_____ PPR _____*120*_____ RRR _____*30*_____ PRI _____*varies*_____ QRS _____*0.12*_____
INTERPRETATION _____*complete A-V block*_____

Figure 5–16.   PPI _____*regular*_____ RRI _____*regular*_____ PPR _____*120*_____ RRR _____*60*_____ PRI _____*0.22*_____ QRS _____*0.12*_____
INTERPRETATION _____*second degree A-V block Type II, 2:1 conduction*_____

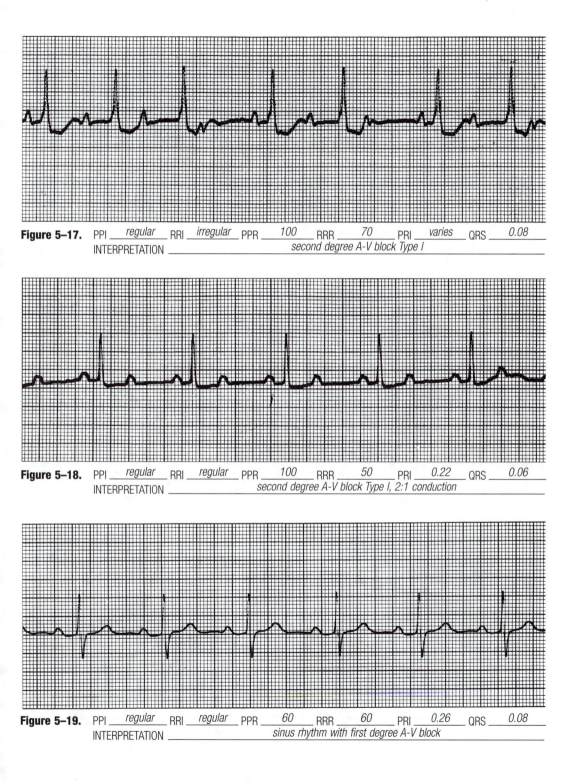

Figure 5–17. PPI _regular_ RRI _irregular_ PPR _100_ RRR _70_ PRI _varies_ QRS _0.08_
INTERPRETATION _second degree A-V block Type I_

Figure 5–18. PPI _regular_ RRI _regular_ PPR _100_ RRR _50_ PRI _0.22_ QRS _0.06_
INTERPRETATION _second degree A-V block Type I, 2:1 conduction_

Figure 5–19. PPI _regular_ RRI _regular_ PPR _60_ RRR _60_ PRI _0.26_ QRS _0.08_
INTERPRETATION _sinus rhythm with first degree A-V block_

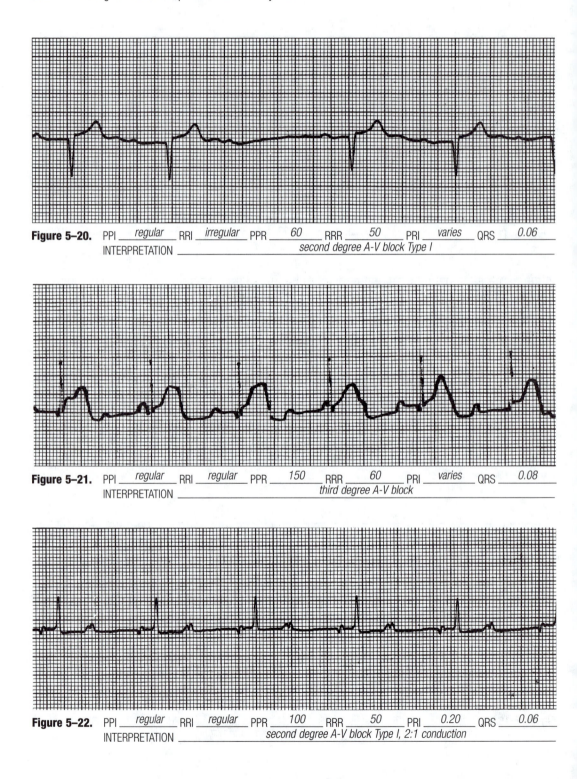

Figure 5–20. PPI ___*regular*___ RRI ___*irregular*___ PPR ___*60*___ RRR ___*50*___ PRI ___*varies*___ QRS ___*0.06*___
INTERPRETATION _____*second degree A-V block Type I*_____

Figure 5–21. PPI ___*regular*___ RRI ___*regular*___ PPR ___*150*___ RRR ___*60*___ PRI ___*varies*___ QRS ___*0.08*___
INTERPRETATION _____*third degree A-V block*_____

Figure 5–22. PPI ___*regular*___ RRI ___*regular*___ PPR ___*100*___ RRR ___*50*___ PRI ___*0.20*___ QRS ___*0.06*___
INTERPRETATION _____*second degree A-V block Type I, 2:1 conduction*_____

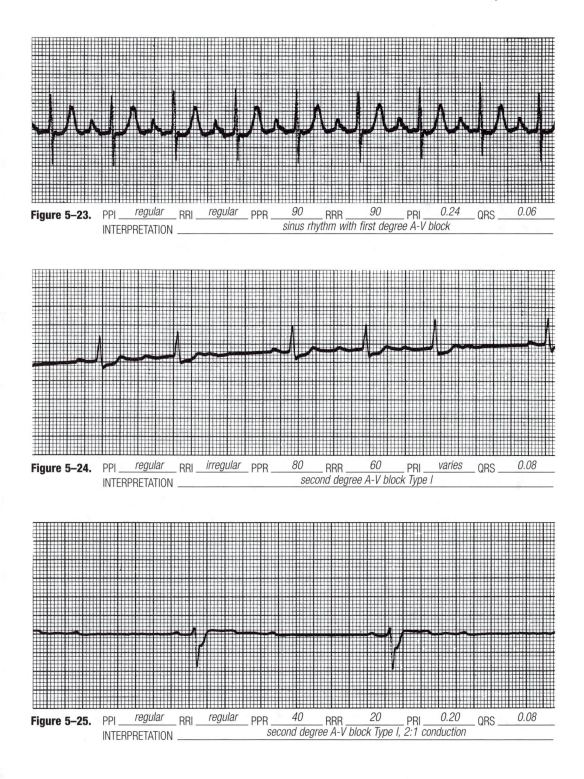

Figure 5–23. PPI _regular_ RRI _regular_ PPR _90_ RRR _90_ PRI _0.24_ QRS _0.06_
INTERPRETATION _sinus rhythm with first degree A-V block_

Figure 5–24. PPI _regular_ RRI _irregular_ PPR _80_ RRR _60_ PRI _varies_ QRS _0.08_
INTERPRETATION _second degree A-V block Type I_

Figure 5–25. PPI _regular_ RRI _regular_ PPR _40_ RRR _20_ PRI _0.20_ QRS _0.08_
INTERPRETATION _second degree A-V block Type I, 2:1 conduction_

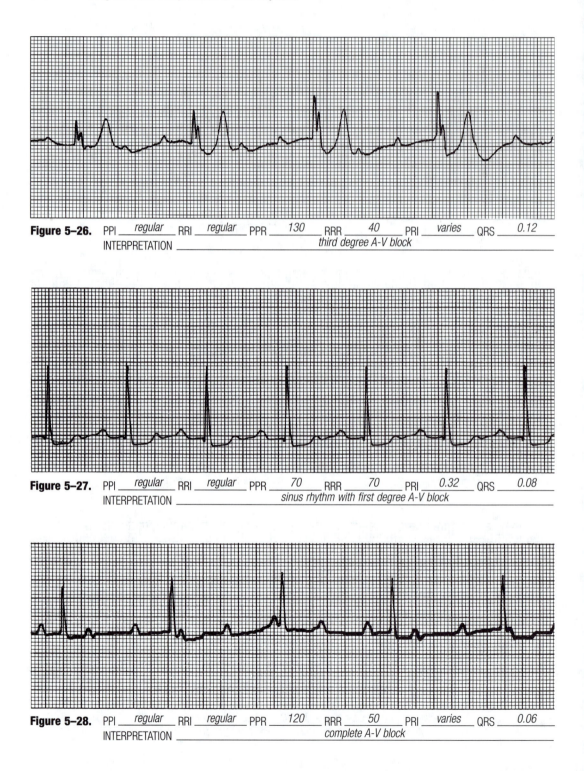

Figure 5–26. PPI _____regular_____ RRI _____regular_____ PPR _____130_____ RRR _____40_____ PRI _____varies_____ QRS _____0.12_____
INTERPRETATION _____third degree A-V block_____

Figure 5–27. PPI _____regular_____ RRI _____regular_____ PPR _____70_____ RRR _____70_____ PRI _____0.32_____ QRS _____0.08_____
INTERPRETATION _____sinus rhythm with first degree A-V block_____

Figure 5–28. PPI _____regular_____ RRI _____regular_____ PPR _____120_____ RRR _____50_____ PRI _____varies_____ QRS _____0.06_____
INTERPRETATION _____complete A-V block_____

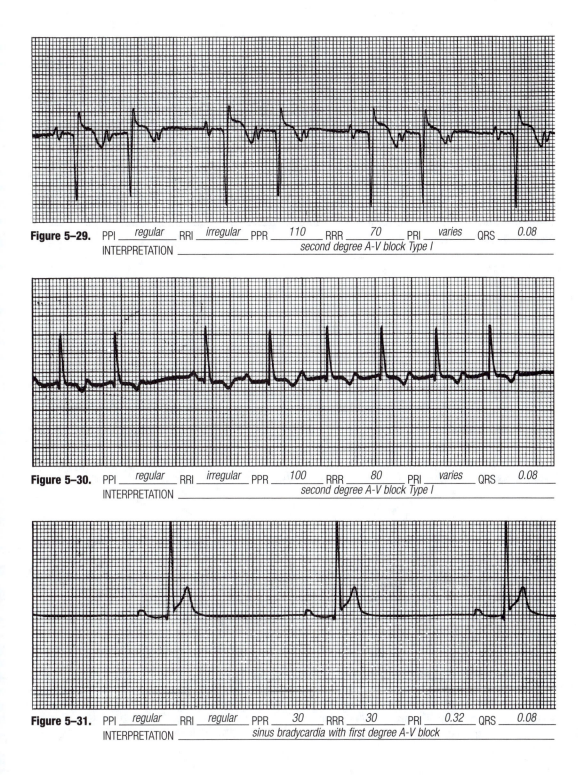

Figure 5–29. PPI _regular_ RRI _irregular_ PPR _110_ RRR _70_ PRI _varies_ QRS _0.08_
INTERPRETATION _____ second degree A-V block Type I _____

Figure 5–30. PPI _regular_ RRI _irregular_ PPR _100_ RRR _80_ PRI _varies_ QRS _0.08_
INTERPRETATION _____ second degree A-V block Type I _____

Figure 5–31. PPI _regular_ RRI _regular_ PPR _30_ RRR _30_ PRI _0.32_ QRS _0.08_
INTERPRETATION _____ sinus bradycardia with first degree A-V block _____

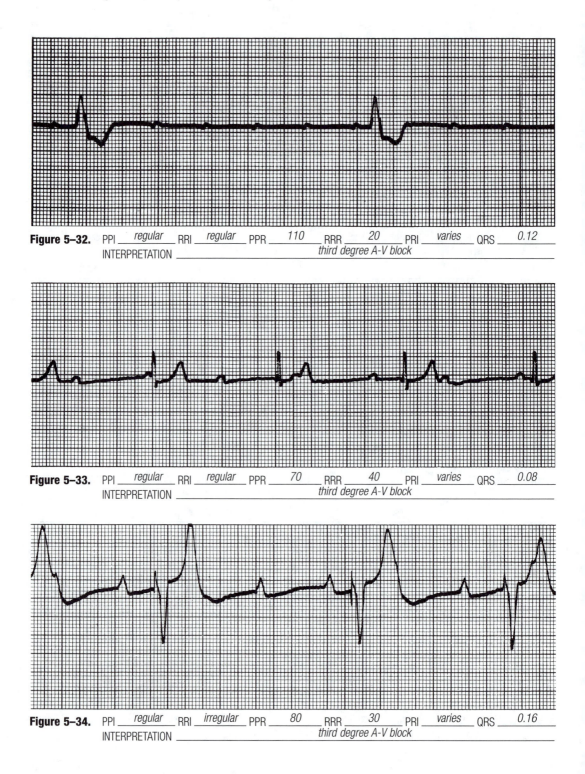

Figure 5–32. PPI _regular_ RRI _regular_ PPR _110_ RRR _20_ PRI _varies_ QRS _0.12_
INTERPRETATION _____ third degree A-V block _____

Figure 5–33. PPI _regular_ RRI _regular_ PPR _70_ RRR _40_ PRI _varies_ QRS _0.08_
INTERPRETATION _____ third degree A-V block _____

Figure 5–34. PPI _regular_ RRI _irregular_ PPR _80_ RRR _30_ PRI _varies_ QRS _0.16_
INTERPRETATION _____ third degree A-V block _____

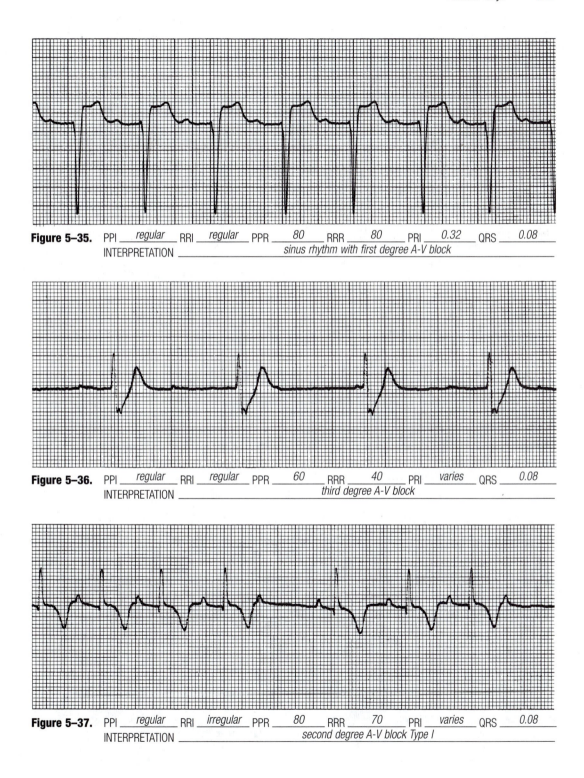

Figure 5–35. PPI ___regular___ RRI ___regular___ PPR ___80___ RRR ___80___ PRI ___0.32___ QRS ___0.08___
INTERPRETATION _____ sinus rhythm with first degree A-V block _____

Figure 5–36. PPI ___regular___ RRI ___regular___ PPR ___60___ RRR ___40___ PRI ___varies___ QRS ___0.08___
INTERPRETATION _____ third degree A-V block _____

Figure 5–37. PPI ___regular___ RRI ___irregular___ PPR ___80___ RRR ___70___ PRI ___varies___ QRS ___0.08___
INTERPRETATION _____ second degree A-V block Type I _____

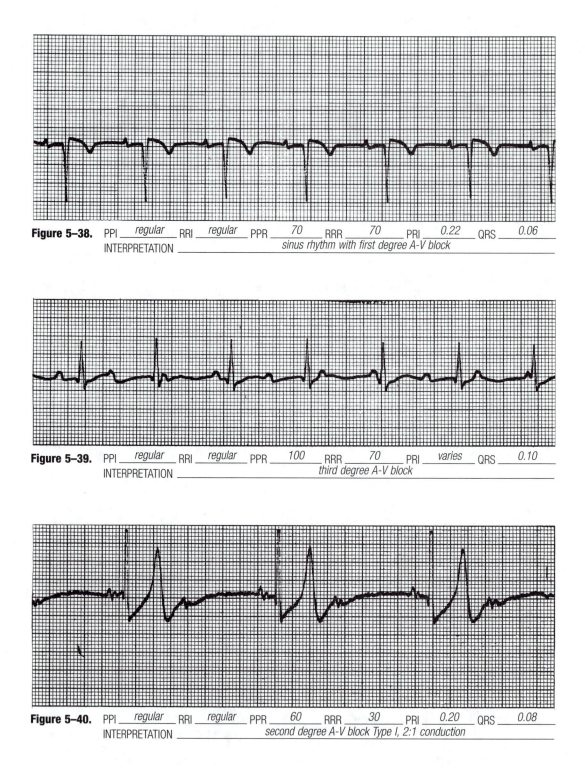

Figure 5–38.   PPI _____*regular*_____ RRI _____*regular*_____ PPR _____*70*_____ RRR _____*70*_____ PRI _____*0.22*_____ QRS _____*0.06*_____
INTERPRETATION _____*sinus rhythm with first degree A-V block*_____

Figure 5–39.   PPI _____*regular*_____ RRI _____*regular*_____ PPR _____*100*_____ RRR _____*70*_____ PRI _____*varies*_____ QRS _____*0.10*_____
INTERPRETATION _____*third degree A-V block*_____

Figure 5–40.   PPI _____*regular*_____ RRI _____*regular*_____ PPR _____*60*_____ RRR _____*30*_____ PRI _____*0.20*_____ QRS _____*0.08*_____
INTERPRETATION _____*second degree A-V block Type I, 2:1 conduction*_____

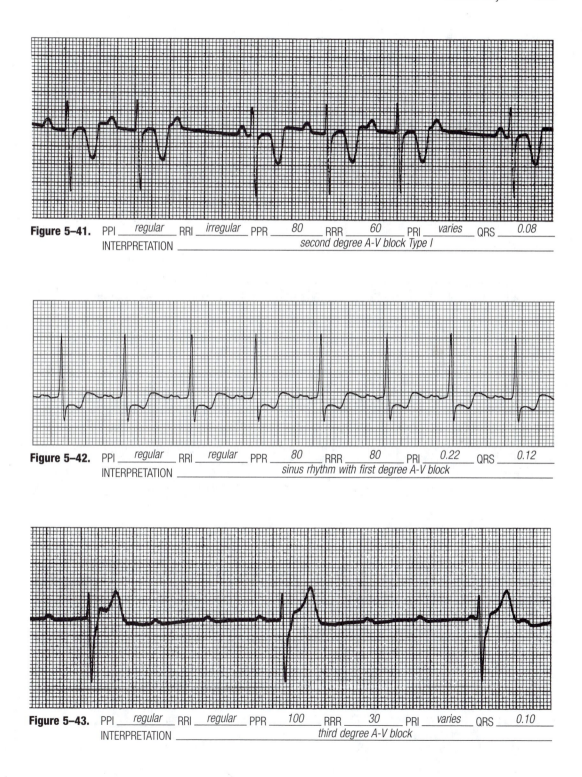

Figure 5–41. PPI ___*regular*___ RRI ___*irregular*___ PPR ___*80*___ RRR ___*60*___ PRI ___*varies*___ QRS ___*0.08*___
INTERPRETATION _____*second degree A-V block Type I*_____

Figure 5–42. PPI ___*regular*___ RRI ___*regular*___ PPR ___*80*___ RRR ___*80*___ PRI ___*0.22*___ QRS ___*0.12*___
INTERPRETATION _____*sinus rhythm with first degree A-V block*_____

Figure 5–43. PPI ___*regular*___ RRI ___*regular*___ PPR ___*100*___ RRR ___*30*___ PRI ___*varies*___ QRS ___*0.10*___
INTERPRETATION _____*third degree A-V block*_____

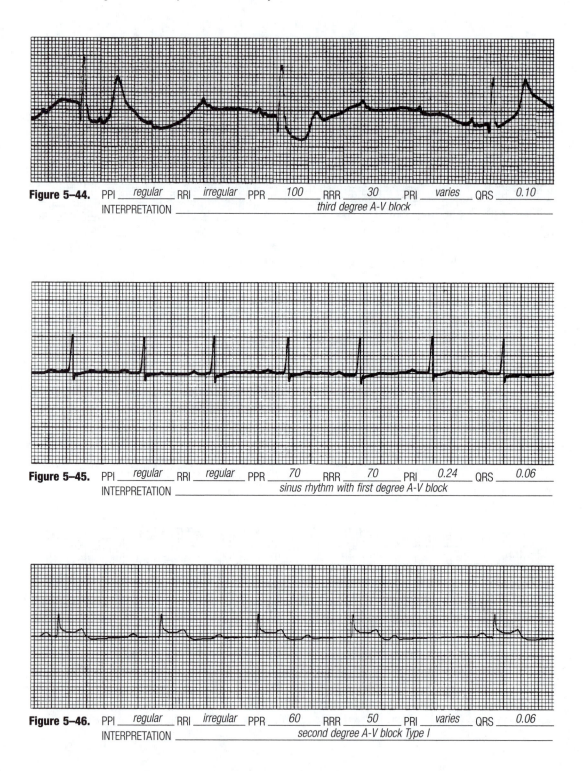

Figure 5–44. PPI _regular_ RRI _irregular_ PPR _100_ RRR _30_ PRI _varies_ QRS _0.10_
INTERPRETATION _third degree A-V block_

Figure 5–45. PPI _regular_ RRI _regular_ PPR _70_ RRR _70_ PRI _0.24_ QRS _0.06_
INTERPRETATION _sinus rhythm with first degree A-V block_

Figure 5–46. PPI _regular_ RRI _irregular_ PPR _60_ RRR _50_ PRI _varies_ QRS _0.06_
INTERPRETATION _second degree A-V block Type I_

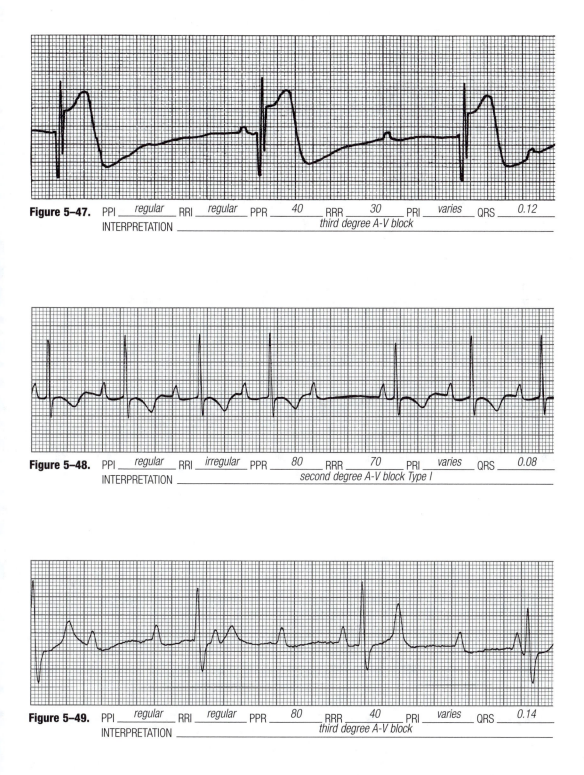

Figure 5–47. PPI __*regular*__ RRI __*regular*__ PPR __*40*__ RRR __*30*__ PRI __*varies*__ QRS __*0.12*__
INTERPRETATION _____*third degree A-V block*_____

Figure 5–48. PPI __*regular*__ RRI __*irregular*__ PPR __*80*__ RRR __*70*__ PRI __*varies*__ QRS __*0.08*__
INTERPRETATION _____*second degree A-V block Type I*_____

Figure 5–49. PPI __*regular*__ RRI __*regular*__ PPR __*80*__ RRR __*40*__ PRI __*varies*__ QRS __*0.14*__
INTERPRETATION _____*third degree A-V block*_____

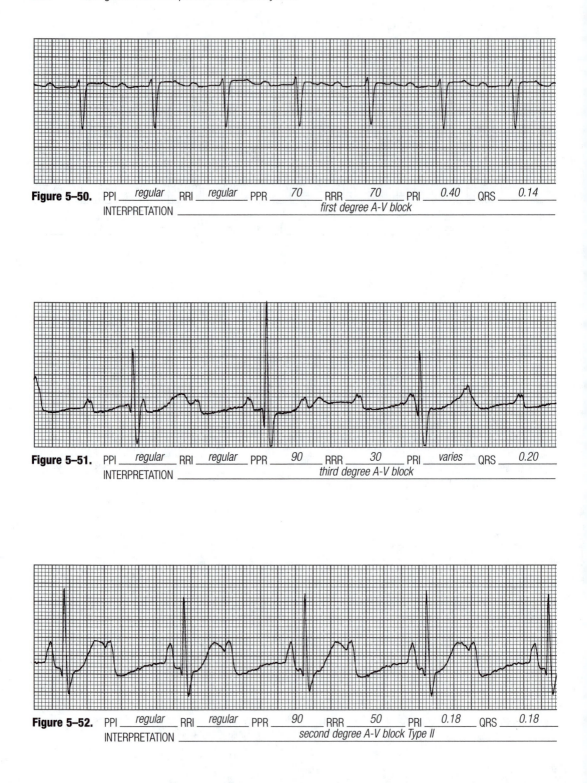

Figure 5–50. PPI ___*regular*___ RRI ___*regular*___ PPR ___70___ RRR ___70___ PRI ___0.40___ QRS ___0.14___
INTERPRETATION _____*first degree A-V block*_____

Figure 5–51. PPI ___*regular*___ RRI ___*regular*___ PPR ___90___ RRR ___30___ PRI ___*varies*___ QRS ___0.20___
INTERPRETATION _____*third degree A-V block*_____

Figure 5–52. PPI ___*regular*___ RRI ___*regular*___ PPR ___90___ RRR ___50___ PRI ___0.18___ QRS ___0.18___
INTERPRETATION _____*second degree A-V block Type II*_____

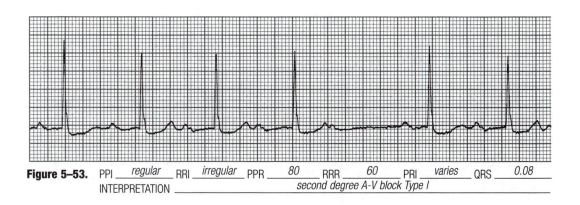

Figure 5–53. PPI __*regular*__ RRI __*irregular*__ PPR __*80*__ RRR __*60*__ PRI __*varies*__ QRS __*0.08*__

INTERPRETATION _____ *second degree A-V block Type I* _____

CHAPTER 6

Answer Key—Matching

1.	e	10.	p	19.	d	28.	f	37.	g
2.	r	11.	o	20.	h	29.	q	38.	h, m
3.	a	12.	p	21.	l, m	30.	d	39.	k
4.	k	13.	o	22.	a	31.	i	40.	k
5.	h	14.	p	23.	c	32.	f	41.	l
6.	b	15.	d	24.	g	33.	d	42.	e, g, h, m
7.	m	16.	d	25.	k	34.	i		
8.	l	17.	d	26.	b	35.	e		
9.	i	18.	d	27.	l	36.	j		

Answer Key—ECG Practice Strips

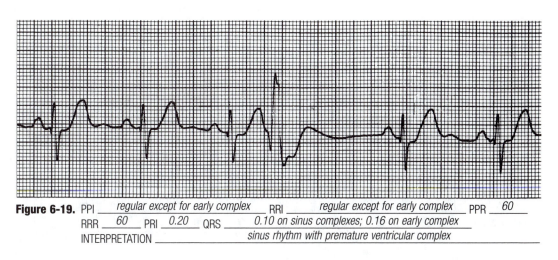

Figure 6-19. PPI __*regular except for early complex*__ RRI __*regular except for early complex*__ PPR __*60*__

RRR __*60*__ PRI __*0.20*__ QRS __*0.10 on sinus complexes; 0.16 on early complex*__

INTERPRETATION _____ *sinus rhythm with premature ventricular complex* _____

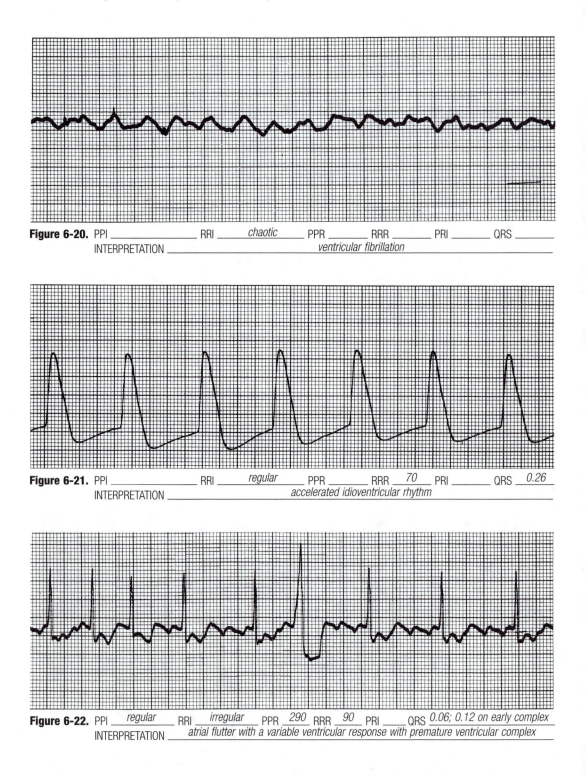

Figure 6-20. PPI _____ RRI _____*chaotic*_____ PPR _____ RRR _____ PRI _____ QRS _____
INTERPRETATION _____*ventricular fibrillation*_____

Figure 6-21. PPI _____ RRI _____*regular*_____ PPR _____ RRR _*70*_ PRI _____ QRS _*0.26*_
INTERPRETATION _____*accelerated idioventricular rhythm*_____

Figure 6-22. PPI _*regular*_ RRI _*irregular*_ PPR _*290*_ RRR _*90*_ PRI _____ QRS *0.06; 0.12 on early complex*
INTERPRETATION _____*atrial flutter with a variable ventricular response with premature ventricular complex*

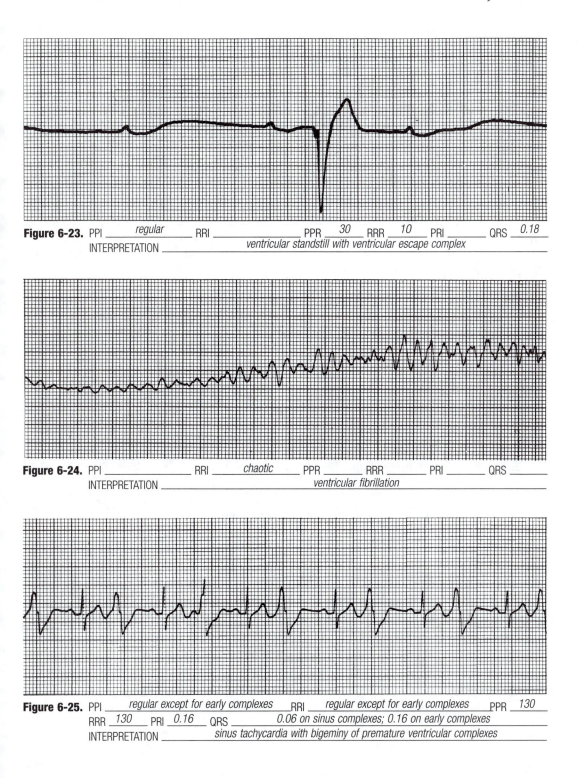

Figure 6-23. PPI _____ *regular* _____ RRI _____ PPR _*30*_ RRR _*10*_ PRI _____ QRS _*0.18*_
INTERPRETATION _____ *ventricular standstill with ventricular escape complex* _____

Figure 6-24. PPI _____ RRI _____ *chaotic* _____ PPR _____ RRR _____ PRI _____ QRS _____
INTERPRETATION _____ *ventricular fibrillation* _____

Figure 6-25. PPI _____ *regular except for early complexes* _____ RRI _____ *regular except for early complexes* _____ PPR _*130*_
RRR _*130*_ PRI _*0.16*_ QRS _____ *0.06 on sinus complexes; 0.16 on early complexes* _____
INTERPRETATION _____ *sinus tachycardia with bigeminy of premature ventricular complexes* _____

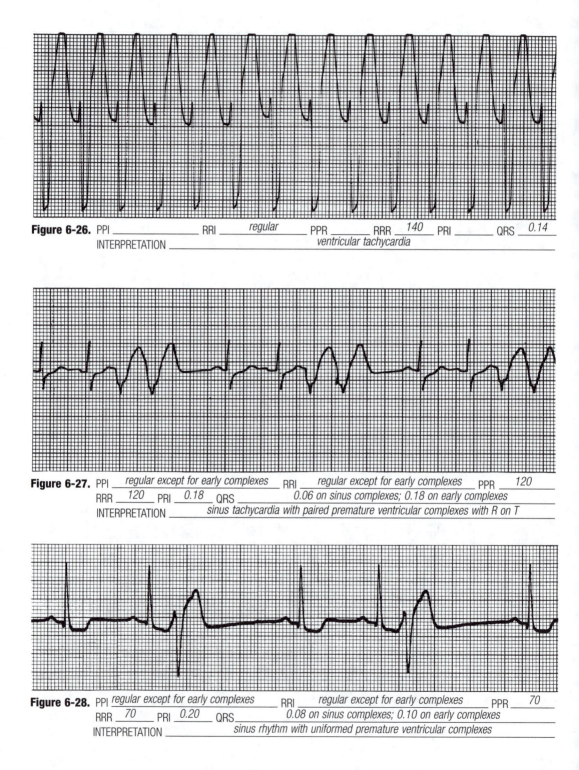

Figure 6-26. PPI _____ RRI ___*regular*___ PPR _____ RRR __*140*__ PRI _____ QRS __*0.14*__
INTERPRETATION _____*ventricular tachycardia*_____

Figure 6-27. PPI __*regular except for early complexes*__ RRI __*regular except for early complexes*__ PPR __*120*__
RRR __*120*__ PRI __*0.18*__ QRS _____*0.06 on sinus complexes; 0.18 on early complexes*_____
INTERPRETATION _____*sinus tachycardia with paired premature ventricular complexes with R on T*_____

Figure 6-28. PPI __*regular except for early complexes*__ RRI __*regular except for early complexes*__ PPR __*70*__
RRR __*70*__ PRI __*0.20*__ QRS _____*0.08 on sinus complexes; 0.10 on early complexes*_____
INTERPRETATION _____*sinus rhythm with uniformed premature ventricular complexes*_____

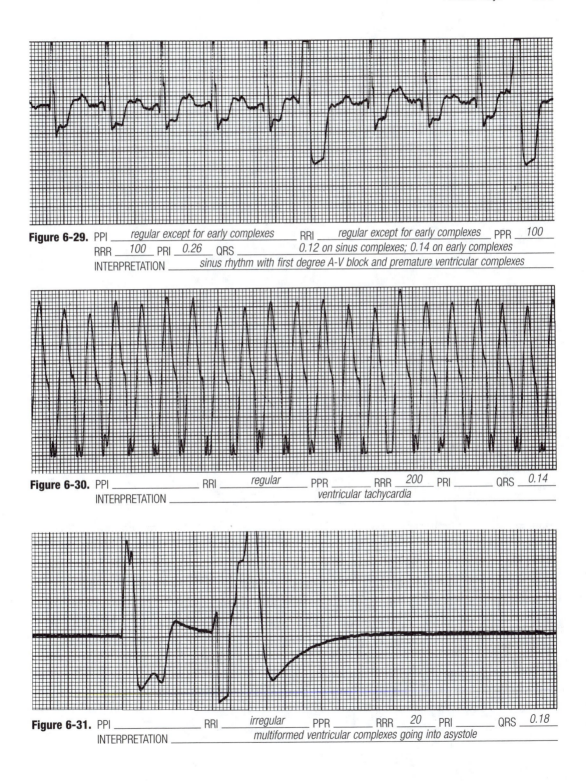

Figure 6-29. PPI _____regular except for early complexes_____ RRI _____regular except for early complexes_____ PPR ___100___
RRR ___100___ PRI _0.26_ QRS _____0.12 on sinus complexes; 0.14 on early complexes_____
INTERPRETATION _____sinus rhythm with first degree A-V block and premature ventricular complexes_____

Figure 6-30. PPI _____ RRI _____regular_____ PPR _____ RRR ___200___ PRI _____ QRS __0.14__
INTERPRETATION _____ventricular tachycardia_____

Figure 6-31. PPI _____ RRI _____irregular_____ PPR _____ RRR ___20___ PRI _____ QRS __0.18__
INTERPRETATION _____multiformed ventricular complexes going into asystole_____

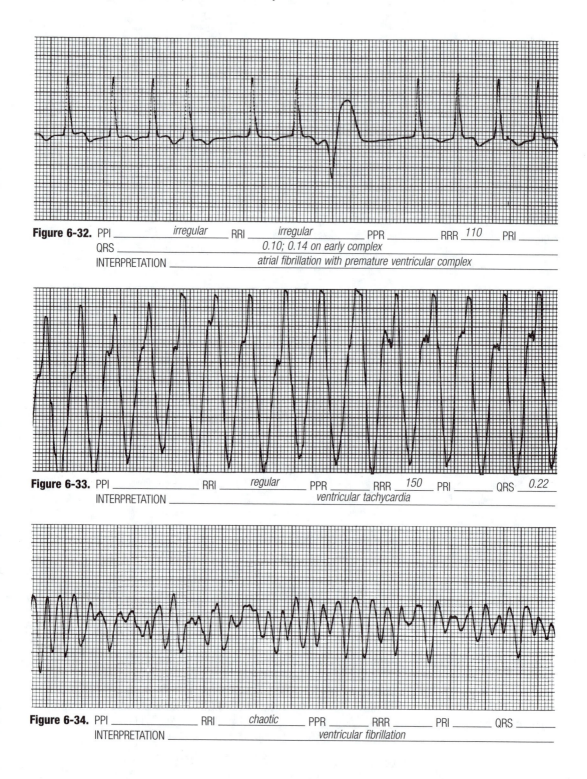

Figure 6-32. PPI _____ _irregular_ _____ RRI _____ _irregular_ _____ PPR _____ RRR _110_ PRI _____
QRS _____ _0.10; 0.14 on early complex_
INTERPRETATION _____ _atrial fibrillation with premature ventricular complex_

Figure 6-33. PPI _____ RRI _____ _regular_ _____ PPR _____ RRR _150_ PRI _____ QRS _0.22_
INTERPRETATION _____ _ventricular tachycardia_

Figure 6-34. PPI _____ RRI _____ _chaotic_ _____ PPR _____ RRR _____ PRI _____ QRS _____
INTERPRETATION _____ _ventricular fibrillation_

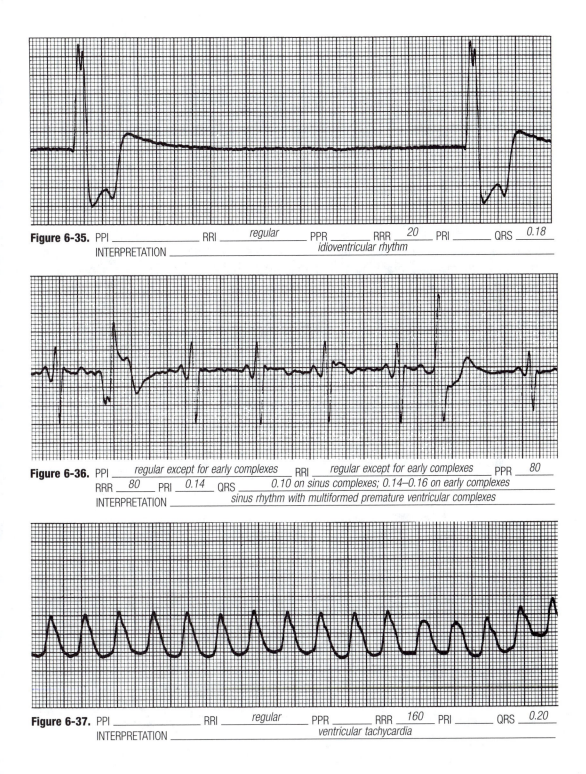

Figure 6-35. PPI _____ RRI ____ *regular* ____ PPR _____ RRR __*20*__ PRI _____ QRS __*0.18*__

INTERPRETATION _____*idioventricular rhythm*_____

Figure 6-36. PPI ___*regular except for early complexes*___ RRI ___*regular except for early complexes*___ PPR __*80*__

RRR __*80*__ PRI __*0.14*__ QRS _____*0.10 on sinus complexes; 0.14–0.16 on early complexes*_____

INTERPRETATION _____*sinus rhythm with multiformed premature ventricular complexes*_____

Figure 6-37. PPI _____ RRI ____ *regular* ____ PPR _____ RRR __*160*__ PRI _____ QRS __*0.20*__

INTERPRETATION _____*ventricular tachycardia*_____

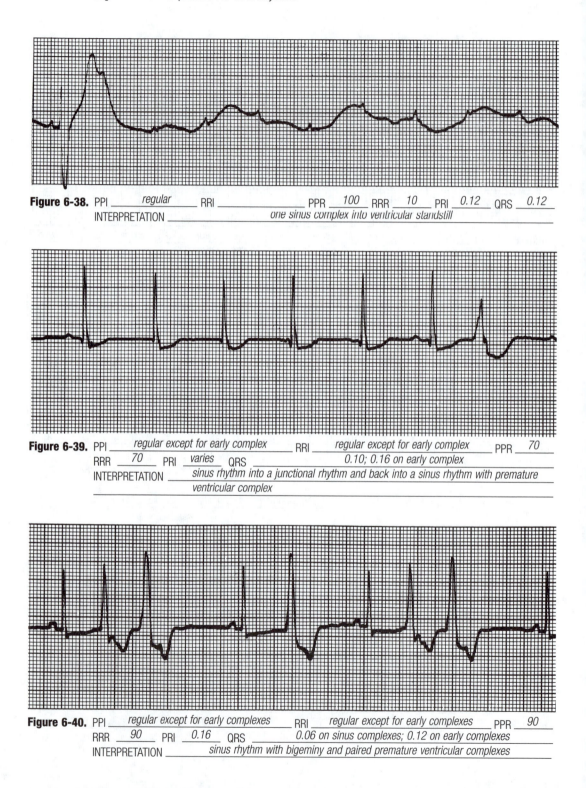

Figure 6-38. PPI _____*regular*_____ RRI _____ PPR __*100*__ RRR ___*10*___ PRI _*0.12*_ QRS _*0.12*_
INTERPRETATION _____*one sinus complex into ventricular standstill*_____

Figure 6-39. PPI _____*regular except for early complex*_____ RRI ____*regular except for early complex*____ PPR __*70*__
RRR __*70*__ PRI _*varies*_ QRS _____*0.10; 0.16 on early complex*_____
INTERPRETATION _____*sinus rhythm into a junctional rhythm and back into a sinus rhythm with premature*_____
_____*ventricular complex*_____

Figure 6-40. PPI ___*regular except for early complexes*___ RRI ___*regular except for early complexes*___ PPR __*90*__
RRR __*90*__ PRI _*0.16*_ QRS _____*0.06 on sinus complexes; 0.12 on early complexes*_____
INTERPRETATION _____*sinus rhythm with bigeminy and paired premature ventricular complexes*_____

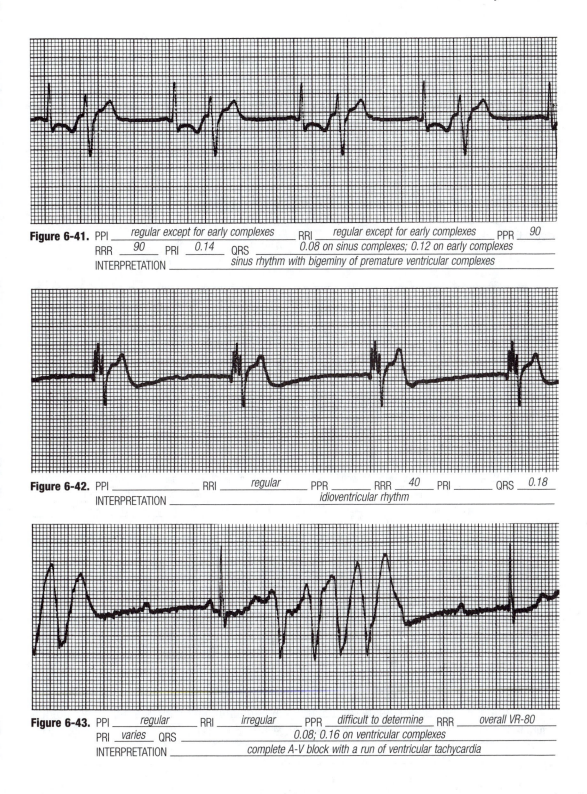

Figure 6-41. PPI _regular except for early complexes_ RRI _regular except for early complexes_ PPR _90_
RRR _90_ PRI _0.14_ QRS _0.08 on sinus complexes; 0.12 on early complexes_
INTERPRETATION _sinus rhythm with bigeminy of premature ventricular complexes_

Figure 6-42. PPI ___ RRI _regular_ PPR ___ RRR _40_ PRI ___ QRS _0.18_
INTERPRETATION _idioventricular rhythm_

Figure 6-43. PPI _regular_ RRI _irregular_ PPR _difficult to determine_ RRR _overall VR-80_
PRI _varies_ QRS _0.08; 0.16 on ventricular complexes_
INTERPRETATION _complete A-V block with a run of ventricular tachycardia_

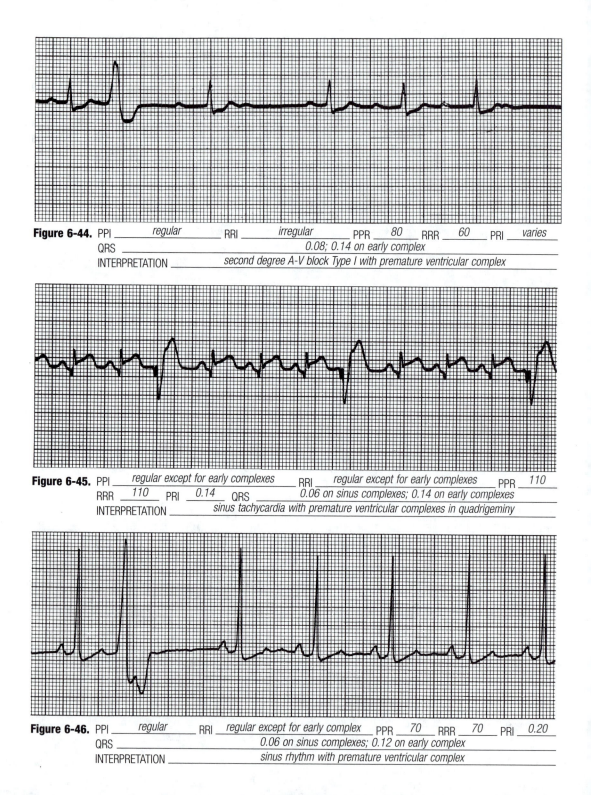

Figure 6-44. PPI _____ *regular* _____ RRI _____ *irregular* _____ PPR __ *80* __ RRR __ *60* __ PRI ___ *varies*
QRS _____ *0.08; 0.14 on early complex* _____
INTERPRETATION _____ *second degree A-V block Type I with premature ventricular complex* _____

Figure 6-45. PPI ___ *regular except for early complexes* ___ RRI ___ *regular except for early complexes* ___ PPR __ *110*
RRR __ *110* __ PRI __ *0.14* __ QRS _____ *0.06 on sinus complexes; 0.14 on early complexes* _____
INTERPRETATION _____ *sinus tachycardia with premature ventricular complexes in quadrigeminy* _____

Figure 6-46. PPI _____ *regular* _____ RRI ___ *regular except for early complex* ___ PPR __ *70* __ RRR __ *70* __ PRI __ *0.20*
QRS _____ *0.06 on sinus complexes; 0.12 on early complex* _____
INTERPRETATION _____ *sinus rhythm with premature ventricular complex* _____

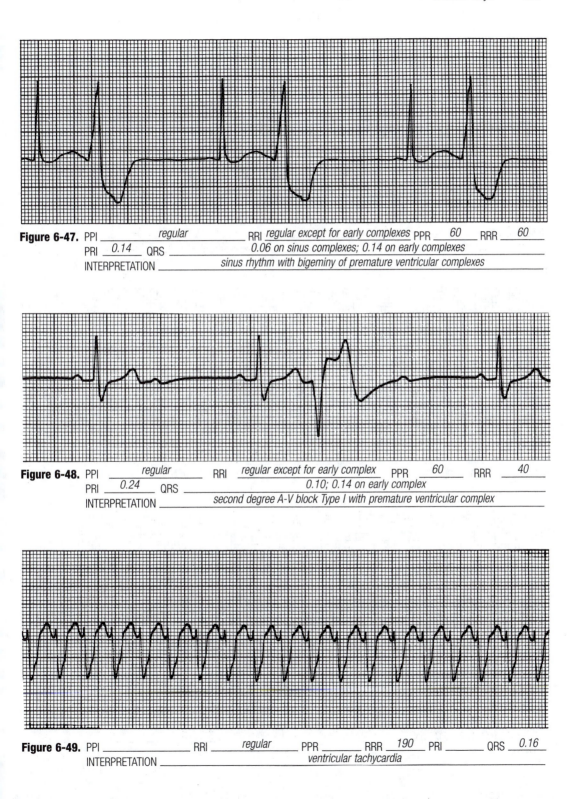

Figure 6-47. PPI _____ _regular_ _____ RRI _regular except for early complexes_ PPR __60__ RRR __60__
PRI _0.14_ QRS _____ 0.06 on sinus complexes; 0.14 on early complexes _____
INTERPRETATION _____ _sinus rhythm with bigeminy of premature ventricular complexes_ _____

Figure 6-48. PPI _____ _regular_ _____ RRI _regular except for early complex_ PPR __60__ RRR __40__
PRI _0.24_ QRS _____ 0.10; 0.14 on early complex _____
INTERPRETATION _____ _second degree A-V block Type I with premature ventricular complex_ _____

Figure 6-49. PPI _____ RRI _____ _regular_ _____ PPR _____ RRR __190__ PRI _____ QRS _0.16_
INTERPRETATION _____ _ventricular tachycardia_ _____

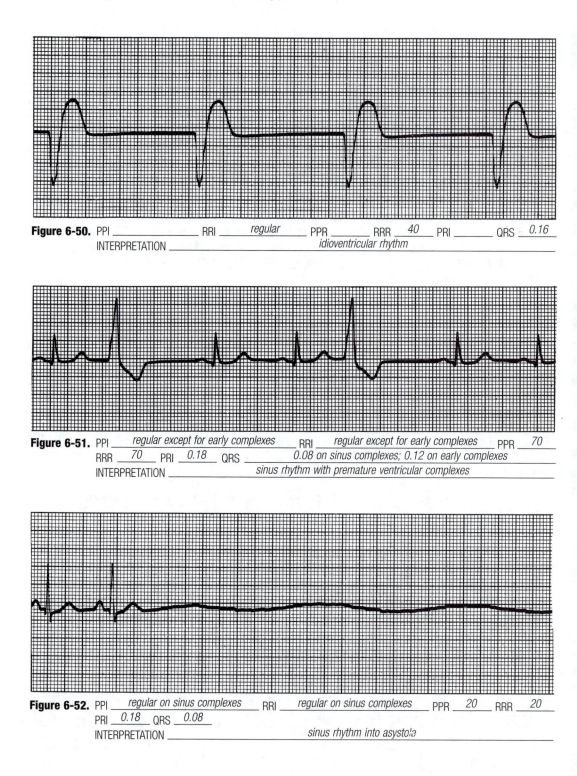

Figure 6-50. PPI _____ RRI ____*regular*____ PPR _____ RRR __*40*__ PRI _____ QRS __*0.16*__
INTERPRETATION _____*idioventricular rhythm*_____

Figure 6-51. PPI ____*regular except for early complexes*____ RRI ____*regular except for early complexes*____ PPR __*70*__
RRR __*70*__ PRI __*0.18*__ QRS _____*0.08 on sinus complexes; 0.12 on early complexes*_____
INTERPRETATION _____*sinus rhythm with premature ventricular complexes*_____

Figure 6-52. PPI ____*regular on sinus complexes*____ RRI ____*regular on sinus complexes*____ PPR __*20*__ RRR __*20*__
PRI __*0.18*__ QRS __*0.08*__
INTERPRETATION _____*sinus rhythm into asystole*_____

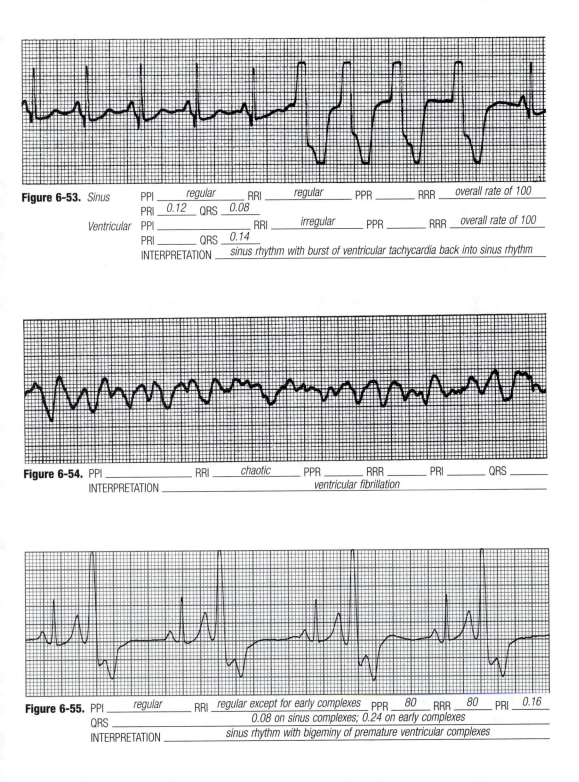

Figure 6-53. *Sinus*   PPI ____*regular*____ RRI ____*regular*____ PPR _____ RRR ___*overall rate of 100*___
PRI _*0.12*_ QRS _*0.08*_

Ventricular   PPI _____ RRI ____*irregular*____ PPR _____ RRR ___*overall rate of 100*___
PRI _____ QRS _*0.14*_

INTERPRETATION ___*sinus rhythm with burst of ventricular tachycardia back into sinus rhythm*___

Figure 6-54. PPI _____ RRI ____*chaotic*____ PPR _____ RRR _____ PRI _____ QRS _____
INTERPRETATION _____*ventricular fibrillation*_____

Figure 6-55. PPI ____*regular*____ RRI ___*regular except for early complexes*___ PPR _*80*_ RRR _*80*_ PRI _*0.16*_
QRS _____*0.08 on sinus complexes; 0.24 on early complexes*_____
INTERPRETATION _____*sinus rhythm with bigeminy of premature ventricular complexes*_____

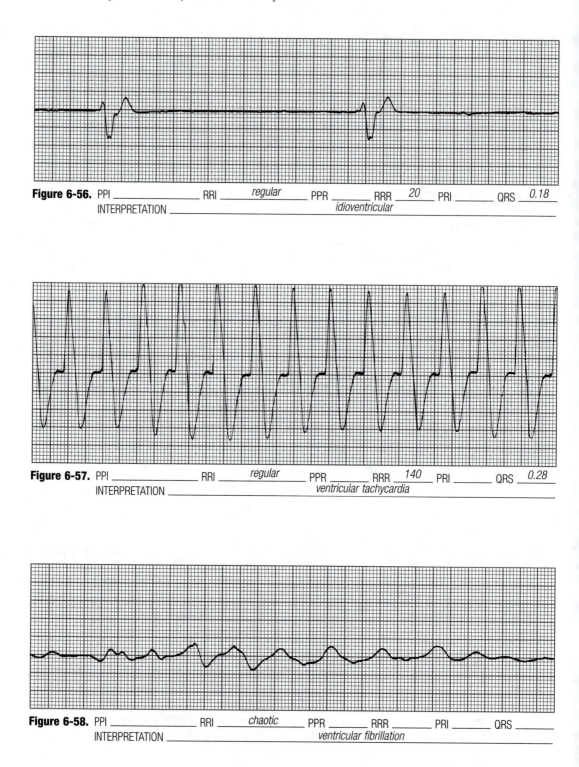

Figure 6-56. PPI _____ RRI _____*regular*_____ PPR _____ RRR __*20*__ PRI _____ QRS __*0.18*__
INTERPRETATION _____*idioventricular*_____

Figure 6-57. PPI _____ RRI _____*regular*_____ PPR _____ RRR __*140*__ PRI _____ QRS __*0.28*__
INTERPRETATION _____*ventricular tachycardia*_____

Figure 6-58. PPI _____ RRI _____*chaotic*_____ PPR _____ RRR _____ PRI _____ QRS _____
INTERPRETATION _____*ventricular fibrillation*_____

CHAPTER 7

Answer Key—Matching

1.	d	6.	b	10.	g	14.	g	18.	c
2.	e, f	7.	b	11.	i	15.	f	19.	b
3.	i	8.	c	12.	k	16.	g	20.	c
4.	o	9.	n	13.	c	17.	e	21.	j
5.	b								

Answer Key—ECG Practice Strips

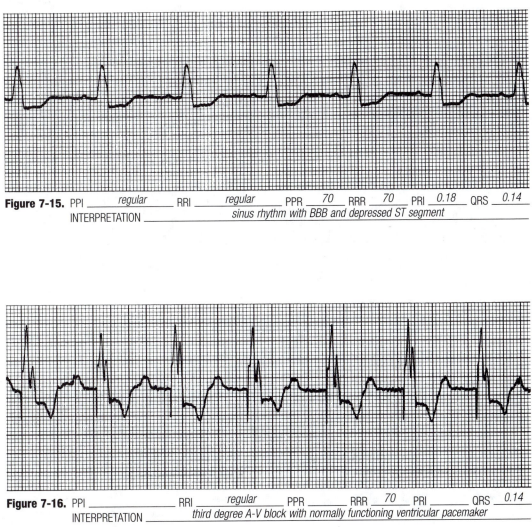

Figure 7-15. PPI _____ *regular* _____ RRI _____ *regular* _____ PPR __ *70* __ RRR __ *70* __ PRI _0.18_ QRS _0.14_
INTERPRETATION _____ *sinus rhythm with BBB and depressed ST segment* _____

Figure 7-16. PPI _____ RRI _____ *regular* _____ PPR _____ RRR __ *70* __ PRI _____ QRS _0.14_
INTERPRETATION _____ *third degree A-V block with normally functioning ventricular pacemaker* _____

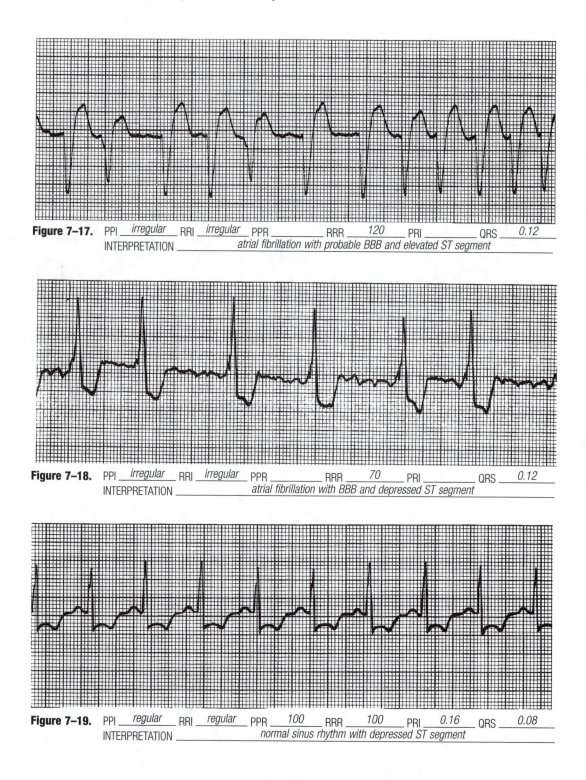

Figure 7–17.   PPI ___*irregular*___ RRI ___*irregular*___ PPR _____ RRR ___*120*___ PRI _____ QRS ___*0.12*___
INTERPRETATION _____*atrial fibrillation with probable BBB and elevated ST segment*_____

Figure 7–18.   PPI ___*irregular*___ RRI ___*irregular*___ PPR _____ RRR ___*70*___ PRI _____ QRS ___*0.12*___
INTERPRETATION _____*atrial fibrillation with BBB and depressed ST segment*_____

Figure 7–19.   PPI ___*regular*___ RRI ___*regular*___ PPR ___*100*___ RRR ___*100*___ PRI ___*0.16*___ QRS ___*0.08*___
INTERPRETATION _____*normal sinus rhythm with depressed ST segment*_____

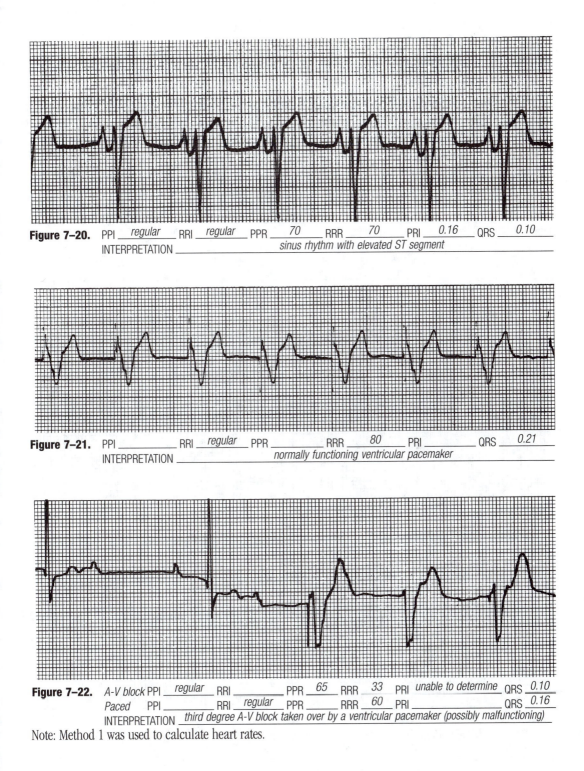

Figure 7–20. PPI _regular_ RRI _regular_ PPR _70_ RRR _70_ PRI _0.16_ QRS _0.10_
INTERPRETATION _sinus rhythm with elevated ST segment_

Figure 7–21. PPI _____ RRI _regular_ PPR _____ RRR _80_ PRI _____ QRS _0.21_
INTERPRETATION _normally functioning ventricular pacemaker_

Figure 7–22. _A-V block_ PPI _regular_ RRI _____ PPR _65_ RRR _33_ PRI _unable to determine_ QRS _0.10_
Paced PPI _____ RRI _regular_ PPR _____ RRR _60_ PRI _____ QRS _0.16_
INTERPRETATION _third degree A-V block taken over by a ventricular pacemaker (possibly malfunctioning)_

Note: Method 1 was used to calculate heart rates.

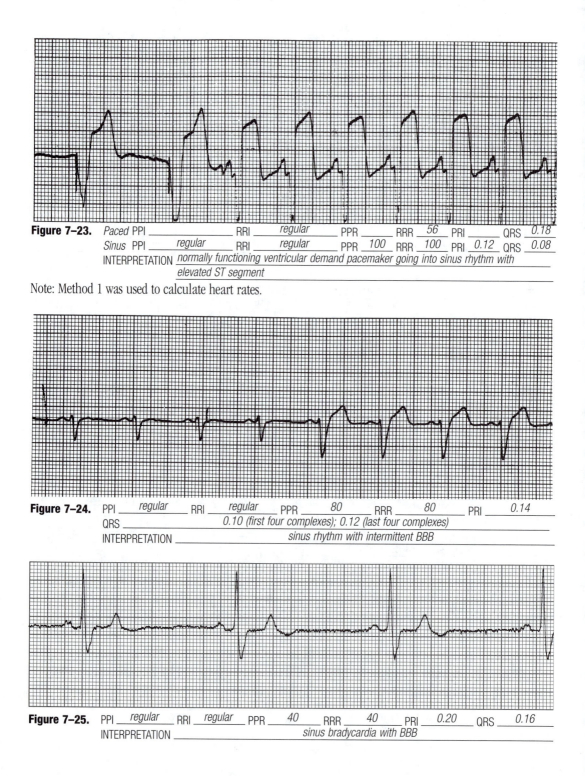

Figure 7–23. *Paced* PPI _____ RRI ___*regular*___ PPR _____ RRR _*56*_ PRI _____ QRS _*0.18*_
Sinus PPI ___*regular*___ RRI ___*regular*___ PPR _*100*_ RRR _*100*_ PRI _*0.12*_ QRS _*0.08*_
INTERPRETATION *normally functioning ventricular demand pacemaker going into sinus rhythm with*
elevated ST segment

Note: Method 1 was used to calculate heart rates.

Figure 7–24. PPI ___*regular*___ RRI ___*regular*___ PPR _*80*_ RRR _*80*_ PRI _*0.14*_
QRS _____*0.10 (first four complexes); 0.12 (last four complexes)*_____
INTERPRETATION _____*sinus rhythm with intermittent BBB*_____

Figure 7–25. PPI ___*regular*___ RRI ___*regular*___ PPR _*40*_ RRR _*40*_ PRI _*0.20*_ QRS _*0.16*_
INTERPRETATION _____*sinus bradycardia with BBB*_____

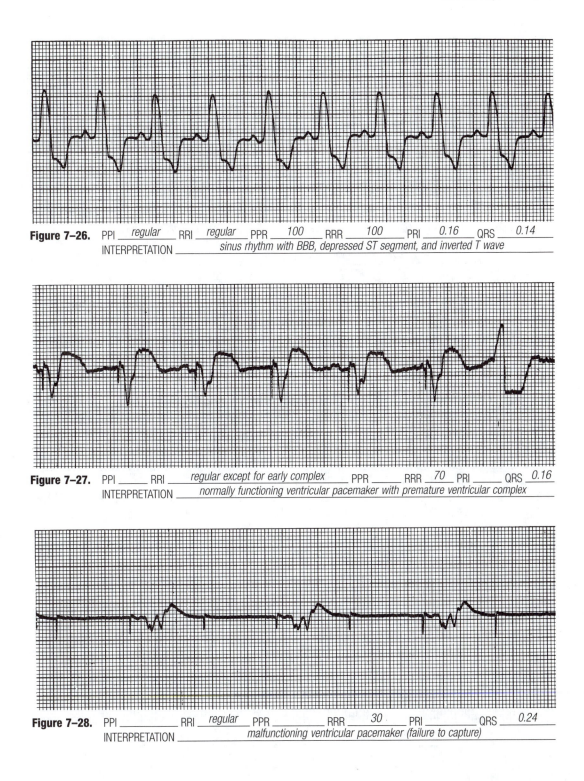

Figure 7–26. PPI _regular_ RRI _regular_ PPR _100_ RRR _100_ PRI _0.16_ QRS _0.14_
INTERPRETATION _sinus rhythm with BBB, depressed ST segment, and inverted T wave_

Figure 7–27. PPI _____ RRI _regular except for early complex_ PPR _____ RRR _70_ PRI _____ QRS _0.16_
INTERPRETATION _normally functioning ventricular pacemaker with premature ventricular complex_

Figure 7–28. PPI _____ RRI _regular_ PPR _____ RRR _30_ PRI _____ QRS _0.24_
INTERPRETATION _malfunctioning ventricular pacemaker (failure to capture)_

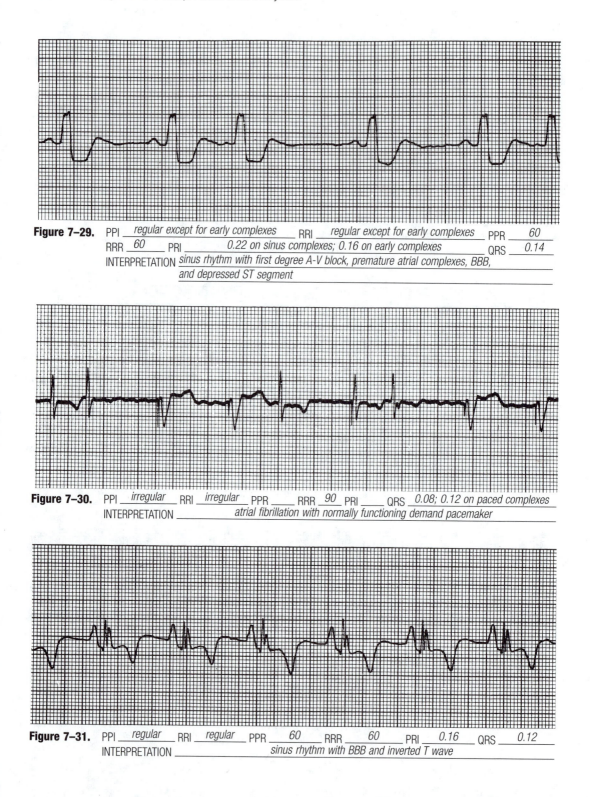

Figure 7–29. PPI ___regular except for early complexes___ RRI ___regular except for early complexes___ PPR ___60___
RRR ___60___ PRI ___0.22 on sinus complexes; 0.16 on early complexes___ QRS ___0.14___
INTERPRETATION _sinus rhythm with first degree A-V block, premature atrial complexes, BBB,_
and depressed ST segment

Figure 7–30. PPI ___irregular___ RRI ___irregular___ PPR _____ RRR ___90___ PRI _____ QRS ___0.08; 0.12 on paced complexes___
INTERPRETATION ___atrial fibrillation with normally functioning demand pacemaker___

Figure 7–31. PPI ___regular___ RRI ___regular___ PPR ___60___ RRR ___60___ PRI ___0.16___ QRS ___0.12___
INTERPRETATION ___sinus rhythm with BBB and inverted T wave___

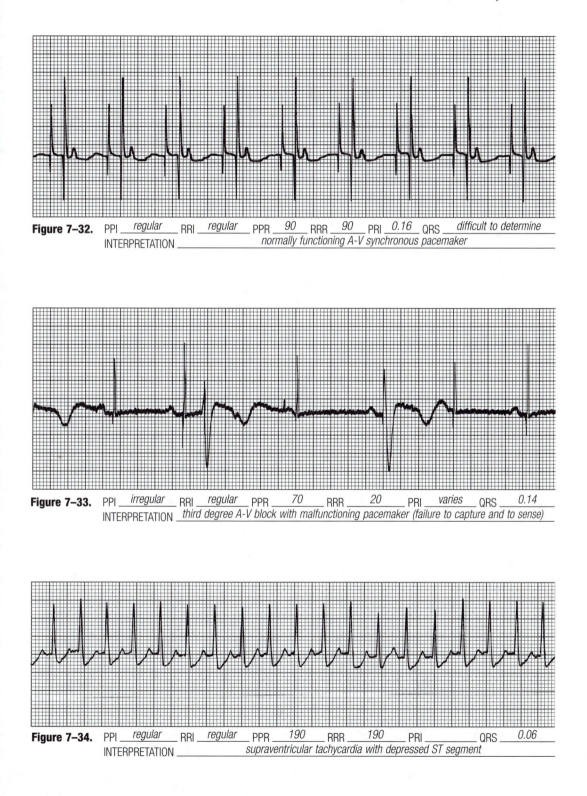

Figure 7–32. PPI _____regular_____ RRI _____regular_____ PPR ___90___ RRR ___90___ PRI ___0.16___ QRS _____difficult to determine_____
INTERPRETATION _____normally functioning A-V synchronous pacemaker_____

Figure 7–33. PPI _____irregular_____ RRI _____regular_____ PPR ___70___ RRR ___20___ PRI _____varies_____ QRS ___0.14___
INTERPRETATION _____third degree A-V block with malfunctioning pacemaker (failure to capture and to sense)_____

Figure 7–34. PPI _____regular_____ RRI _____regular_____ PPR ___190___ RRR ___190___ PRI _____ QRS ___0.06___
INTERPRETATION _____supraventricular tachycardia with depressed ST segment_____

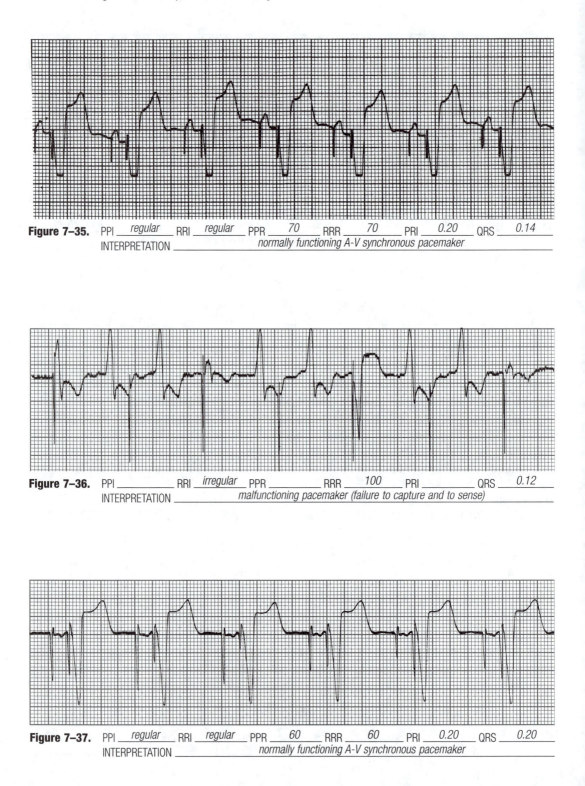

Figure 7–35.   PPI _regular_ RRI _regular_ PPR _70_ RRR _70_ PRI _0.20_ QRS _0.14_
INTERPRETATION _normally functioning A-V synchronous pacemaker_

Figure 7–36.   PPI _____ RRI _irregular_ PPR _____ RRR _100_ PRI _____ QRS _0.12_
INTERPRETATION _malfunctioning pacemaker (failure to capture and to sense)_

Figure 7–37.   PPI _regular_ RRI _regular_ PPR _60_ RRR _60_ PRI _0.20_ QRS _0.20_
INTERPRETATION _normally functioning A-V synchronous pacemaker_

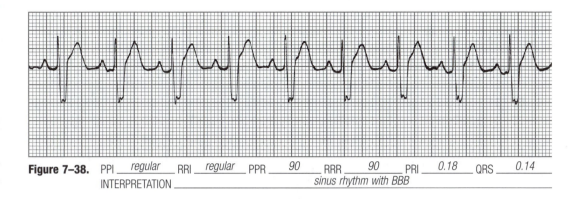

Figure 7–38. PPI ___regular___ RRI ___regular___ PPR ___90___ RRR ___90___ PRI ___0.18___ QRS ___0.14___
INTERPRETATION _____ sinus rhythm with BBB _____

CHAPTER 8

Answer Key—Review 1

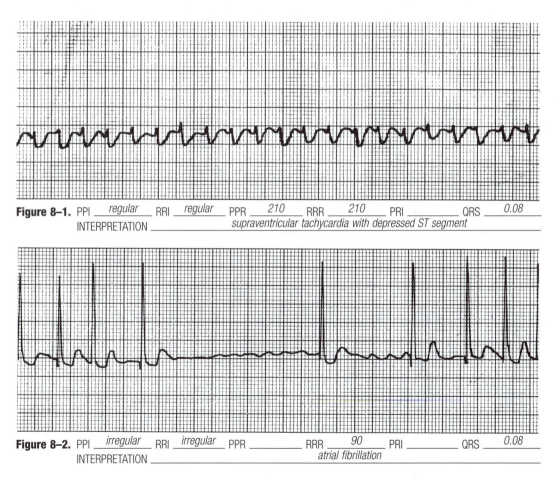

Figure 8–1. PPI ___regular___ RRI ___regular___ PPR ___210___ RRR ___210___ PRI _____ QRS ___0.08___
INTERPRETATION _____ supraventricular tachycardia with depressed ST segment _____

Figure 8–2. PPI ___irregular___ RRI ___irregular___ PPR _____ RRR ___90___ PRI _____ QRS ___0.08___
INTERPRETATION _____ atrial fibrillation _____

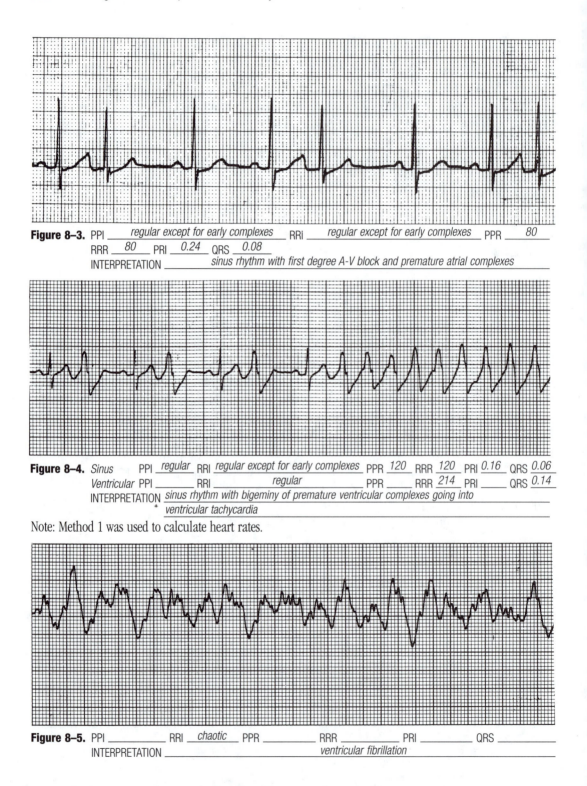

Figure 8–3. PPI ___*regular except for early complexes*___ RRI ___*regular except for early complexes*___ PPR ___*80*___
RRR ___*80*___ PRI ___*0.24*___ QRS ___*0.08*___
INTERPRETATION ___*sinus rhythm with first degree A-V block and premature atrial complexes*___

Figure 8–4. *Sinus* PPI ___*regular*___ RRI ___*regular except for early complexes*___ PPR ___*120*___ RRR ___*120*___ PRI ___*0.16*___ QRS ___*0.06*___
Ventricular PPI _____ RRI ___*regular*___ PPR _____ RRR ___*214*___ PRI _____ QRS ___*0.14*___
INTERPRETATION ___*sinus rhythm with bigeminy of premature ventricular complexes going into*___
___*ventricular tachycardia*___

Note: Method 1 was used to calculate heart rates.

Figure 8–5. PPI _____ RRI ___*chaotic*___ PPR _____ RRR _____ PRI _____ QRS _____
INTERPRETATION _____*ventricular fibrillation*_____

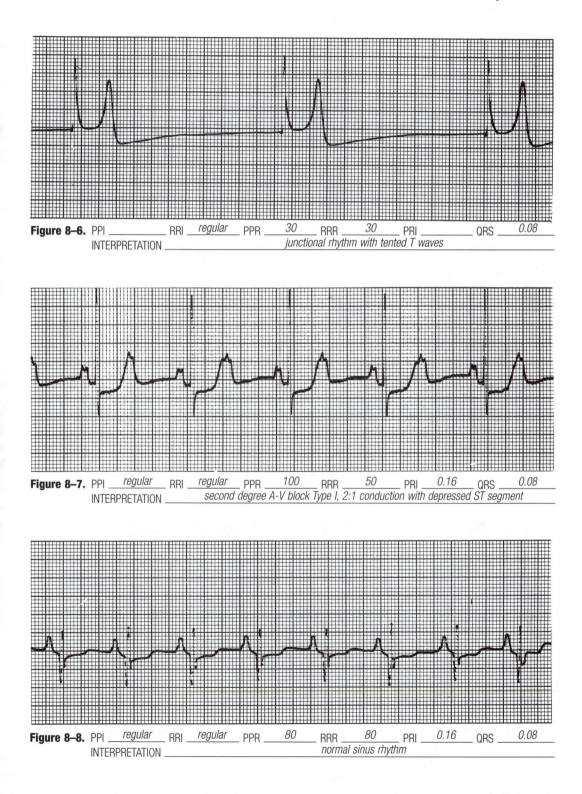

Figure 8–6. PPI _____ RRI _*regular*_ PPR _*30*_ RRR _*30*_ PRI _____ QRS _*0.08*_
INTERPRETATION _____ *junctional rhythm with tented T waves* _____

Figure 8–7. PPI _*regular*_ RRI _*regular*_ PPR _*100*_ RRR _*50*_ PRI _*0.16*_ QRS _*0.08*_
INTERPRETATION _____ *second degree A-V block Type I, 2:1 conduction with depressed ST segment*

Figure 8–8. PPI _*regular*_ RRI _*regular*_ PPR _*80*_ RRR _*80*_ PRI _*0.16*_ QRS _*0.08*_
INTERPRETATION _____ *normal sinus rhythm* _____

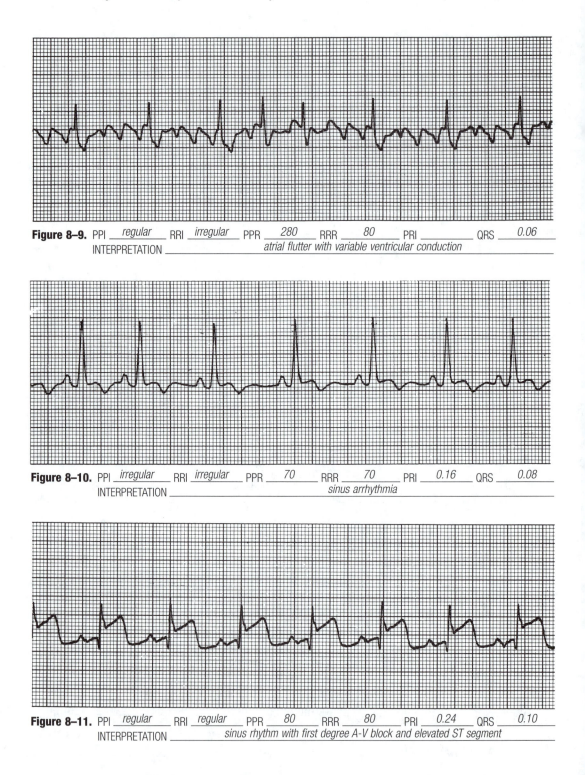

Figure 8–9. PPI ___regular___ RRI ___irregular___ PPR ___280___ RRR ___80___ PRI _____ QRS ___0.06___
INTERPRETATION _____ *atrial flutter with variable ventricular conduction* _____

Figure 8–10. PPI ___irregular___ RRI ___irregular___ PPR ___70___ RRR ___70___ PRI ___0.16___ QRS ___0.08___
INTERPRETATION _____ *sinus arrhythmia* _____

Figure 8–11. PPI ___regular___ RRI ___regular___ PPR ___80___ RRR ___80___ PRI ___0.24___ QRS ___0.10___
INTERPRETATION _____ *sinus rhythm with first degree A-V block and elevated ST segment* _____

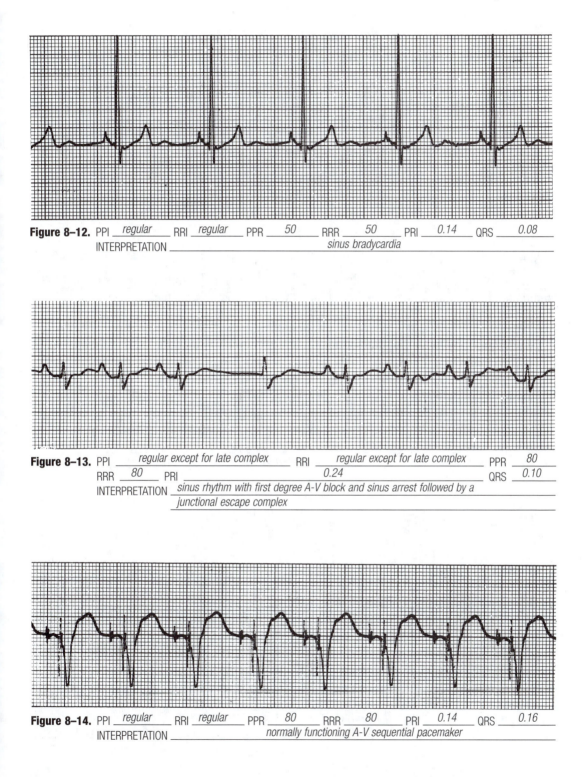

Figure 8–12. PPI ___*regular*___ RRI ___*regular*___ PPR ___*50*___ RRR ___*50*___ PRI ___*0.14*___ QRS ___*0.08*___
INTERPRETATION _____*sinus bradycardia*_____

Figure 8–13. PPI _____*regular except for late complex*_____ RRI _____*regular except for late complex*_____ PPR ___*80*___
RRR ___*80*___ PRI _____*0.24*_____ QRS ___*0.10*___
INTERPRETATION ___*sinus rhythm with first degree A-V block and sinus arrest followed by a*___
___*junctional escape complex*___

Figure 8–14. PPI ___*regular*___ RRI ___*regular*___ PPR ___*80*___ RRR ___*80*___ PRI ___*0.14*___ QRS ___*0.16*___
INTERPRETATION _____*normally functioning A-V sequential pacemaker*_____

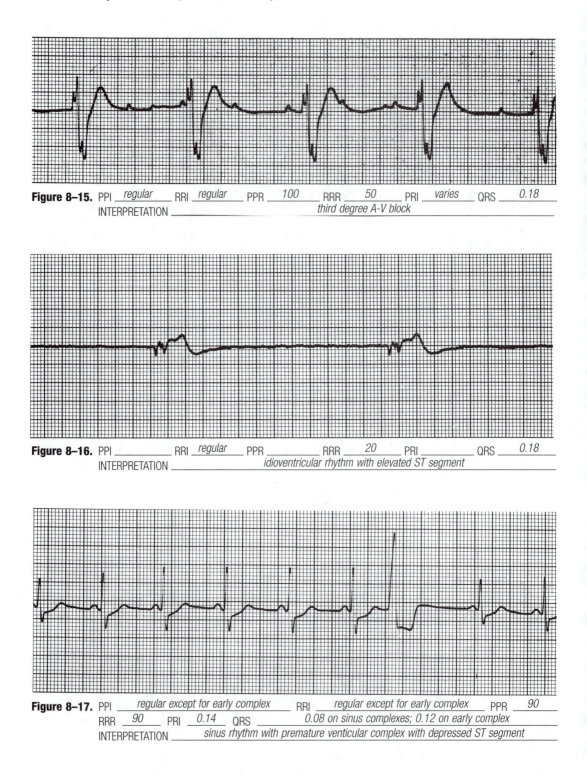

Figure 8–15. PPI _regular_ RRI _regular_ PPR _100_ RRR _50_ PRI _varies_ QRS _0.18_
INTERPRETATION _____ *third degree A-V block* _____

Figure 8–16. PPI _____ RRI _regular_ PPR _____ RRR _20_ PRI _____ QRS _0.18_
INTERPRETATION _____ *idioventricular rhythm with elevated ST segment* _____

Figure 8–17. PPI _____ *regular except for early complex* _____ RRI _____ *regular except for early complex* _____ PPR _90_
RRR _90_ PRI _0.14_ QRS _____ *0.08 on sinus complexes; 0.12 on early complex* _____
INTERPRETATION _____ *sinus rhythm with premature ventricular complex with depressed ST segment*

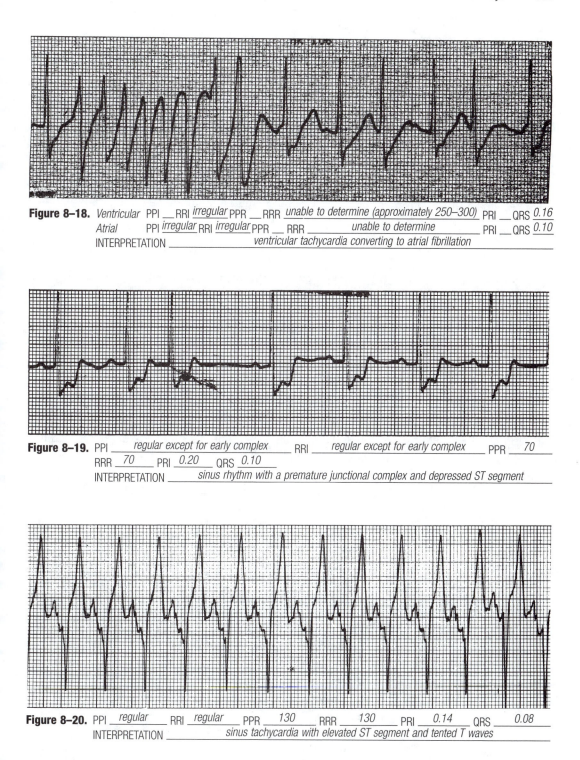

Figure 8–18. *Ventricular* PPI __ RRI *irregular* PPR __ RRR *unable to determine (approximately 250–300)* PRI __ QRS *0.16*
Atrial PPI *irregular* RRI *irregular* PPR __ RRR *unable to determine* PRI __ QRS *0.10*
INTERPRETATION *ventricular tachycardia converting to atrial fibrillation*

Figure 8–19. PPI *regular except for early complex* RRI *regular except for early complex* PPR *70*
RRR *70* PRI *0.20* QRS *0.10*
INTERPRETATION *sinus rhythm with a premature junctional complex and depressed ST segment*

Figure 8–20. PPI *regular* RRI *regular* PPR *130* RRR *130* PRI *0.14* QRS *0.08*
INTERPRETATION *sinus tachycardia with elevated ST segment and tented T waves*

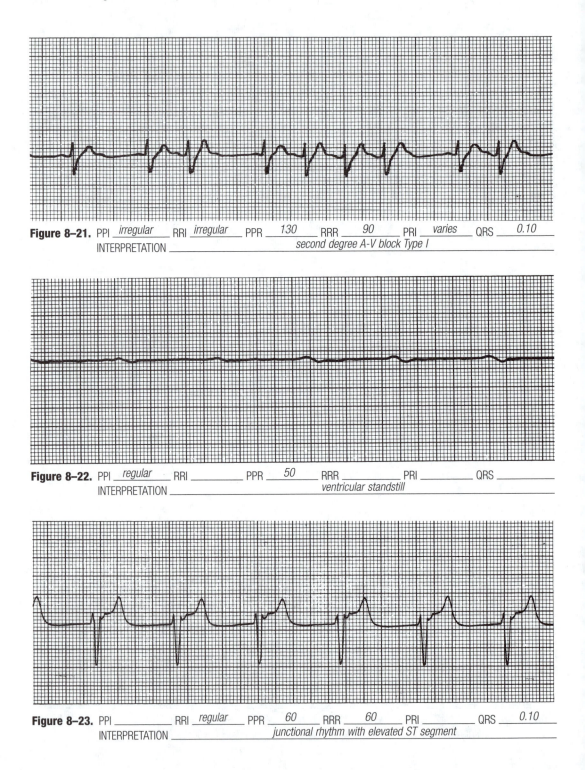

Figure 8–21. PPI _irregular_ RRI _irregular_ PPR _130_ RRR _90_ PRI _varies_ QRS _0.10_
INTERPRETATION _____ second degree A-V block Type I _____

Figure 8–22. PPI _regular_ RRI _____ PPR _50_ RRR _____ PRI _____ QRS _____
INTERPRETATION _____ ventricular standstill _____

Figure 8–23. PPI _____ RRI _regular_ PPR _60_ RRR _60_ PRI _____ QRS _0.10_
INTERPRETATION _____ junctional rhythm with elevated ST segment _____

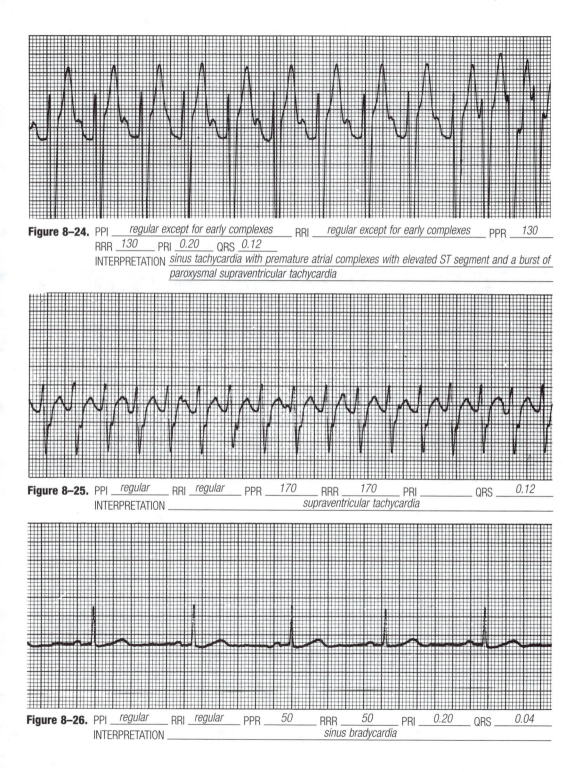

Figure 8–24. PPI ___regular except for early complexes___ RRI ___regular except for early complexes___ PPR ___130___
RRR ___130___ PRI ___0.20___ QRS ___0.12___
INTERPRETATION ___sinus tachycardia with premature atrial complexes with elevated ST segment and a burst of paroxysmal supraventricular tachycardia___

Figure 8–25. PPI ___regular___ RRI ___regular___ PPR ___170___ RRR ___170___ PRI _____ QRS ___0.12___
INTERPRETATION ___supraventricular tachycardia___

Figure 8–26. PPI ___regular___ RRI ___regular___ PPR ___50___ RRR ___50___ PRI ___0.20___ QRS ___0.04___
INTERPRETATION ___sinus bradycardia___

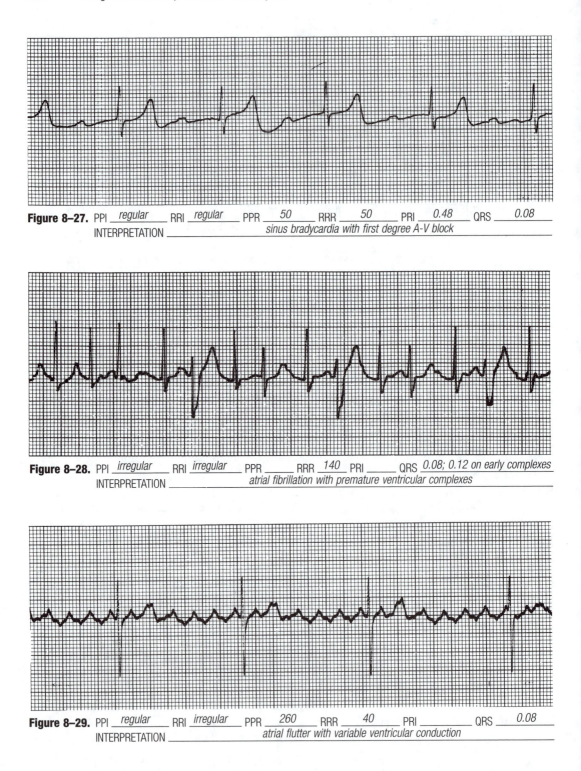

Figure 8–27. PPI _regular_ RRI _regular_ PPR _50_ RRR _50_ PRI _0.48_ QRS _0.08_
INTERPRETATION _sinus bradycardia with first degree A-V block_

Figure 8–28. PPI _irregular_ RRI _irregular_ PPR _____ RRR _140_ PRI _____ QRS _0.08; 0.12 on early complexes_
INTERPRETATION _atrial fibrillation with premature ventricular complexes_

Figure 8–29. PPI _regular_ RRI _irregular_ PPR _260_ RRR _40_ PRI _____ QRS _0.08_
INTERPRETATION _atrial flutter with variable ventricular conduction_

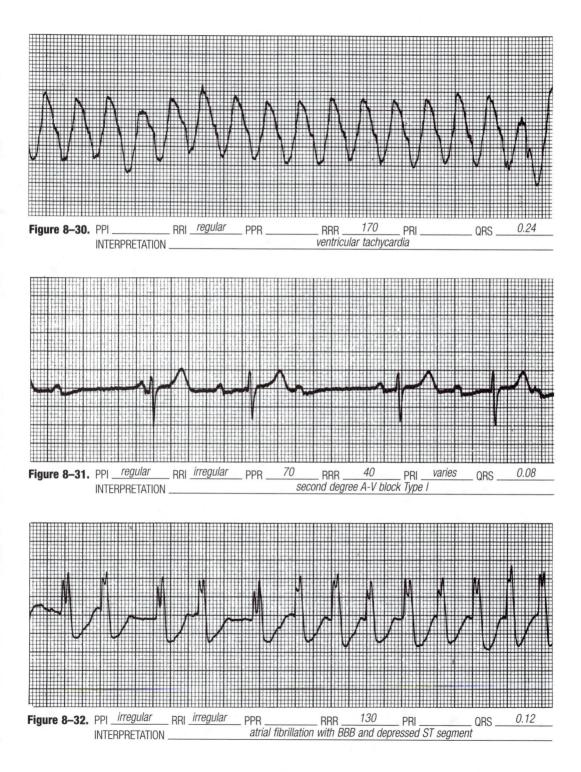

Figure 8–30. PPI _____ RRI _regular_ PPR _____ RRR _170_ PRI _____ QRS _0.24_
INTERPRETATION _____ _ventricular tachycardia_ _____

Figure 8–31. PPI _regular_ RRI _irregular_ PPR _70_ RRR _40_ PRI _varies_ QRS _0.08_
INTERPRETATION _____ _second degree A-V block Type I_ _____

Figure 8–32. PPI _irregular_ RRI _irregular_ PPR _____ RRR _130_ PRI _____ QRS _0.12_
INTERPRETATION _____ _atrial fibrillation with BBB and depressed ST segment_ _____

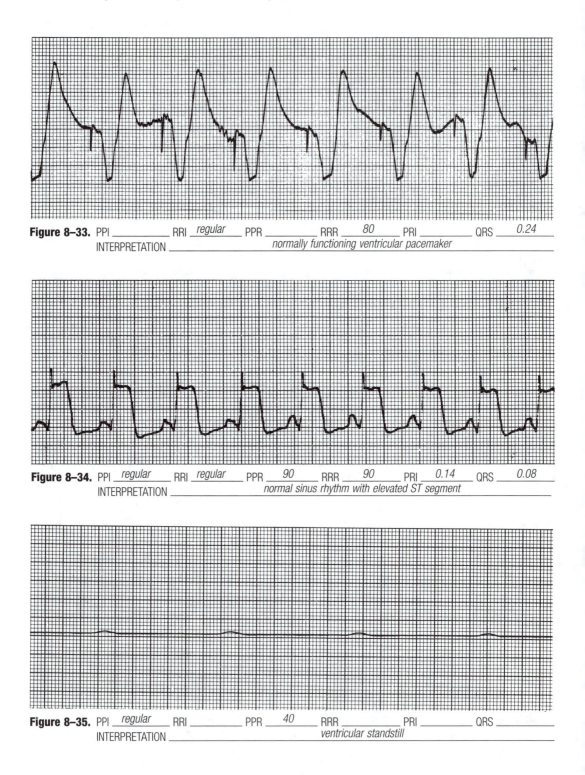

Figure 8–33. PPI _____ RRI _*regular*_ PPR _____ RRR ___*80*___ PRI _____ QRS ___*0.24*___
INTERPRETATION _____ *normally functioning ventricular pacemaker* _____

Figure 8–34. PPI _*regular*_ RRI _*regular*_ PPR ___*90*___ RRR ___*90*___ PRI ___*0.14*___ QRS ___*0.08*___
INTERPRETATION _____ *normal sinus rhythm with elevated ST segment* _____

Figure 8–35. PPI _*regular*_ RRI _____ PPR ___*40*___ RRR _____ PRI _____ QRS _____
INTERPRETATION _____ *ventricular standstill* _____

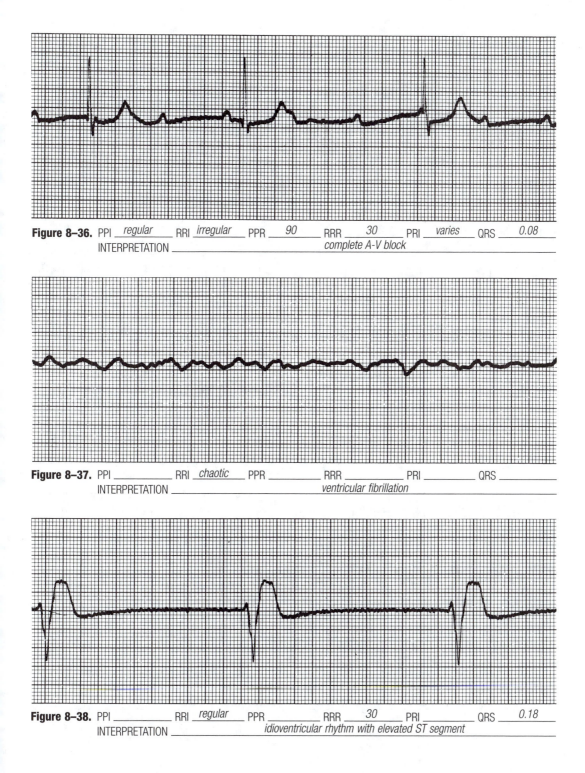

Figure 8–36. PPI _regular_ RRI _irregular_ PPR _90_ RRR _30_ PRI _varies_ QRS _0.08_
INTERPRETATION _complete A-V block_

Figure 8–37. PPI _____ RRI _chaotic_ PPR _____ RRR _____ PRI _____ QRS _____
INTERPRETATION _ventricular fibrillation_

Figure 8–38. PPI _____ RRI _regular_ PPR _____ RRR _30_ PRI _____ QRS _0.18_
INTERPRETATION _idioventricular rhythm with elevated ST segment_

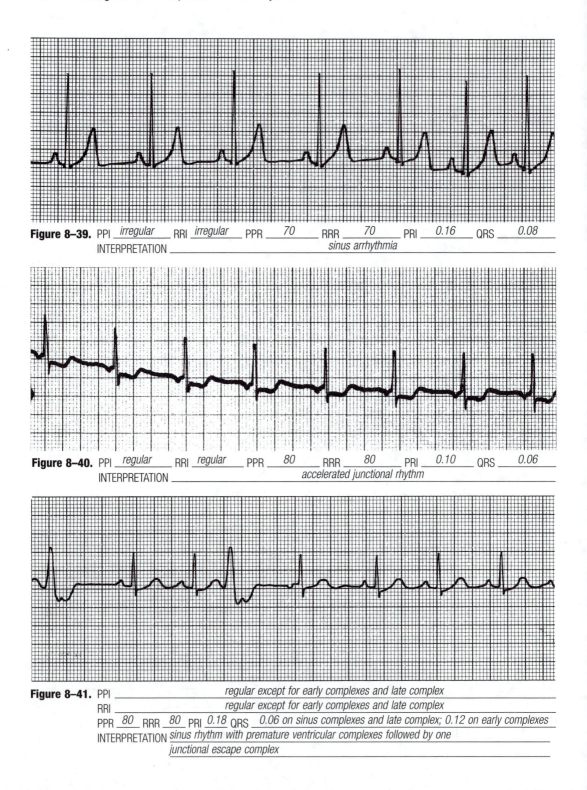

Figure 8–39. PPI _irregular_ RRI _irregular_ PPR _70_ RRR _70_ PRI _0.16_ QRS _0.08_
INTERPRETATION _____ _sinus arrhythmia_ _____

Figure 8–40. PPI _regular_ RRI _regular_ PPR _80_ RRR _80_ PRI _0.10_ QRS _0.06_
INTERPRETATION _____ _accelerated junctional rhythm_ _____

Figure 8–41. PPI _____ _regular except for early complexes and late complex_ _____
RRI _____ _regular except for early complexes and late complex_ _____
PPR _80_ RRR _80_ PRI _0.18_ QRS _0.06 on sinus complexes and late complex; 0.12 on early complexes_
INTERPRETATION _sinus rhythm with premature ventricular complexes followed by one_
junctional escape complex

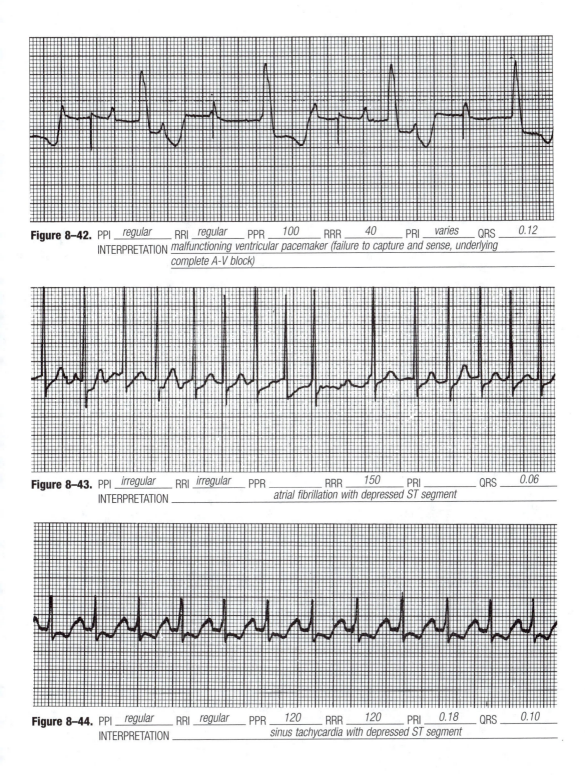

Figure 8–42. PPI _regular_ RRI _regular_ PPR _100_ RRR _40_ PRI _varies_ QRS _0.12_
INTERPRETATION _malfunctioning ventricular pacemaker (failure to capture and sense, underlying_
complete A-V block)

Figure 8–43. PPI _irregular_ RRI _irregular_ PPR _____ RRR _150_ PRI _____ QRS _0.06_
INTERPRETATION _____ atrial fibrillation with depressed ST segment

Figure 8–44. PPI _regular_ RRI _regular_ PPR _120_ RRR _120_ PRI _0.18_ QRS _0.10_
INTERPRETATION _____ sinus tachycardia with depressed ST segment

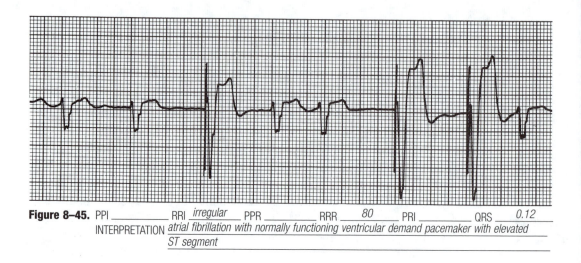

Figure 8–45. PPI _____ RRI _irregular_ PPR _____ RRR __80__ PRI _____ QRS __0.12__

INTERPRETATION _atrial fibrillation with normally functioning ventricular demand pacemaker with elevated_ _ST segment_

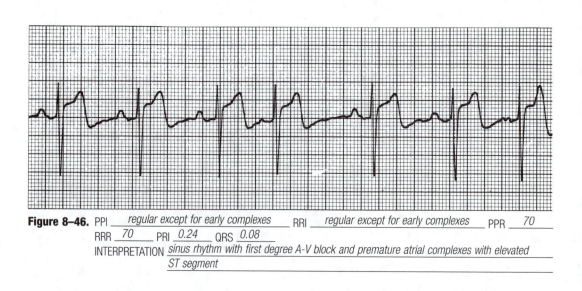

Figure 8–46. PPI __regular except for early complexes__ RRI __regular except for early complexes__ PPR __70__

RRR __70__ PRI __0.24__ QRS __0.08__

INTERPRETATION _sinus rhythm with first degree A-V block and premature atrial complexes with elevated_ _ST segment_

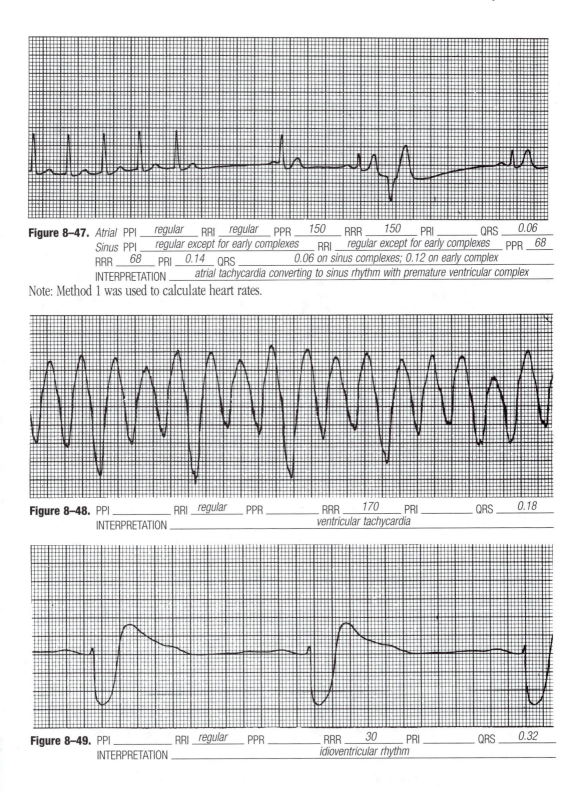

Figure 8–47. *Atrial* PPI _____*regular*_____ RRI _____*regular*_____ PPR _____*150*_____ RRR _____*150*_____ PRI _____ QRS _____*0.06*_____
Sinus PPI _____*regular except for early complexes*_____ RRI _____*regular except for early complexes*_____ PPR _*68*_
RRR _____*68*_____ PRI _*0.14*_ QRS _____*0.06 on sinus complexes; 0.12 on early complex*_____
INTERPRETATION _____*atrial tachycardia converting to sinus rhythm with premature ventricular complex*_____

Note: Method 1 was used to calculate heart rates.

Figure 8–48. PPI _____ RRI _*regular*_ PPR _____ RRR _____*170*_____ PRI _____ QRS _____*0.18*_____
INTERPRETATION _____*ventricular tachycardia*_____

Figure 8–49. PPI _____ RRI _*regular*_ PPR _____ RRR _____*30*_____ PRI _____ QRS _____*0.32*_____
INTERPRETATION _____*idioventricular rhythm*_____

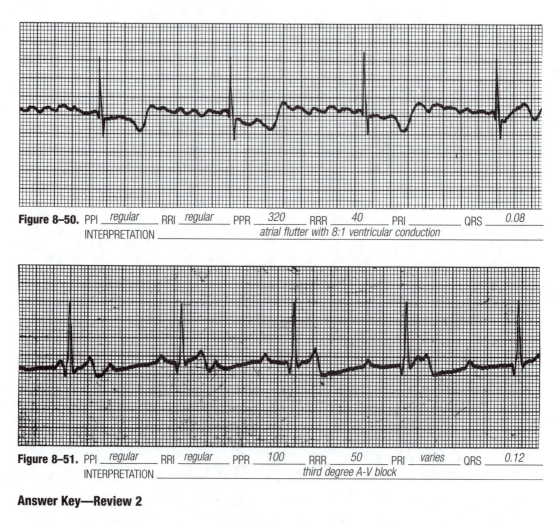

Figure 8–50. PPI ___*regular*___ RRI ___*regular*___ PPR ___320___ RRR ___40___ PRI _____ QRS ___0.08___
INTERPRETATION _____*atrial flutter with 8:1 ventricular conduction*_____

Figure 8–51. PPI ___*regular*___ RRI ___*regular*___ PPR ___100___ RRR ___50___ PRI ___*varies*___ QRS ___0.12___
INTERPRETATION _____*third degree A-V block*_____

Answer Key—Review 2

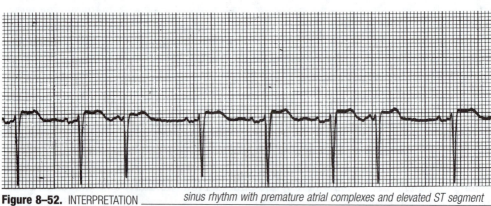

Figure 8–52. INTERPRETATION _____*sinus rhythm with premature atrial complexes and elevated ST segment*_____

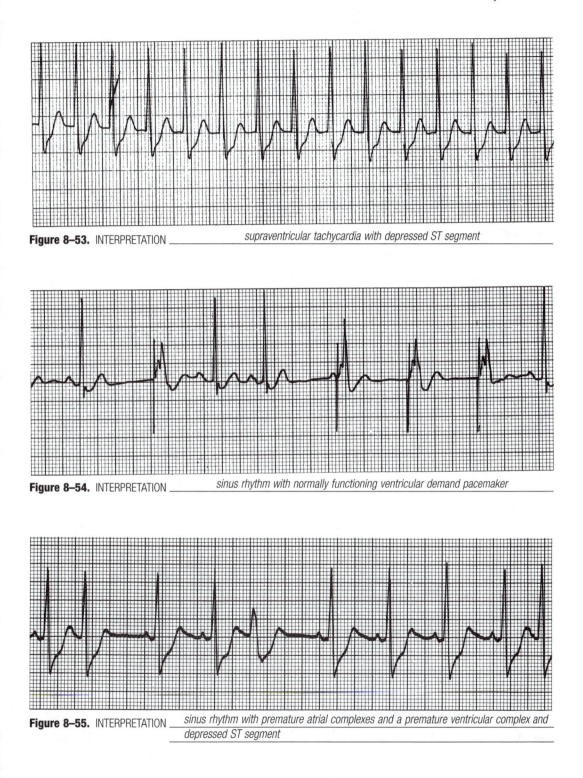

Figure 8–53. INTERPRETATION _____ *supraventricular tachycardia with depressed ST segment*

Figure 8–54. INTERPRETATION _____ *sinus rhythm with normally functioning ventricular demand pacemaker*

Figure 8–55. INTERPRETATION _____ *sinus rhythm with premature atrial complexes and a premature ventricular complex and depressed ST segment*

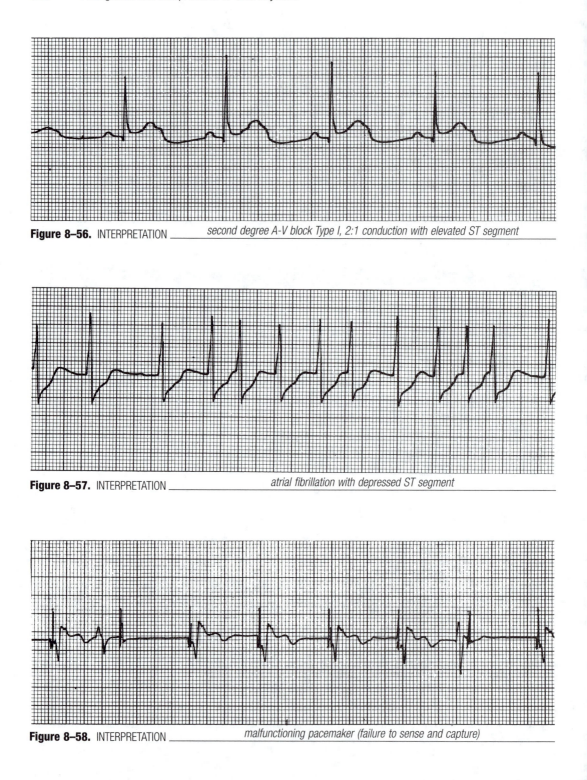

Figure 8–56. INTERPRETATION _____ *second degree A-V block Type I, 2:1 conduction with elevated ST segment*

Figure 8–57. INTERPRETATION _____ *atrial fibrillation with depressed ST segment*

Figure 8–58. INTERPRETATION _____ *malfunctioning pacemaker (failure to sense and capture)*

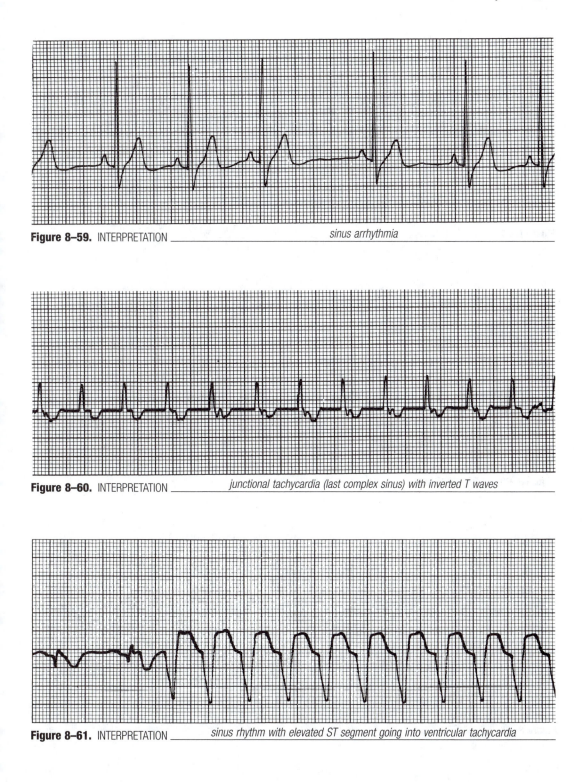

Figure 8–59. INTERPRETATION _____ *sinus arrhythmia* _____

Figure 8–60. INTERPRETATION _____ *junctional tachycardia (last complex sinus) with inverted T waves* _____

Figure 8–61. INTERPRETATION _____ *sinus rhythm with elevated ST segment going into ventricular tachycardia* _____

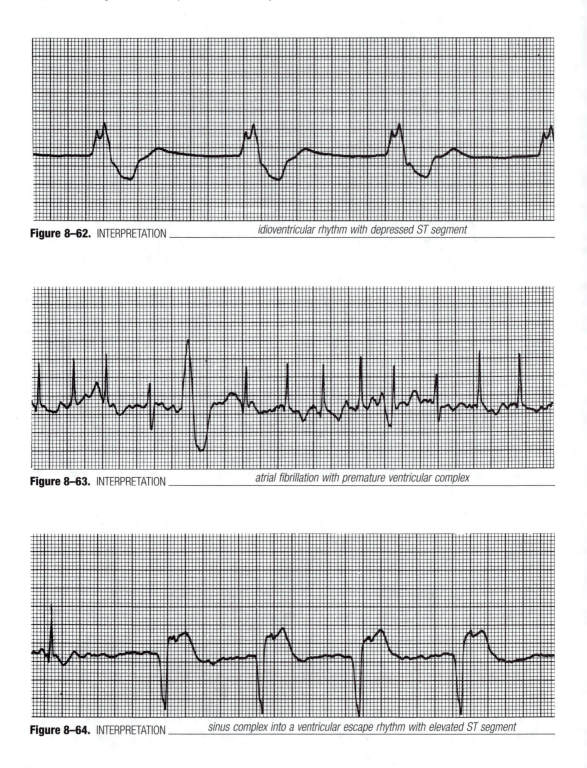

Figure 8–62. INTERPRETATION _____ *idioventricular rhythm with depressed ST segment*

Figure 8–63. INTERPRETATION _____ *atrial fibrillation with premature ventricular complex*

Figure 8–64. INTERPRETATION _____ *sinus complex into a ventricular escape rhythm with elevated ST segment*

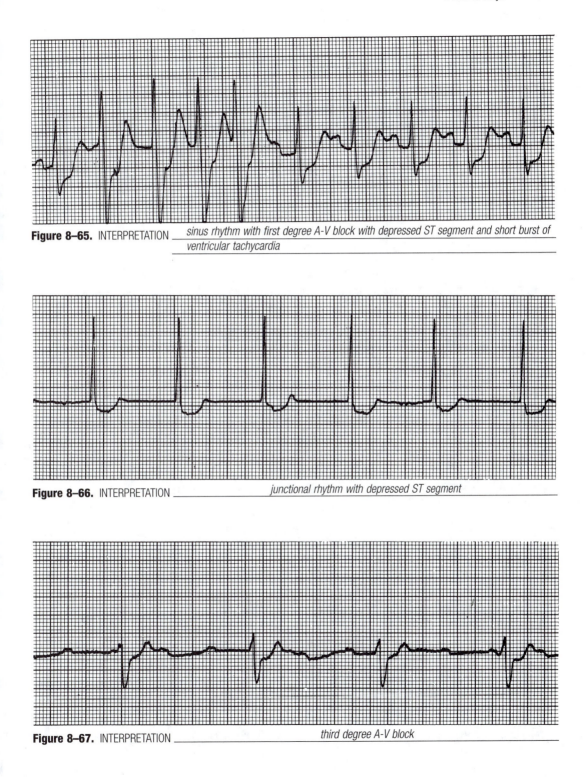

Figure 8–65. INTERPRETATION _sinus rhythm with first degree A-V block with depressed ST segment and short burst of ventricular tachycardia_

Figure 8–66. INTERPRETATION _junctional rhythm with depressed ST segment_

Figure 8–67. INTERPRETATION _third degree A-V block_

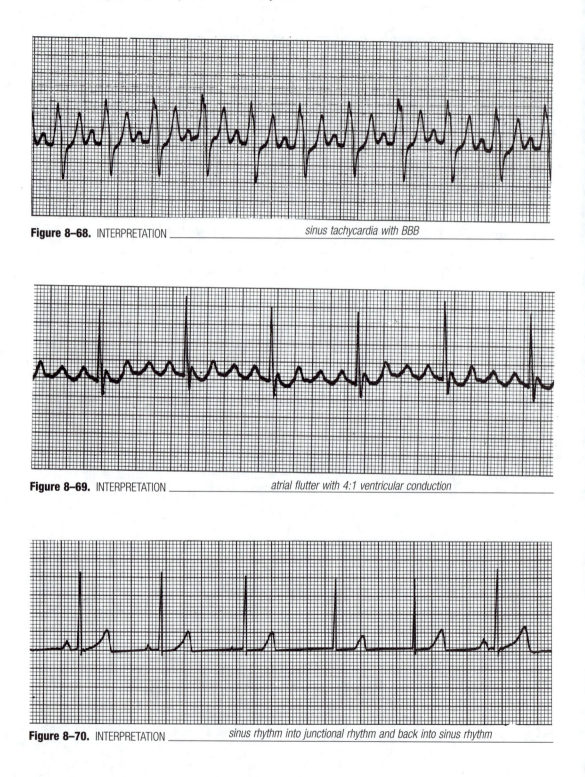

Figure 8–68. INTERPRETATION _____ *sinus tachycardia with BBB*

Figure 8–69. INTERPRETATION _____ *atrial flutter with 4:1 ventricular conduction*

Figure 8–70. INTERPRETATION _____ *sinus rhythm into junctional rhythm and back into sinus rhythm*

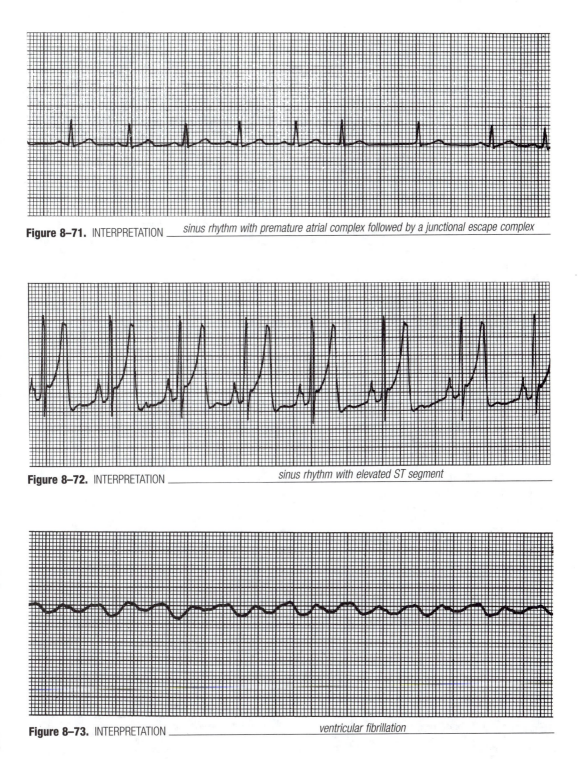

Figure 8–71. INTERPRETATION ___ *sinus rhythm with premature atrial complex followed by a junctional escape complex* ___

Figure 8–72. INTERPRETATION ___ *sinus rhythm with elevated ST segment* ___

Figure 8–73. INTERPRETATION ___ *ventricular fibrillation* ___

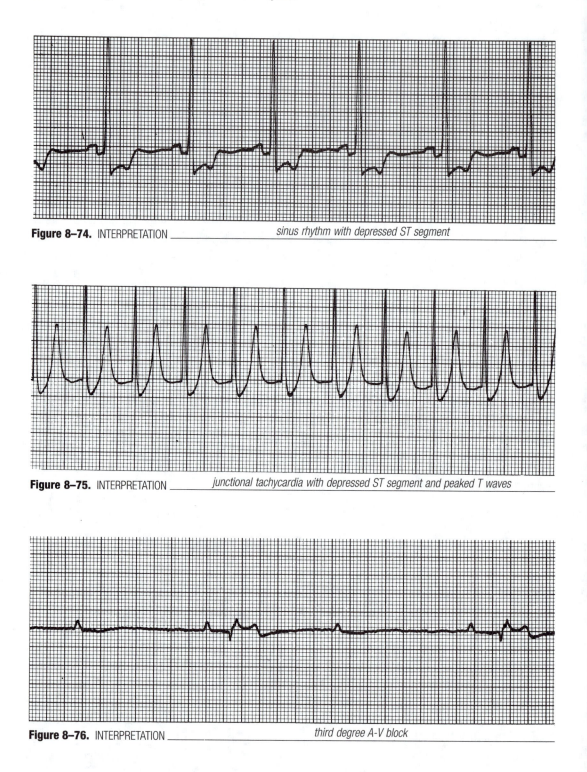

Figure 8–74. INTERPRETATION _____ *sinus rhythm with depressed ST segment*

Figure 8–75. INTERPRETATION _____ *junctional tachycardia with depressed ST segment and peaked T waves*

Figure 8–76. INTERPRETATION _____ *third degree A-V block*

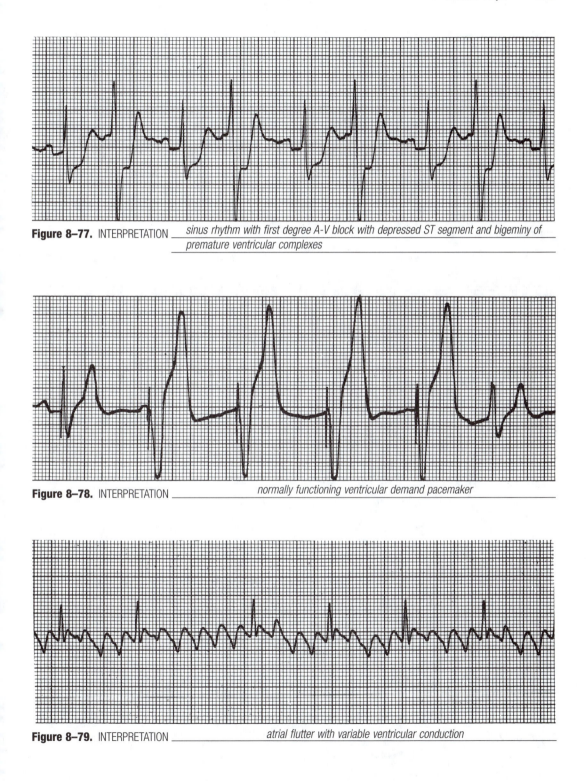

Figure 8–77. INTERPRETATION _sinus rhythm with first degree A-V block with depressed ST segment and bigeminy of premature ventricular complexes_

Figure 8–78. INTERPRETATION _normally functioning ventricular demand pacemaker_

Figure 8–79. INTERPRETATION _atrial flutter with variable ventricular conduction_

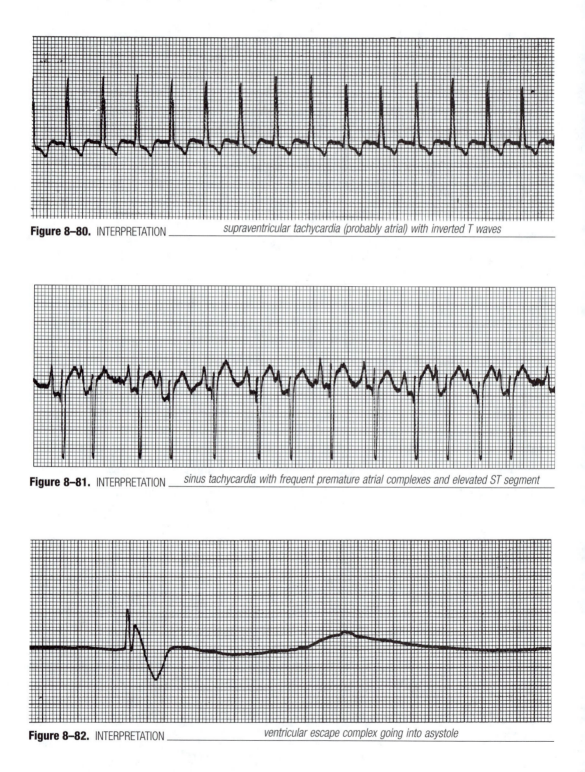

Figure 8–80. INTERPRETATION _____ *supraventricular tachycardia (probably atrial) with inverted T waves*

Figure 8–81. INTERPRETATION _____ *sinus tachycardia with frequent premature atrial complexes and elevated ST segment*

Figure 8–82. INTERPRETATION _____ *ventricular escape complex going into asystole*

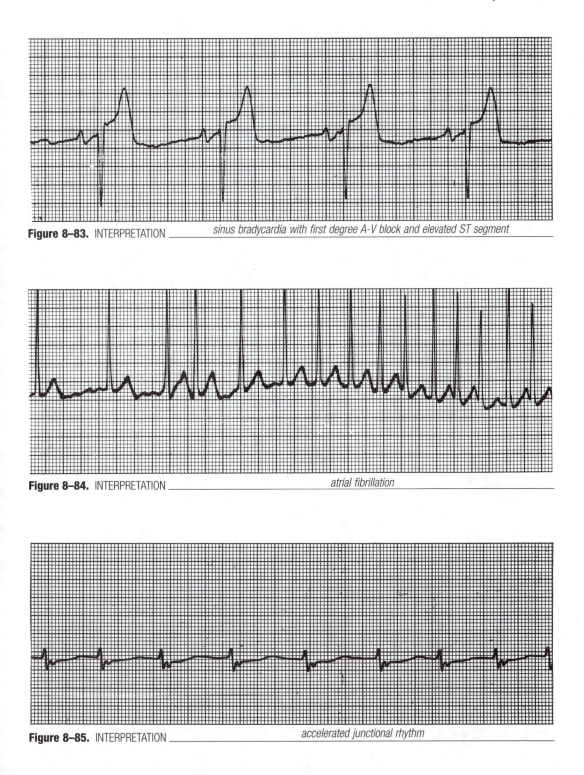

Figure 8–83. INTERPRETATION _____ *sinus bradycardia with first degree A-V block and elevated ST segment* _____

Figure 8–84. INTERPRETATION _____ *atrial fibrillation* _____

Figure 8–85. INTERPRETATION _____ *accelerated junctional rhythm*

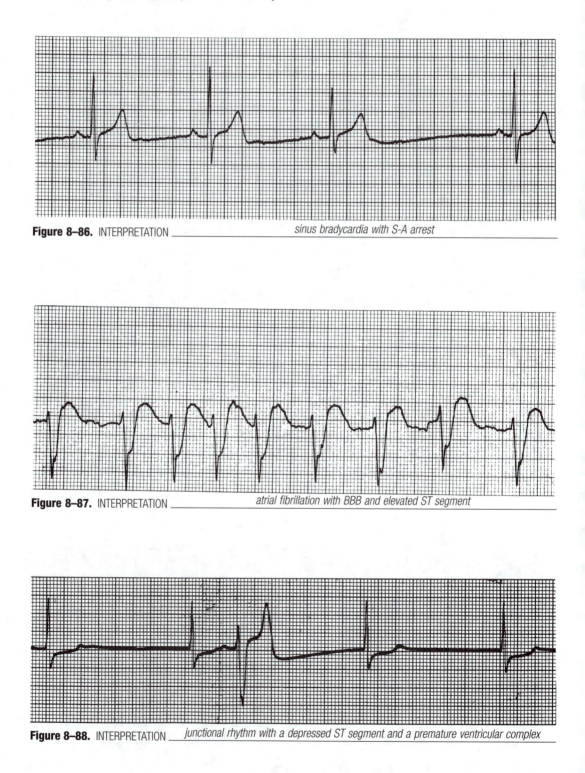

Figure 8–86. INTERPRETATION _____ *sinus bradycardia with S-A arrest*

Figure 8–87. INTERPRETATION _____ *atrial fibrillation with BBB and elevated ST segment*

Figure 8–88. INTERPRETATION _____ *junctional rhythm with a depressed ST segment and a premature ventricular complex*

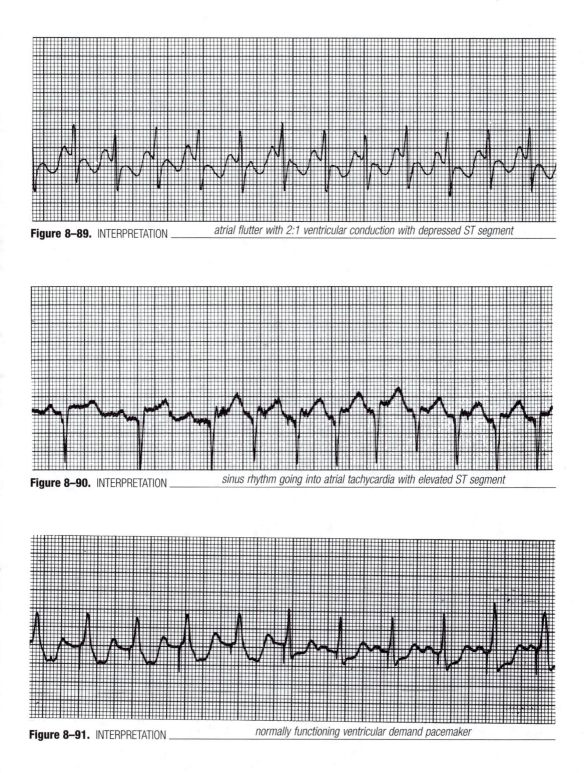

Figure 8–89. INTERPRETATION _____ *atrial flutter with 2:1 ventricular conduction with depressed ST segment*

Figure 8–90. INTERPRETATION _____ *sinus rhythm going into atrial tachycardia with elevated ST segment*

Figure 8–91. INTERPRETATION _____ *normally functioning ventricular demand pacemaker*

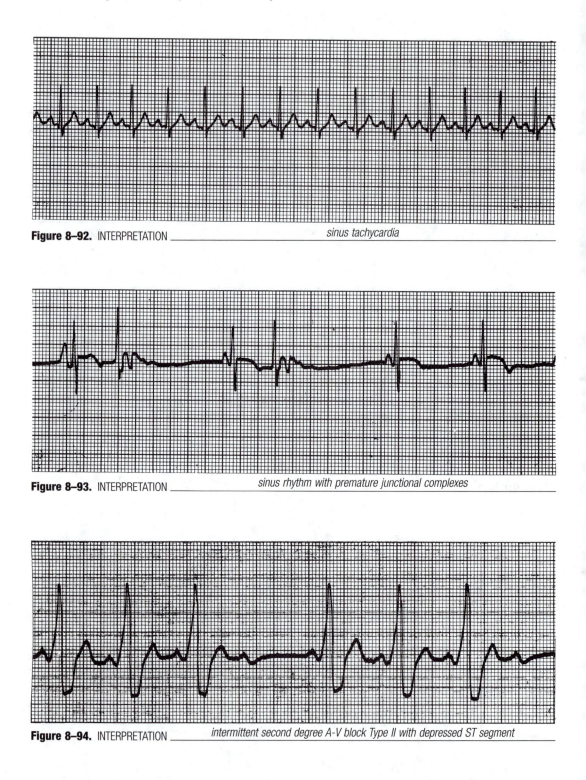

Figure 8–92. INTERPRETATION _____ *sinus tachycardia*

Figure 8–93. INTERPRETATION _____ *sinus rhythm with premature junctional complexes*

Figure 8–94. INTERPRETATION _____ *intermittent second degree A-V block Type II with depressed ST segment*

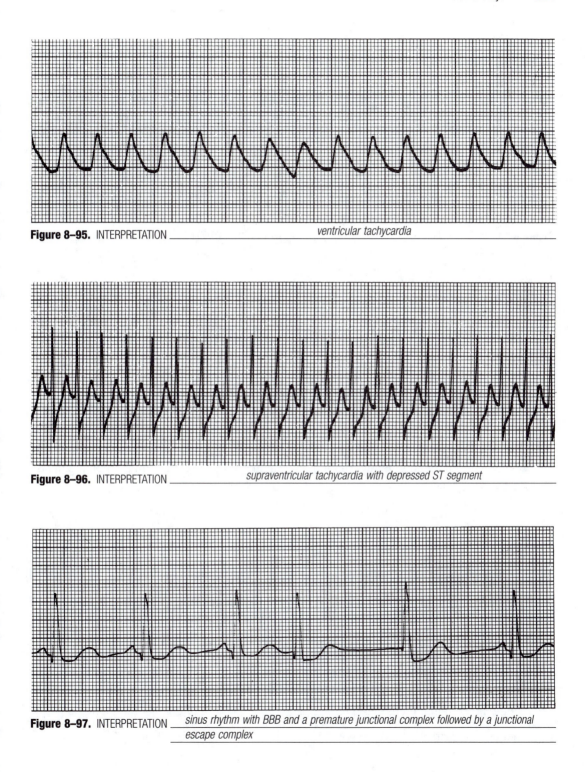

Figure 8–95. INTERPRETATION _____ *ventricular tachycardia* _____

Figure 8–96. INTERPRETATION _____ *supraventricular tachycardia with depressed ST segment* _____

Figure 8–97. INTERPRETATION _____ *sinus rhythm with BBB and a premature junctional complex followed by a junctional escape complex* _____

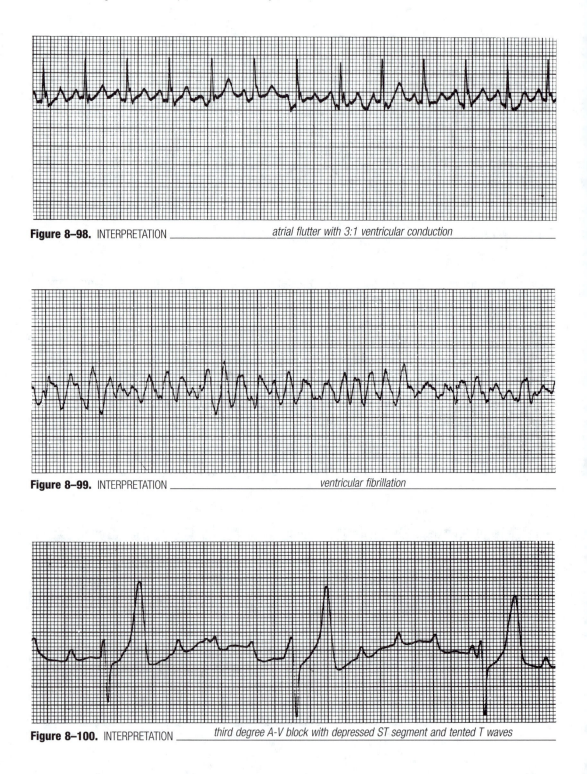

Figure 8–98. INTERPRETATION _____ *atrial flutter with 3:1 ventricular conduction* _____

Figure 8–99. INTERPRETATION _____ *ventricular fibrillation* _____

Figure 8–100. INTERPRETATION _____ *third degree A-V block with depressed ST segment and tented T waves*

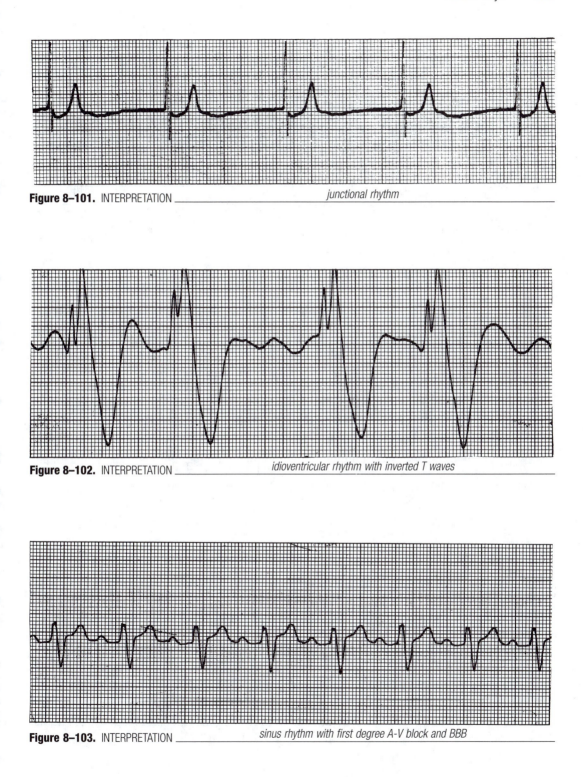

Figure 8–101. INTERPRETATION _____ *junctional rhythm* _____

Figure 8–102. INTERPRETATION _____ *idioventricular rhythm with inverted T waves* _____

Figure 8–103. INTERPRETATION _____ *sinus rhythm with first degree A-V block and BBB* _____

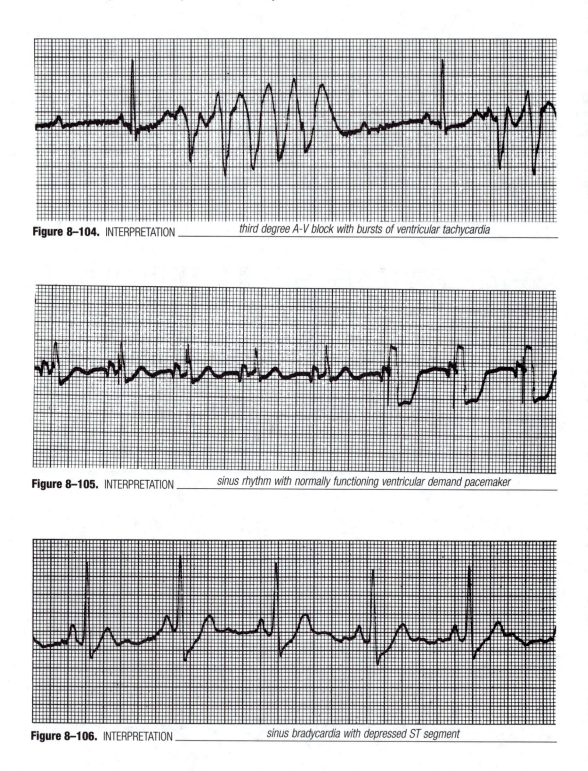

Figure 8–104. INTERPRETATION _____ *third degree A-V block with bursts of ventricular tachycardia*

Figure 8–105. INTERPRETATION _____ *sinus rhythm with normally functioning ventricular demand pacemaker*

Figure 8–106. INTERPRETATION _____ *sinus bradycardia with depressed ST segment*

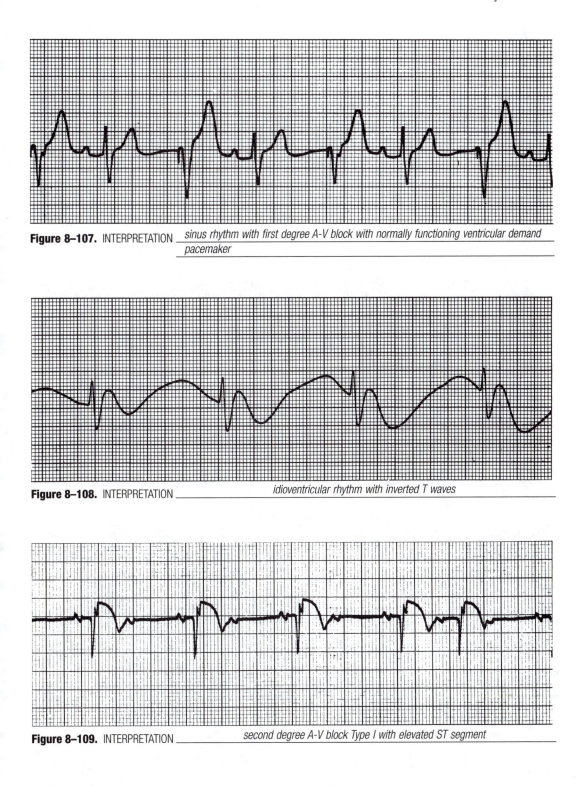

Figure 8–107. INTERPRETATION *sinus rhythm with first degree A-V block with normally functioning ventricular demand pacemaker*

Figure 8–108. INTERPRETATION *idioventricular rhythm with inverted T waves*

Figure 8–109. INTERPRETATION *second degree A-V block Type I with elevated ST segment*

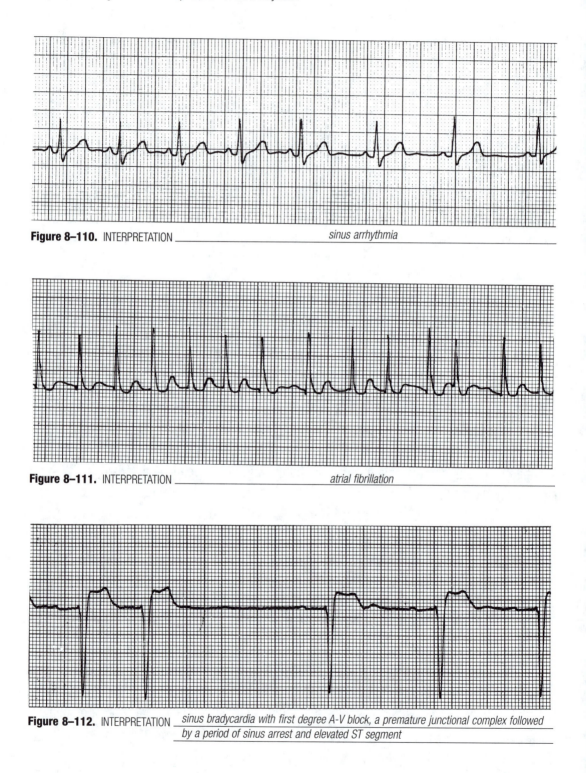

Figure 8–110. INTERPRETATION _____ *sinus arrhythmia*

Figure 8–111. INTERPRETATION _____ *atrial fibrillation*

Figure 8–112. INTERPRETATION *sinus bradycardia with first degree A-V block, a premature junctional complex followed by a period of sinus arrest and elevated ST segment*

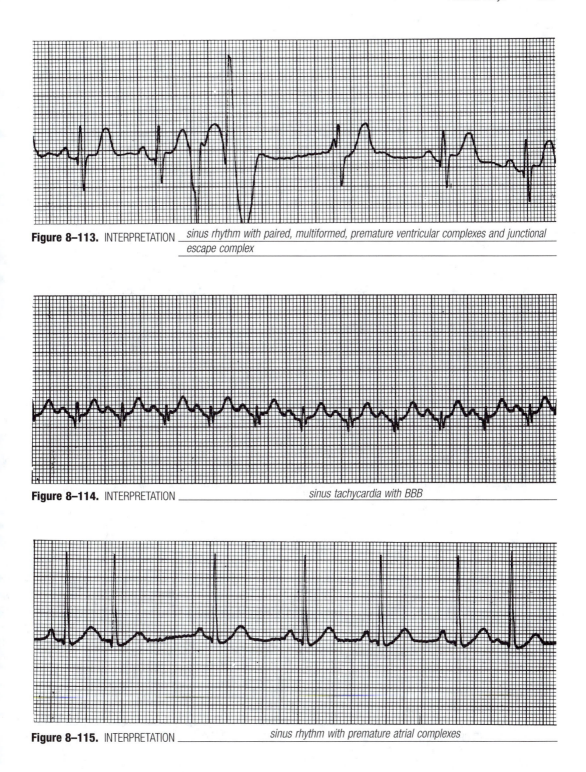

Figure 8–113. INTERPRETATION *sinus rhythm with paired, multiformed, premature ventricular complexes and junctional escape complex*

Figure 8–114. INTERPRETATION *sinus tachycardia with BBB*

Figure 8–115. INTERPRETATION *sinus rhythm with premature atrial complexes*

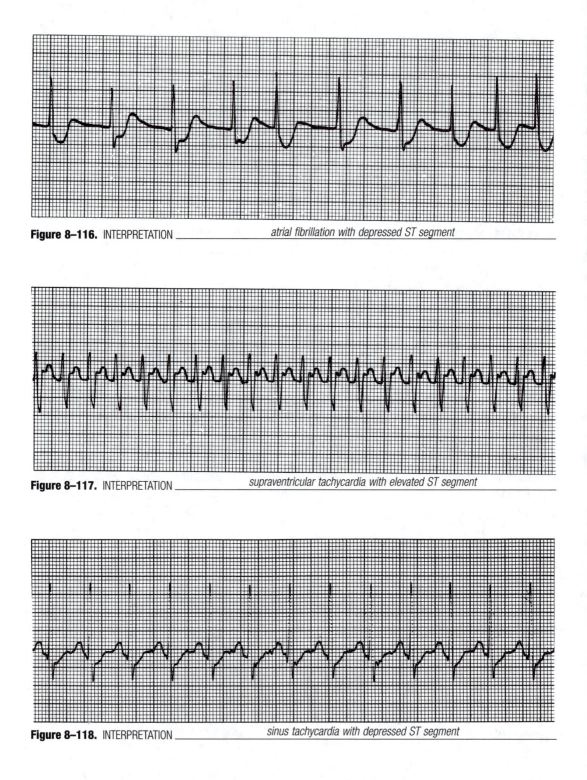

Figure 8–116. INTERPRETATION _____ *atrial fibrillation with depressed ST segment*

Figure 8–117. INTERPRETATION _____ *supraventricular tachycardia with elevated ST segment*

Figure 8–118. INTERPRETATION _____ *sinus tachycardia with depressed ST segment*

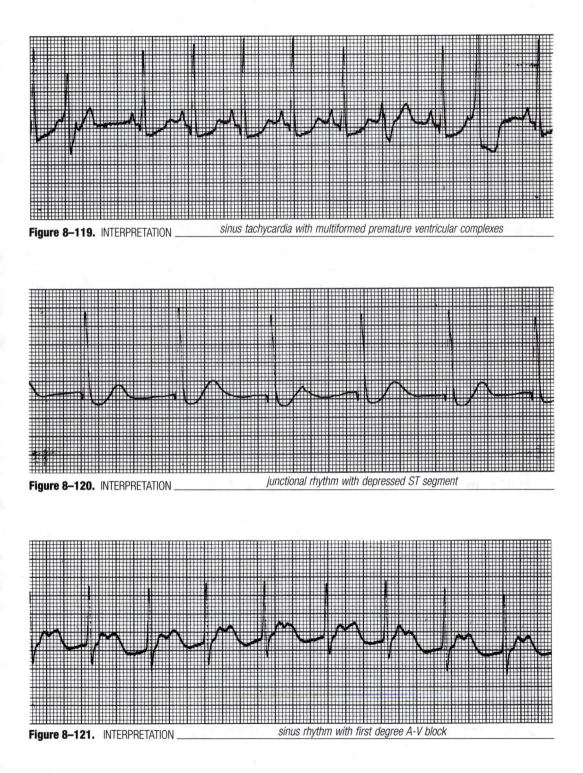

Figure 8–119. INTERPRETATION _____ *sinus tachycardia with multiformed premature ventricular complexes*

Figure 8–120. INTERPRETATION _____ *junctional rhythm with depressed ST segment*

Figure 8–121. INTERPRETATION _____ *sinus rhythm with first degree A-V block*

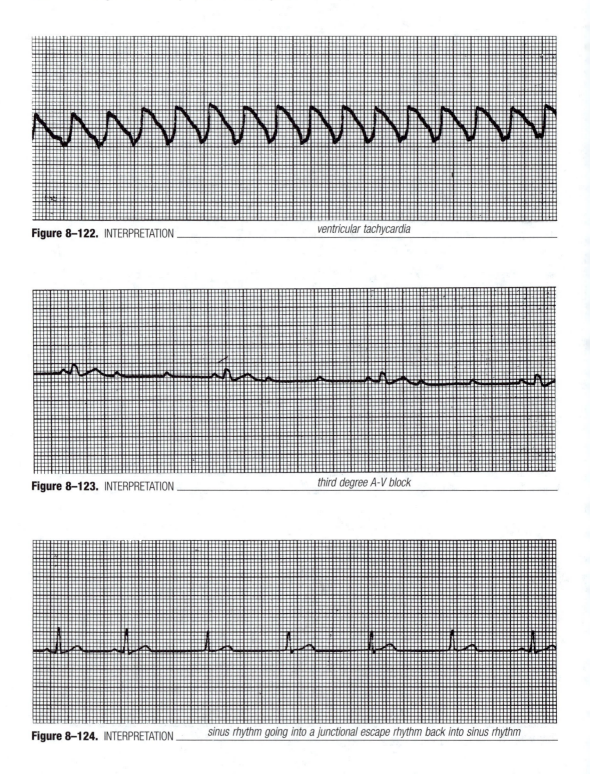

Figure 8–122. INTERPRETATION _____ *ventricular tachycardia* _____

Figure 8–123. INTERPRETATION _____ *third degree A-V block* _____

Figure 8–124. INTERPRETATION _____ *sinus rhythm going into a junctional escape rhythm back into sinus rhythm* _____

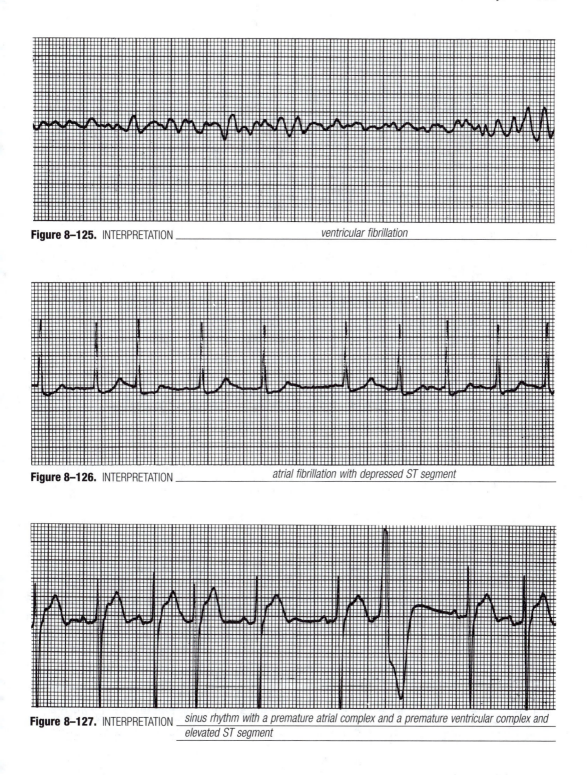

Figure 8–125. INTERPRETATION _____ *ventricular fibrillation* _____

Figure 8–126. INTERPRETATION _____ *atrial fibrillation with depressed ST segment* _____

Figure 8–127. INTERPRETATION _____ *sinus rhythm with a premature atrial complex and a premature ventricular complex and elevated ST segment* _____

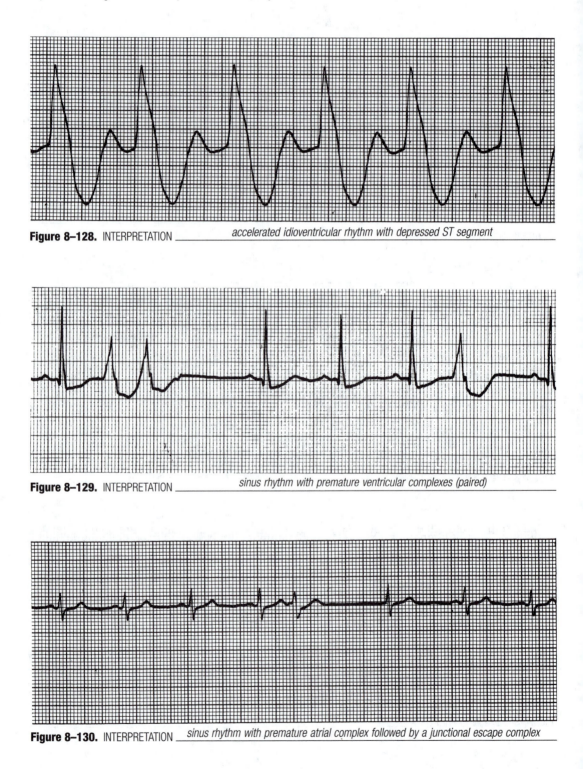

Figure 8–128. INTERPRETATION ___*accelerated idioventricular rhythm with depressed ST segment*___

Figure 8–129. INTERPRETATION ___*sinus rhythm with premature ventricular complexes (paired)*___

Figure 8–130. INTERPRETATION ___*sinus rhythm with premature atrial complex followed by a junctional escape complex*___

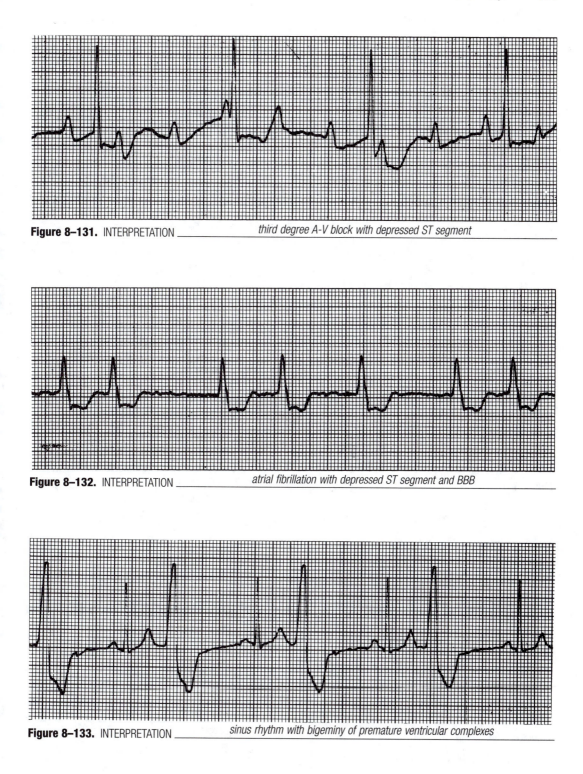

Figure 8–131. INTERPRETATION _____ *third degree A-V block with depressed ST segment*

Figure 8–132. INTERPRETATION _____ *atrial fibrillation with depressed ST segment and BBB*

Figure 8–133. INTERPRETATION _____ *sinus rhythm with bigeminy of premature ventricular complexes*

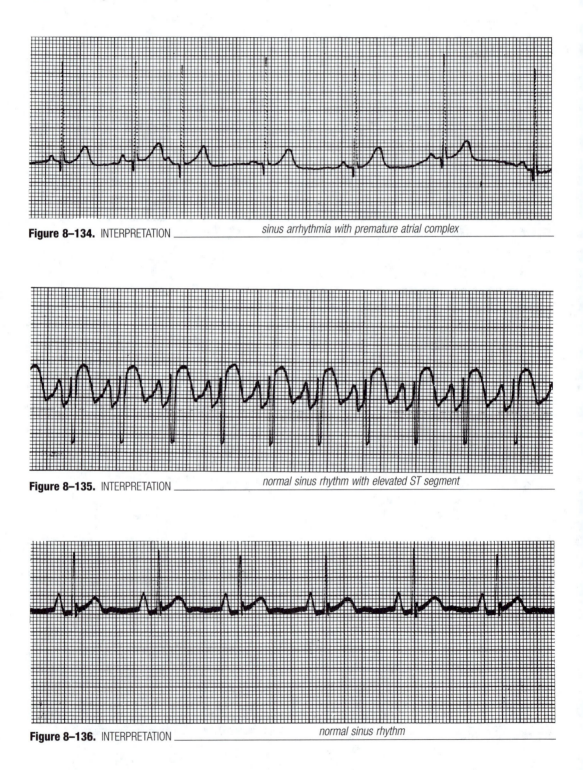

Figure 8–134. INTERPRETATION _____ *sinus arrhythmia with premature atrial complex*

Figure 8–135. INTERPRETATION _____ *normal sinus rhythm with elevated ST segment*

Figure 8–136. INTERPRETATION _____ *normal sinus rhythm*

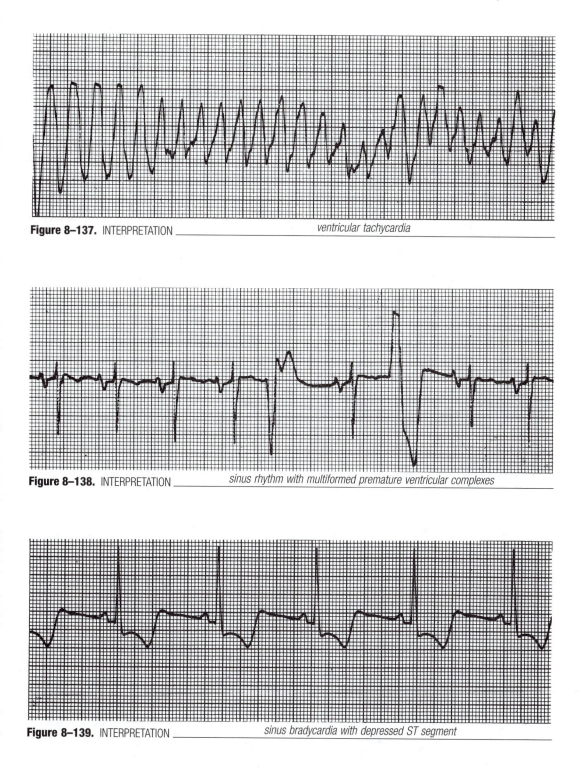

Figure 8–137. INTERPRETATION _____ *ventricular tachycardia*

Figure 8–138. INTERPRETATION _____ *sinus rhythm with multiformed premature ventricular complexes*

Figure 8–139. INTERPRETATION _____ *sinus bradycardia with depressed ST segment*

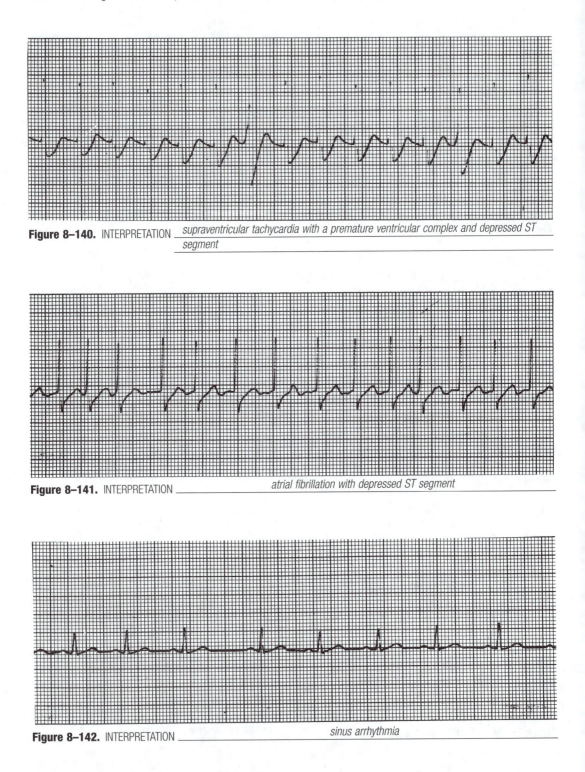

Figure 8–140. INTERPRETATION _supraventricular tachycardia with a premature ventricular complex and depressed ST segment_

Figure 8–141. INTERPRETATION _____ _atrial fibrillation with depressed ST segment_

Figure 8–142. INTERPRETATION _____ _sinus arrhythmia_

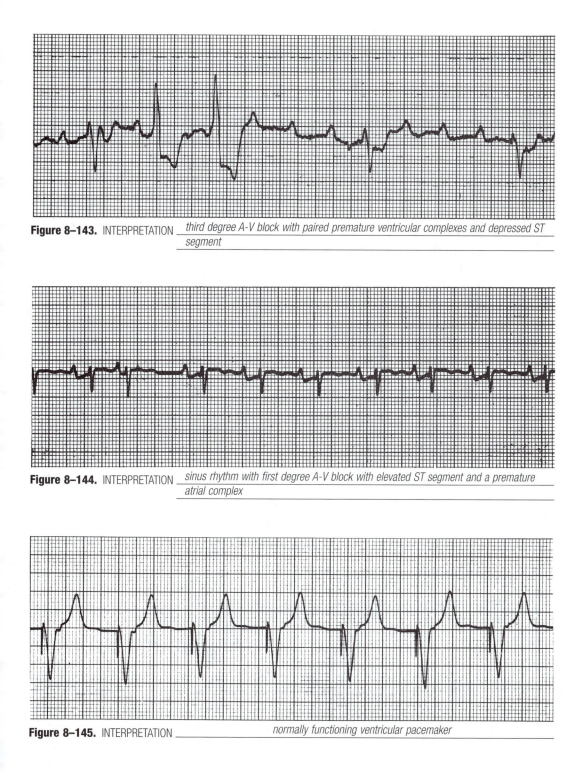

Figure 8–143. INTERPRETATION _third degree A-V block with paired premature ventricular complexes and depressed ST segment_

Figure 8–144. INTERPRETATION _sinus rhythm with first degree A-V block with elevated ST segment and a premature atrial complex_

Figure 8–145. INTERPRETATION _normally functioning ventricular pacemaker_

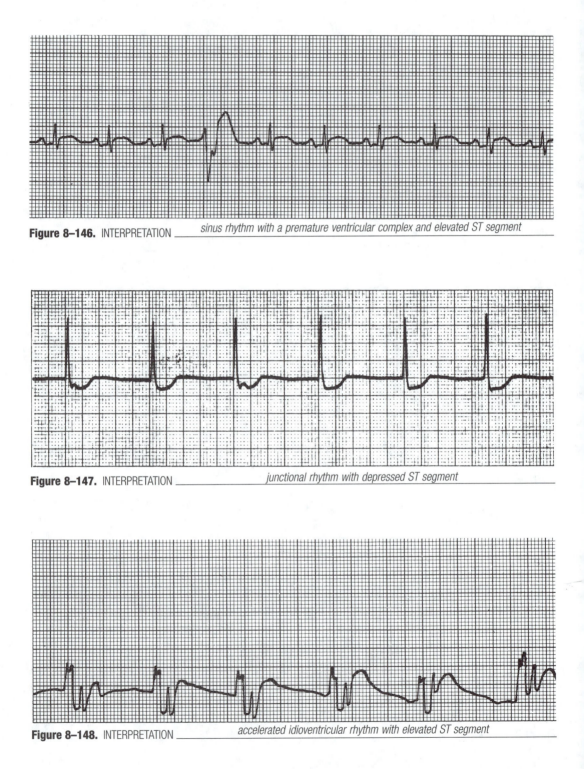

Figure 8–146. INTERPRETATION _____ *sinus rhythm with a premature ventricular complex and elevated ST segment*

Figure 8–147. INTERPRETATION _____ *junctional rhythm with depressed ST segment*

Figure 8–148. INTERPRETATION _____ *accelerated idioventricular rhythm with elevated ST segment*

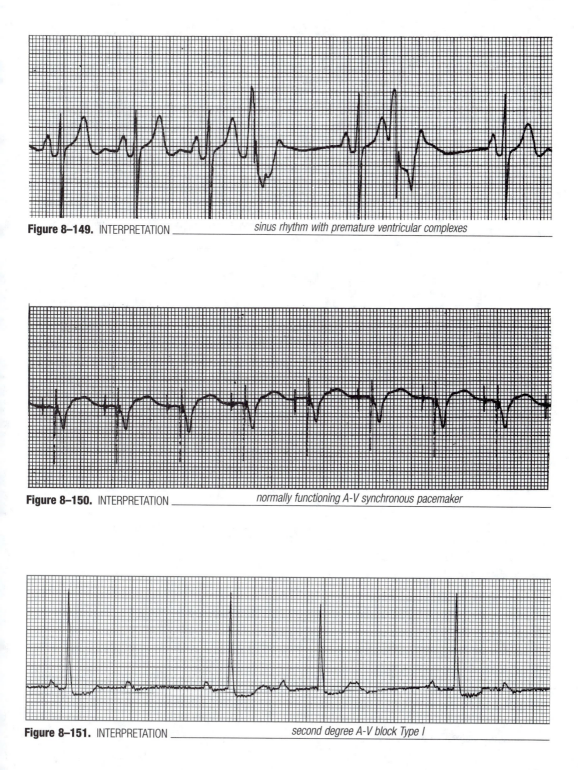

Figure 8–149. INTERPRETATION _____ *sinus rhythm with premature ventricular complexes*

Figure 8–150. INTERPRETATION _____ *normally functioning A-V synchronous pacemaker*

Figure 8–151. INTERPRETATION _____ *second degree A-V block Type I*

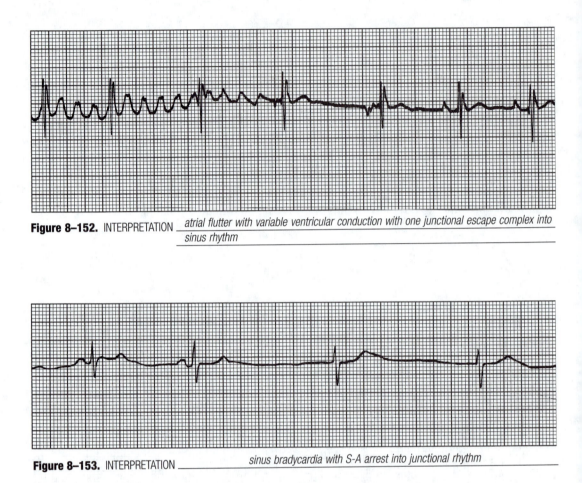

Figure 8–152. INTERPRETATION *atrial flutter with variable ventricular conduction with one junctional escape complex into sinus rhythm*

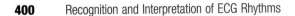

Figure 8–153. INTERPRETATION *sinus bradycardia with S-A arrest into junctional rhythm*

CHAPTER 9

Answer Key—Fill-in

1. a. cause decreased cardiac output
    b. are potentially life threatening
2. a. hypotension
    b. decreased level of consciousness
    c. chest pain
    d. dyspnea
    e. congestive heart failure
3. a. second-degree A-V block Type II
    b. third-degree A-V block

    c. ventricular tachycardia
    d. vetricular fibrillation

4. a. bradycardia
    b. tachycardia
    c. ectopics
    d. cardiac arrest
5. a. slow it down
    b. speed it up
6. suppress

7. viable
8. a. sinus bradycardia
   b. junctional rhythm
   c. A-V blocks
   d. idioventricular rhythm
9. atropine
10. a. transcutanous pacing
    b. dopamine
    c. epinephrine
    d. Isuprel
11. a. second-degree A-V block Type II
    b. complete A-V block
    c. idioventricular rhythm
12. a. junctional tachycardia
    b. atrial flutter
    c. atrial fibrillation
    d. supraventricular tachycardia
    e. sinus tachycardia
13. a. stable
    b. unstable
14. a. vagal maneuvers
    b. adenosine
    c. verapamil
    d. cardioversion
15. cadioversion
16. a. 50
    b. 50
    c. 100
17. sinus tachycardia
18. cause
19. a. fever
    b. pain
    c. shock
    d. anxiety
20. a. accelerated idioventricular
    b. ventricular tachycardia
21. a. stable

b. unstable
c. pulseless
22. a. lidocaine
    b. procainamide
23. cardioversion
24. ventricular fibrillation
25. oxygen
26. a. frequent (more than 6/min)
    b. R on T
    c. multiformed
    d. acute MI
    e. paired, runs
    f. bigeminy, trigeminy
27. a. lidocaine
    b. procainamide
    c. bretylium
28. atropine
29. a. ventricular fibrillation
    b. ventricular tachycardia
    c. asystole
    d. pulseless electrical activity
30. precordial thump
31. a. defibrillation
    b. epinephrine
32. a. transcutanous pacing
    b. epinephrine
    c. atropine
33. a. bradycardia with a rate less than 40/min
    b. idoventricular rhythm without a pulse
    c. tachycardia
34. poor
35. a. hypovolemia
    b. cardiac tamponade
    c. tension pneumothorax
    d. hypoxia
    e. acidosis
36. epinephrine

Answer Key—ECG Practice Strips

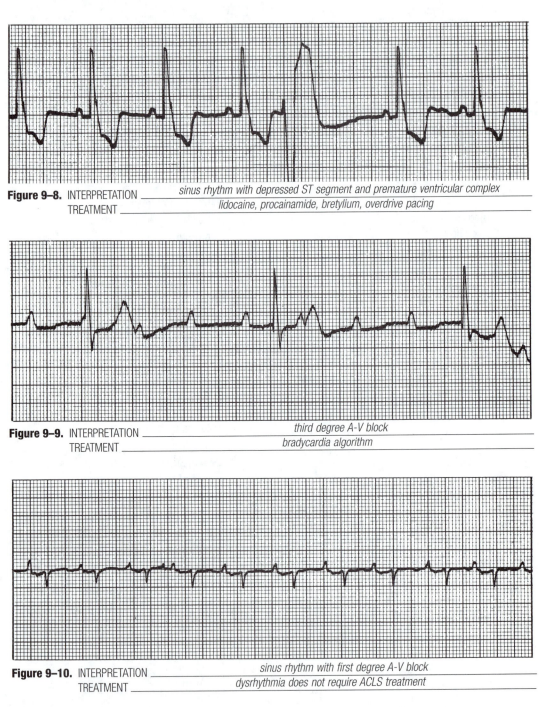

Figure 9–8. INTERPRETATION _____ *sinus rhythm with depressed ST segment and premature ventricular complex*
TREATMENT _____ *lidocaine, procainamide, bretylium, overdrive pacing*

Figure 9–9. INTERPRETATION _____ *third degree A-V block*
TREATMENT _____ *bradycardia algorithm*

Figure 9–10. INTERPRETATION _____ *sinus rhythm with first degree A-V block*
TREATMENT _____ *dysrhythmia does not require ACLS treatment*

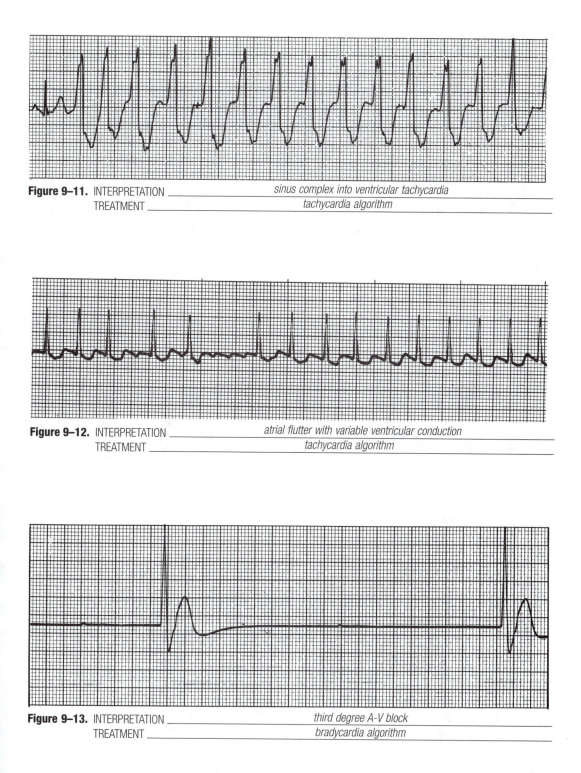

Figure 9–11. INTERPRETATION _____ *sinus complex into ventricular tachycardia*
TREATMENT _____ *tachycardia algorithm*

Figure 9–12. INTERPRETATION _____ *atrial flutter with variable ventricular conduction*
TREATMENT _____ *tachycardia algorithm*

Figure 9–13. INTERPRETATION _____ *third degree A-V block*
TREATMENT _____ *bradycardia algorithm*

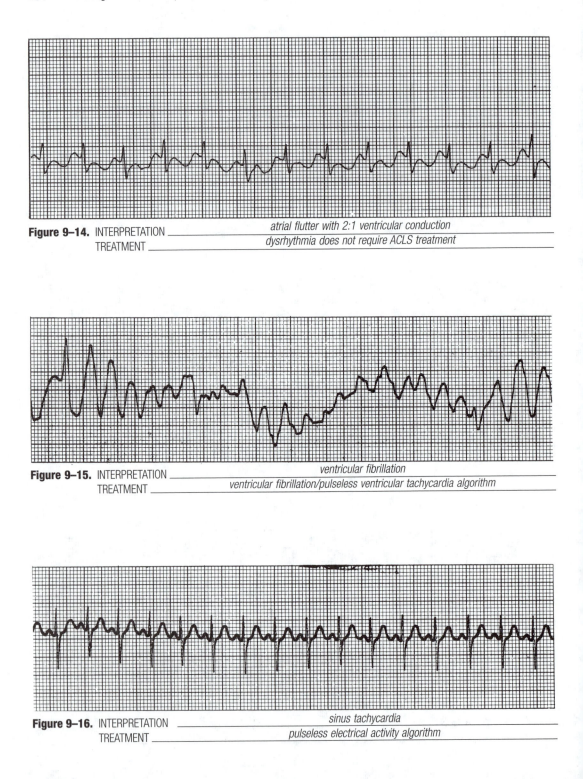

Figure 9–14. INTERPRETATION _____ *atrial flutter with 2:1 ventricular conduction*
TREATMENT _____ *dysrhythmia does not require ACLS treatment*

Figure 9–15. INTERPRETATION _____ *ventricular fibrillation*
TREATMENT _____ *ventricular fibrillation/pulseless ventricular tachycardia algorithm*

Figure 9–16. INTERPRETATION _____ *sinus tachycardia*
TREATMENT _____ *pulseless electrical activity algorithm*

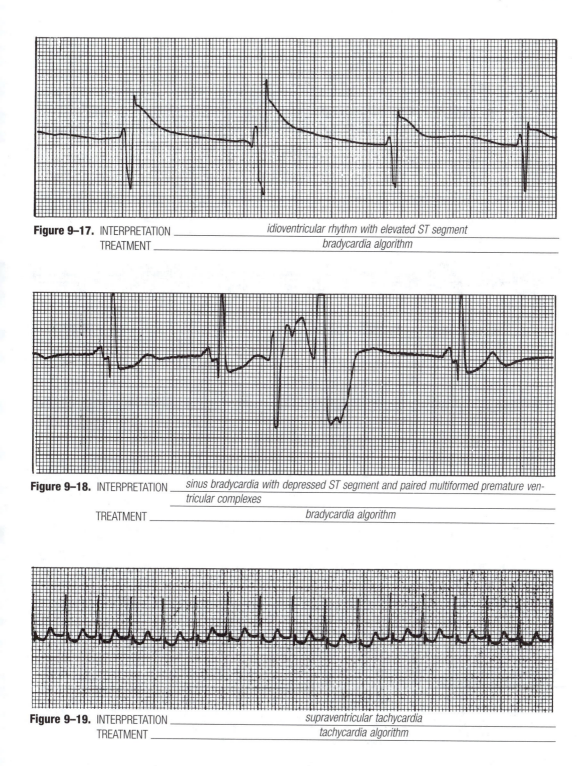

Figure 9–17. INTERPRETATION _____ *idioventricular rhythm with elevated ST segment*

TREATMENT _____ *bradycardia algorithm*

Figure 9–18. INTERPRETATION _____ *sinus bradycardia with depressed ST segment and paired multiformed premature ventricular complexes*

TREATMENT _____ *bradycardia algorithm*

Figure 9–19. INTERPRETATION _____ *supraventricular tachycardia*

TREATMENT _____ *tachycardia algorithm*

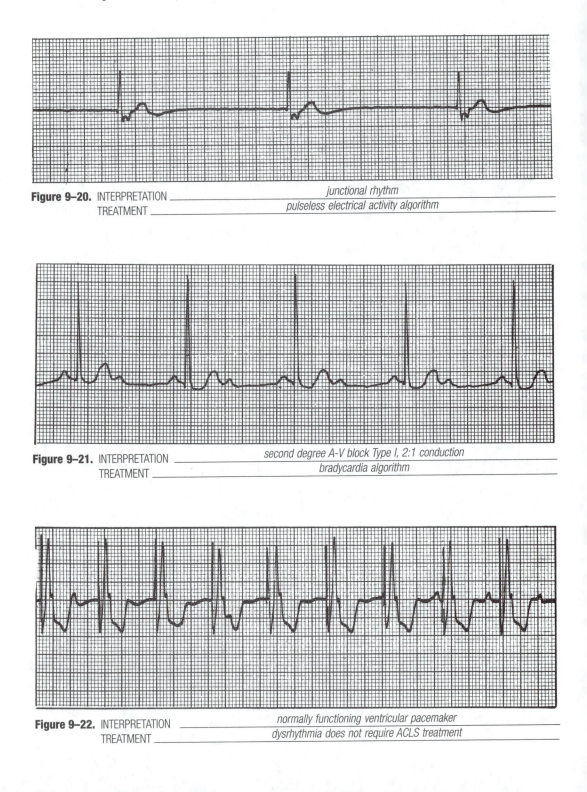

Figure 9–20. INTERPRETATION _____ *junctional rhythm*
TREATMENT _____ *pulseless electrical activity algorithm*

Figure 9–21. INTERPRETATION _____ *second degree A-V block Type I, 2:1 conduction*
TREATMENT _____ *bradycardia algorithm*

Figure 9–22. INTERPRETATION _____ *normally functioning ventricular pacemaker*
TREATMENT _____ *dysrhythmia does not require ACLS treatment*

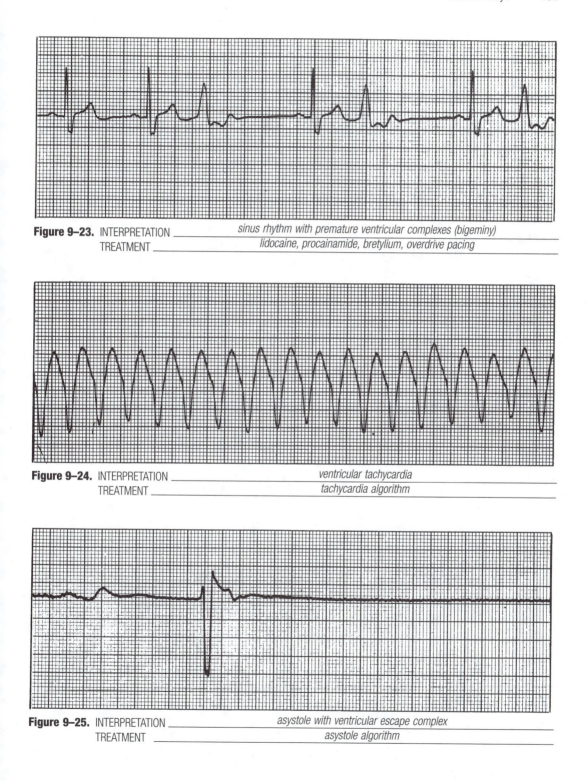

Figure 9–23. INTERPRETATION _____ *sinus rhythm with premature ventricular complexes (bigeminy)*
TREATMENT _____ *lidocaine, procainamide, bretylium, overdrive pacing*

Figure 9–24. INTERPRETATION _____ *ventricular tachycardia*
TREATMENT _____ *tachycardia algorithm*

Figure 9–25. INTERPRETATION _____ *asystole with ventricular escape complex*
TREATMENT _____ *asystole algorithm*

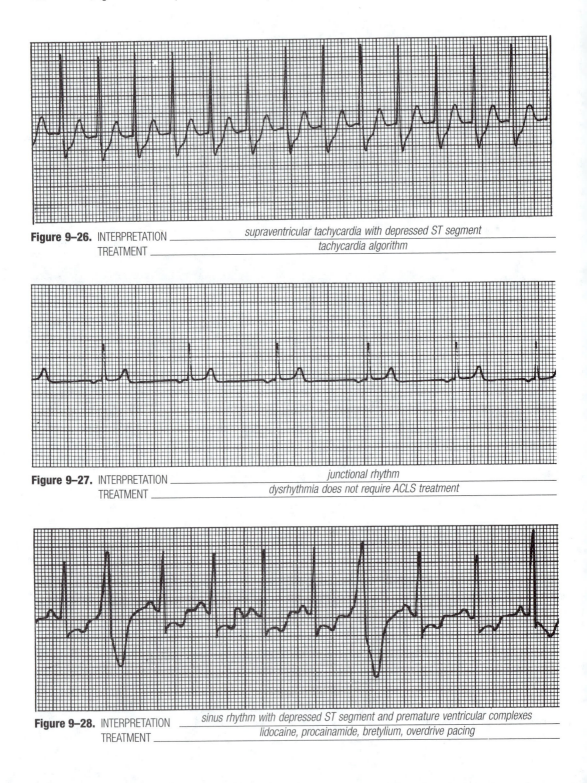

Figure 9–26. INTERPRETATION _____ *supraventricular tachycardia with depressed ST segment*
TREATMENT _____ *tachycardia algorithm*

Figure 9–27. INTERPRETATION _____ *junctional rhythm*
TREATMENT _____ *dysrhythmia does not require ACLS treatment*

Figure 9–28. INTERPRETATION _____ *sinus rhythm with depressed ST segment and premature ventricular complexes*
TREATMENT _____ *lidocaine, procainamide, bretylium, overdrive pacing*

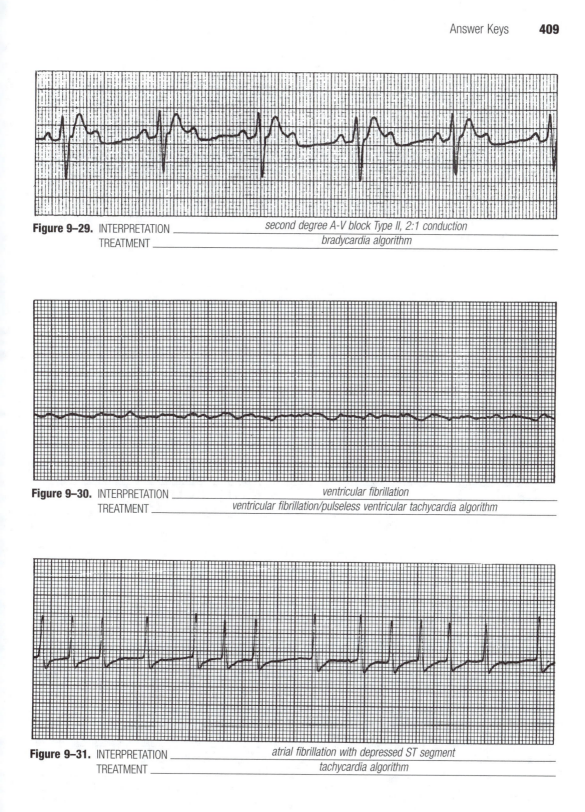

Figure 9–29. INTERPRETATION _____ *second degree A-V block Type II, 2:1 conduction*
TREATMENT _____ *bradycardia algorithm*

Figure 9–30. INTERPRETATION _____ *ventricular fibrillation*
TREATMENT _____ *ventricular fibrillation/pulseless ventricular tachycardia algorithm*

Figure 9–31. INTERPRETATION _____ *atrial fibrillation with depressed ST segment*
TREATMENT _____ *tachycardia algorithm*

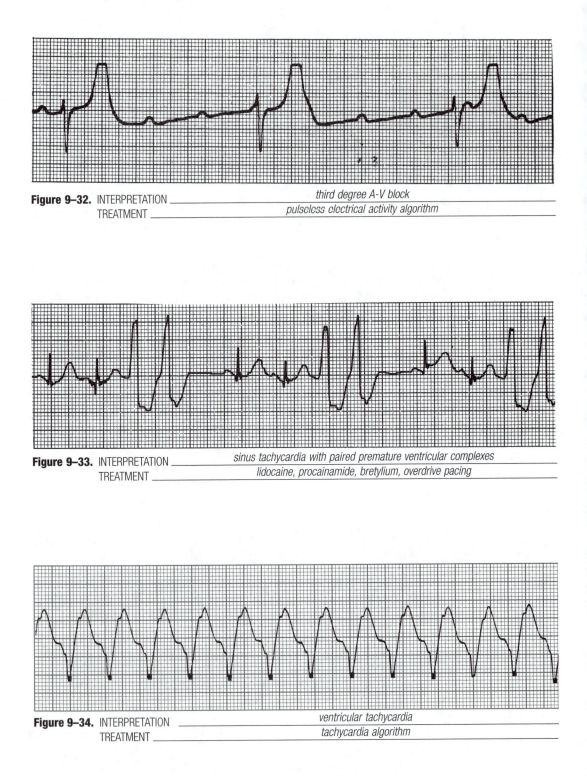

Figure 9–32. INTERPRETATION _____ *third degree A-V block*
TREATMENT _____ *pulseless electrical activity algorithm*

Figure 9–33. INTERPRETATION _____ *sinus tachycardia with paired premature ventricular complexes*
TREATMENT _____ *lidocaine, procainamide, bretylium, overdrive pacing*

Figure 9–34. INTERPRETATION _____ *ventricular tachycardia*
TREATMENT _____ *tachycardia algorithm*

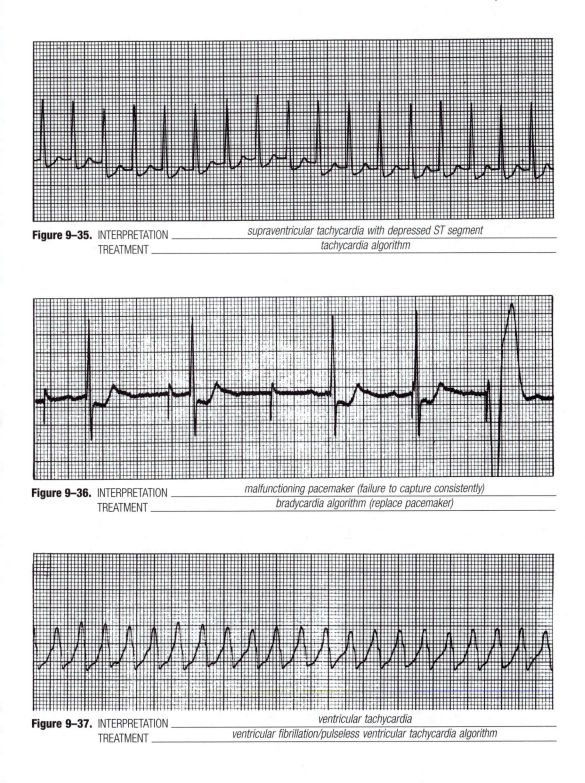

Figure 9–35. INTERPRETATION _____ *supraventricular tachycardia with depressed ST segment*
TREATMENT _____ *tachycardia algorithm*

Figure 9–36. INTERPRETATION _____ *malfunctioning pacemaker (failure to capture consistently)*
TREATMENT _____ *bradycardia algorithm (replace pacemaker)*

Figure 9–37. INTERPRETATION _____ *ventricular tachycardia*
TREATMENT _____ *ventricular fibrillation/pulseless ventricular tachycardia algorithm*

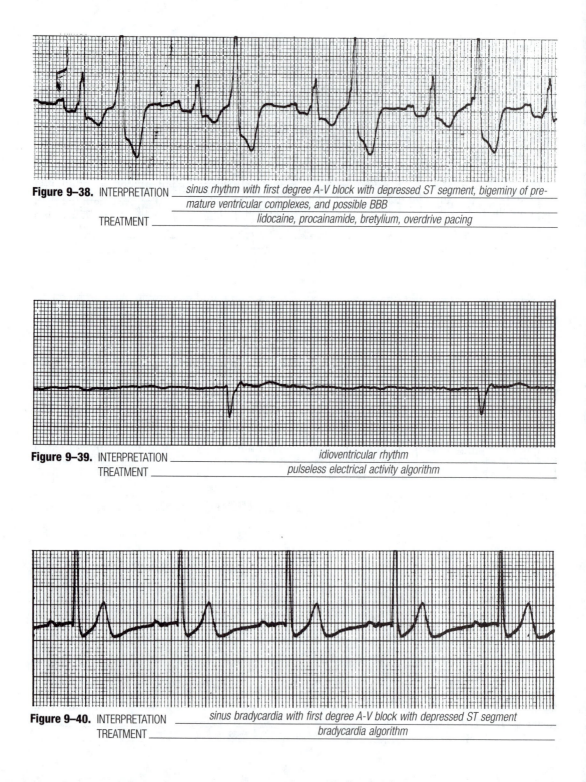

Figure 9–38. INTERPRETATION _sinus rhythm with first degree A-V block with depressed ST segment, bigeminy of premature ventricular complexes, and possible BBB_

TREATMENT _lidocaine, procainamide, bretylium, overdrive pacing_

Figure 9–39. INTERPRETATION _idioventricular rhythm_

TREATMENT _pulseless electrical activity algorithm_

Figure 9–40. INTERPRETATION _sinus bradycardia with first degree A-V block with depressed ST segment_

TREATMENT _bradycardia algorithm_

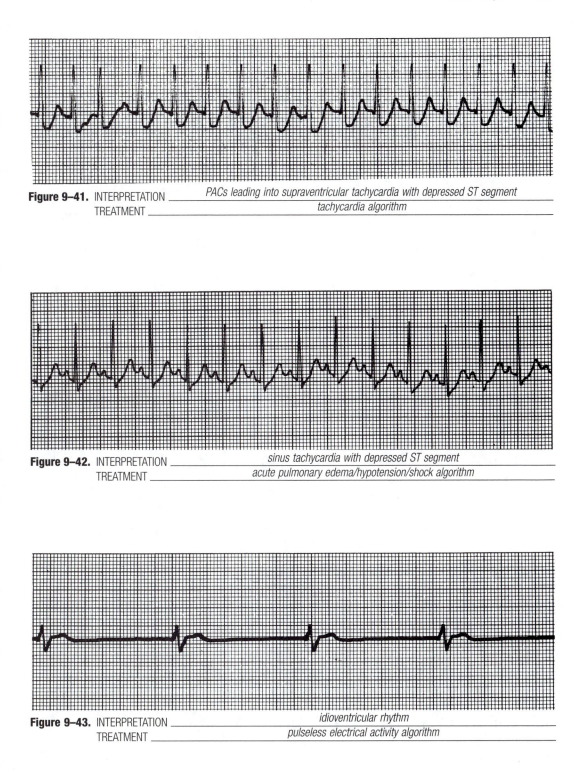

Figure 9–41. INTERPRETATION _____ _PACs leading into supraventricular tachycardia with depressed ST segment_
TREATMENT _____ _tachycardia algorithm_

Figure 9–42. INTERPRETATION _____ _sinus tachycardia with depressed ST segment_
TREATMENT _____ _acute pulmonary edema/hypotension/shock algorithm_

Figure 9–43. INTERPRETATION _____ _idioventricular rhythm_
TREATMENT _____ _pulseless electrical activity algorithm_

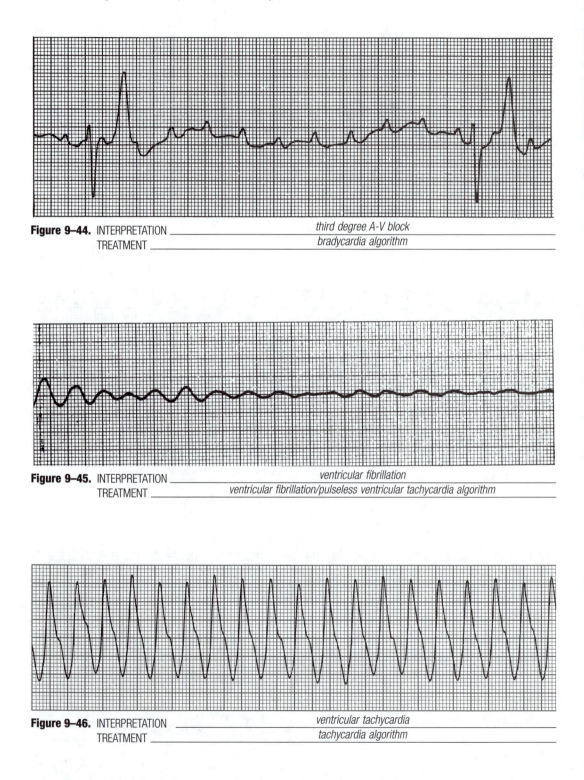

Figure 9–44. INTERPRETATION _____ *third degree A-V block*
TREATMENT _____ *bradycardia algorithm*

Figure 9–45. INTERPRETATION _____ *ventricular fibrillation*
TREATMENT _____ *ventricular fibrillation/pulseless ventricular tachycardia algorithm*

Figure 9–46. INTERPRETATION _____ *ventricular tachycardia*
TREATMENT _____ *tachycardia algorithm*

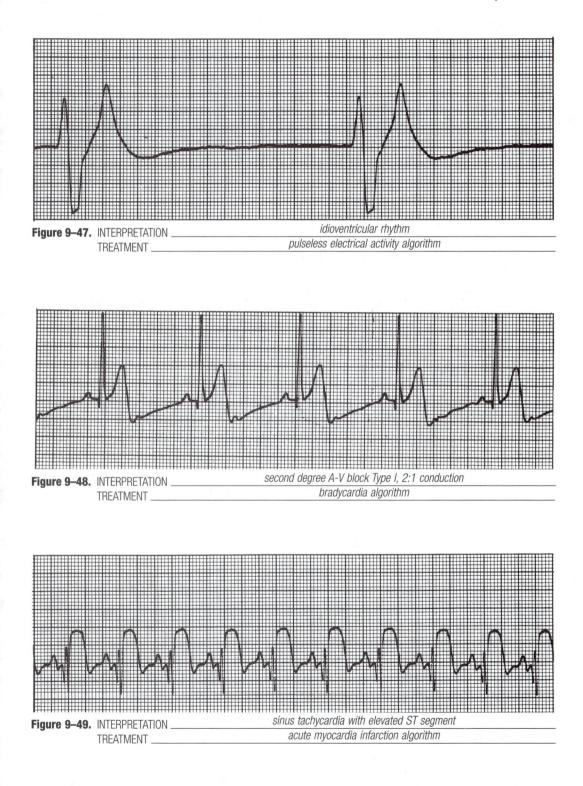

Figure 9–47. INTERPRETATION _____ *idioventricular rhythm*
TREATMENT _____ *pulseless electrical activity algorithm*

Figure 9–48. INTERPRETATION _____ *second degree A-V block Type I, 2:1 conduction*
TREATMENT _____ *bradycardia algorithm*

Figure 9–49. INTERPRETATION _____ *sinus tachycardia with elevated ST segment*
TREATMENT _____ *acute myocardia infarction algorithm*

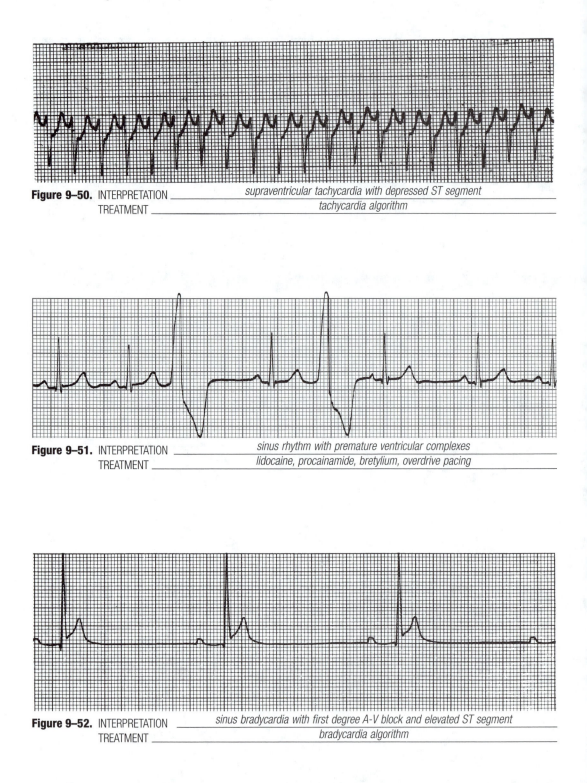

Figure 9–50. INTERPRETATION _____ *supraventricular tachycardia with depressed ST segment*
TREATMENT _____ *tachycardia algorithm*

Figure 9–51. INTERPRETATION _____ *sinus rhythm with premature ventricular complexes*
TREATMENT _____ *lidocaine, procainamide, bretylium, overdrive pacing*

Figure 9–52. INTERPRETATION _____ *sinus bradycardia with first degree A-V block and elevated ST segment*
TREATMENT _____ *bradycardia algorithm*

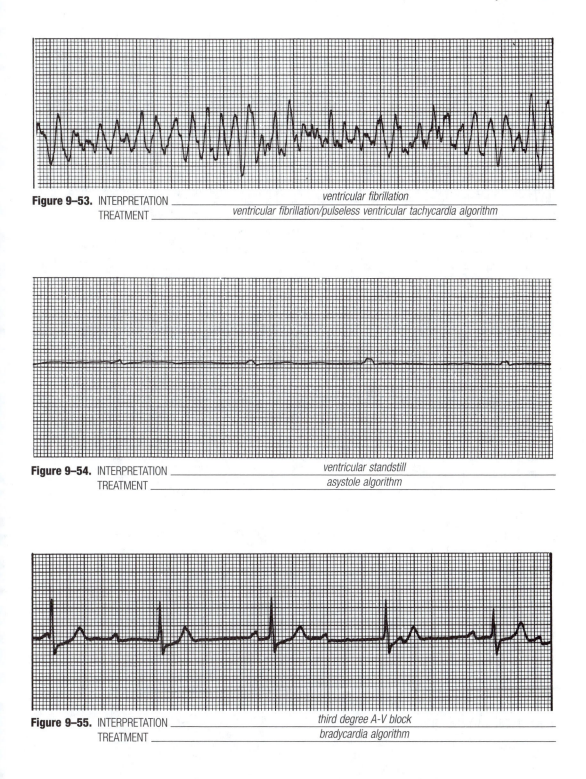

Figure 9–53. INTERPRETATION _____ *ventricular fibrillation*
TREATMENT _____ *ventricular fibrillation/pulseless ventricular tachycardia algorithm*

Figure 9–54. INTERPRETATION _____ *ventricular standstill*
TREATMENT _____ *asystole algorithm*

Figure 9–55. INTERPRETATION _____ *third degree A-V block*
TREATMENT _____ *bradycardia algorithm*

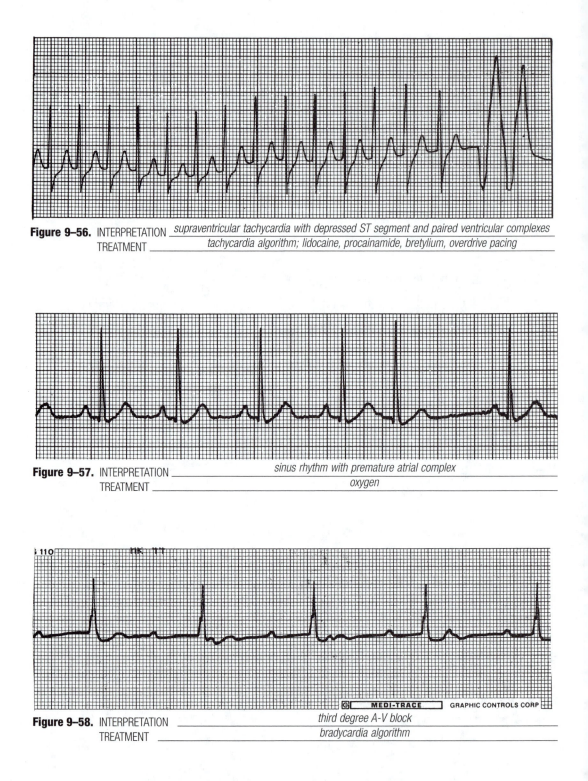

Figure 9–56. INTERPRETATION *supraventricular tachycardia with depressed ST segment and paired ventricular complexes*
TREATMENT *tachycardia algorithm; lidocaine, procainamide, bretylium, overdrive pacing*

Figure 9–57. INTERPRETATION *sinus rhythm with premature atrial complex*
TREATMENT *oxygen*

Figure 9–58. INTERPRETATION *third degree A-V block*
TREATMENT *bradycardia algorithm*

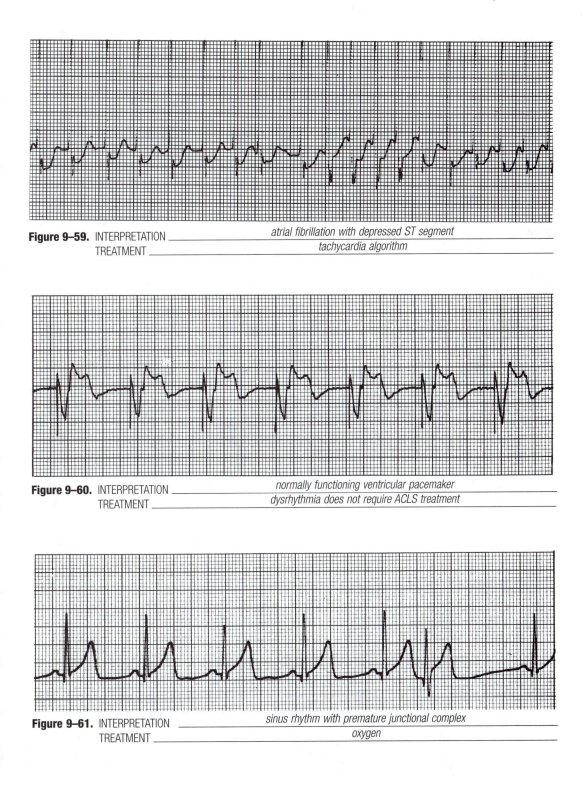

Figure 9–59. INTERPRETATION _____ *atrial fibrillation with depressed ST segment*
TREATMENT _____ *tachycardia algorithm*

Figure 9–60. INTERPRETATION _____ *normally functioning ventricular pacemaker*
TREATMENT _____ *dysrhythmia does not require ACLS treatment*

Figure 9–61. INTERPRETATION _____ *sinus rhythm with premature junctional complex*
TREATMENT _____ *oxygen*

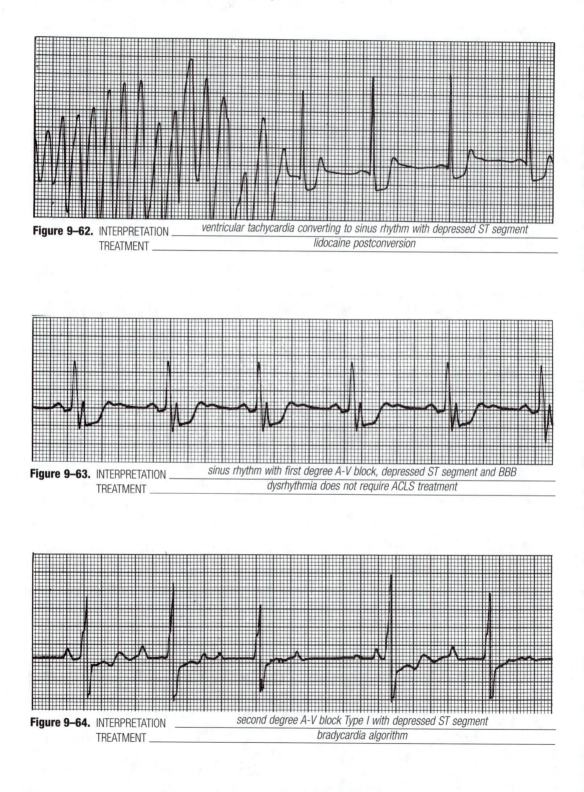

Figure 9–62. INTERPRETATION _____ *ventricular tachycardia converting to sinus rhythm with depressed ST segment*
TREATMENT _____ *lidocaine postconversion*

Figure 9–63. INTERPRETATION _____ *sinus rhythm with first degree A-V block, depressed ST segment and BBB*
TREATMENT _____ *dysrhythmia does not require ACLS treatment*

Figure 9–64. INTERPRETATION _____ *second degree A-V block Type I with depressed ST segment*
TREATMENT _____ *bradycardia algorithm*

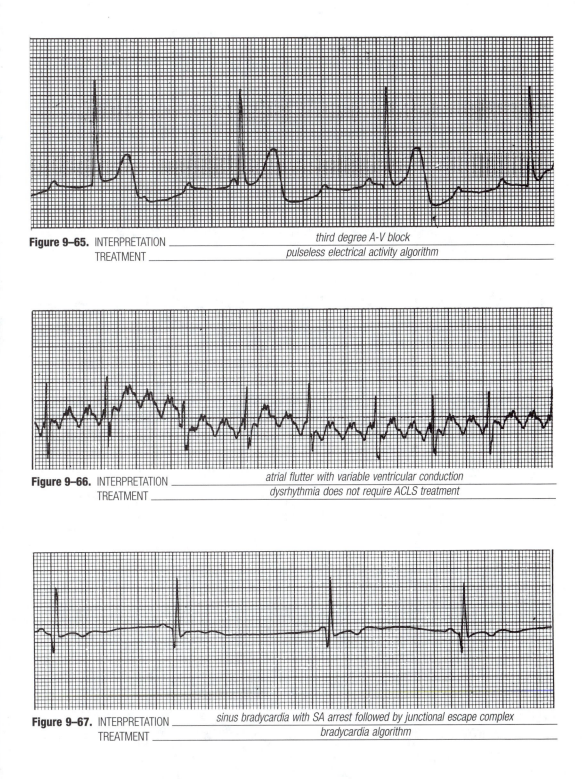

Figure 9–65. INTERPRETATION _____ *third degree A-V block* _____
TREATMENT _____ *pulseless electrical activity algorithm* _____

Figure 9–66. INTERPRETATION _____ *atrial flutter with variable ventricular conduction* _____
TREATMENT _____ *dysrhythmia does not require ACLS treatment* _____

Figure 9–67. INTERPRETATION _____ *sinus bradycardia with SA arrest followed by junctional escape complex* _____
TREATMENT _____ *bradycardia algorithm* _____

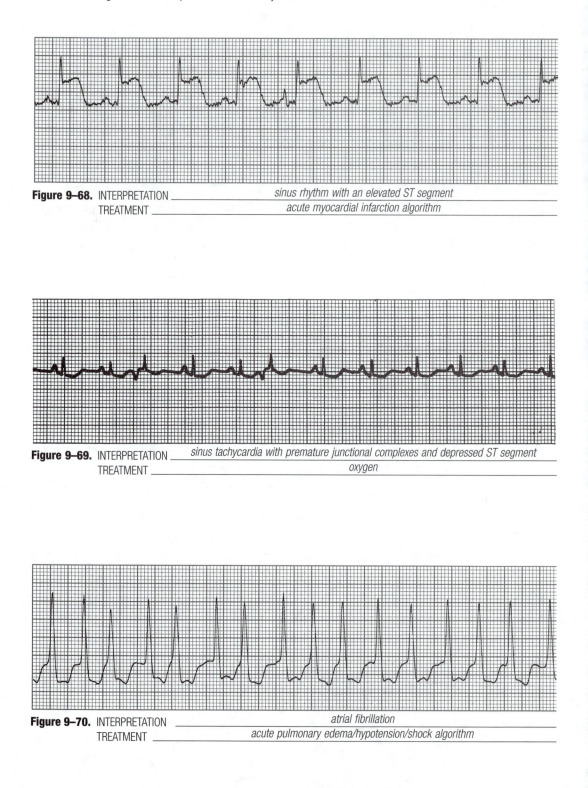

Figure 9–68. INTERPRETATION _____ *sinus rhythm with an elevated ST segment*
TREATMENT _____ *acute myocardial infarction algorithm*

Figure 9–69. INTERPRETATION ____ *sinus tachycardia with premature junctional complexes and depressed ST segment*
TREATMENT _____ *oxygen*

Figure 9–70. INTERPRETATION _____ *atrial fibrillation*
TREATMENT _____ *acute pulmonary edema/hypotension/shock algorithm*

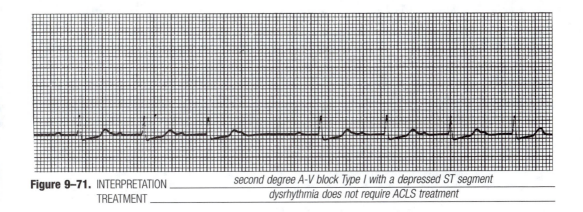

Figure 9–71. INTERPRETATION _____ *second degree A-V block Type I with a depressed ST segment* _____
TREATMENT _____ *dysrhythmia does not require ACLS treatment* _____

Bibliography

Andreoli, KG, et al. *Comprehensive Cardiac Care: A Text for Nurses, Physicians, and Other Health Practitioners.* 6th ed. St. Louis, MO: CV Mosby Co; 1987.

Brandenburg, RD, et al. *Cardiology Fundamentals and Practice.* Chicago: Year Book Medical Publishers, Inc; 1987.

Chung, EK. *Principles of Cardiac Arrhythmias.* 4th ed. Baltimore: Williams & Wilkins Co; 1989.

Conover, MB. *Understanding Electrocardiology.* 7th ed. St. Louis, MO: CV Mosby Company; 1996.

Cummins, Richard O, et al. *Textbook of Advanced Cardiac Life Support.* Dallas, TX: American Heart Association; 1994.

Goldman, MJ. *Principles of Clinical Electrocardiography.* 12th ed. Los Altos, CA: Lange Medical Publications; 1986.

Guyton, AC. *Textbook of Medical Physiology.* 7th ed. Philadelphia: WB Saunders Co; 1986.

Mandel, W. *Cardiac Arrhythmias, Their Mechanisms, Diagnosis, and Management.* 2nd ed. Philadelphia: WB Saunders Co; 1987.

Marriott, HJL. *Practical Electrocardiography.* 9th ed. Baltimore: Williams & Wilkins Co; 1994.

Marriott, HJL, Conover, MB. *Advanced Concepts in Arrhythmias.* 2nd ed. St. Louis, MO: CV Mosby Company; 1989.

Patel, JM, et al. *Arrhythmias—Detection, Treatment, and Cardiac Drugs.* Philadelphia: WB Saunders Co; 1989.

Schlant, Robert C., et al. *Hurst's The Heart.* 8th ed. New York: McGraw-Hill Inc.; 1994.